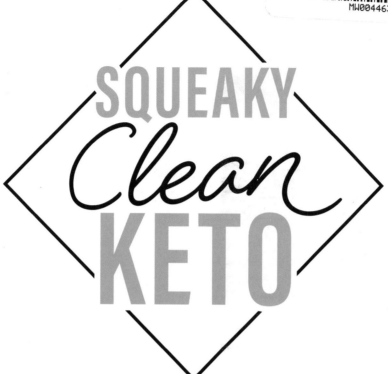

Next Level Keto to Hack Your Health

Mellissa Sevigny

Victory Belt Publishing Inc.
Las Vegas

First Published in 2020 by Victory Belt Publishing Inc.

Copyright © 2020 Mellissa Sevigny

All rights reserved

No part of this publication may be reproduced or distributed in any form or by any means, electronic or mechanical, or stored in a database or retrieval system, without prior written permission from the publisher.

ISBN-13: 978-1-628604-00-9

The author is not a licensed practitioner, physician, or medical professional and offers no medical diagnoses, treatments, suggestions, or counseling. The information presented herein has not been evaluated by the U.S. Food and Drug Administration, and it is not intended to diagnose, treat, cure, or prevent any disease. Full medical clearance from a licensed physician should be obtained before beginning or modifying any diet, exercise, or lifestyle program, and physicians should be informed of all nutritional changes.

The author/owner claims no responsibility to any person or entity for any liability, loss, or damage caused or alleged to be caused directly or indirectly as a result of the use, application, or interpretation of the information presented herein.

Cover Design by Kat Lannom and Justin-Aaron Velasco

Interior Design by Charisse Reyes, Crizalie Olimpo, and Justin-Aaron Velasco

Illustrations by Elita San Juan

Printed in Canada

TC 0322

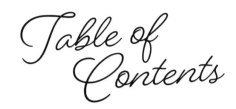

Table of Contents

INTRODUCTION / 4

Welcome to Squeaky Clean Keto! / 5

The SCKC Experiment / 7

The Program (aka the Nuts and Bolts) / 11

Getting Started / 17

Frequently Asked Questions / 26

But First, Coffee: Tips for the Coffee Lover Going Squeaky / 34

Meal Prep Tips / 37

Kitchen Safety / 41

Essential Squeaky Clean Keto Pantry / 44

Kitchen Arsenal / 49

MEAL PLANS / 54

Squeaky Clean Keto Meal Plan / 56

5-Day Keto Soup Diet Plan / 64

THE RECIPES / 68

Basics / 70

Breakfast / 114

Soups, Salads & Wraps / 136

Chicken / 168

Beef / 194

Pork / 218

Seafood / 238

Veggie Mains & Sides / 266

Drinks & Snacks / 312

RESOURCE GUIDE / 344

ALLERGEN INDEX / 346

RECIPE INDEX / 350

DOWNLOADABLE CHARTS / 355

GENERAL INDEX / 356

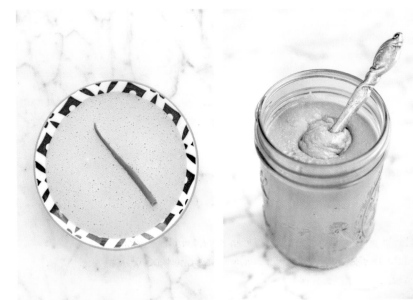

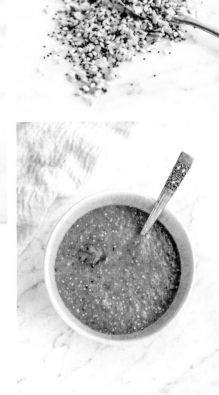

INTRODUCTION

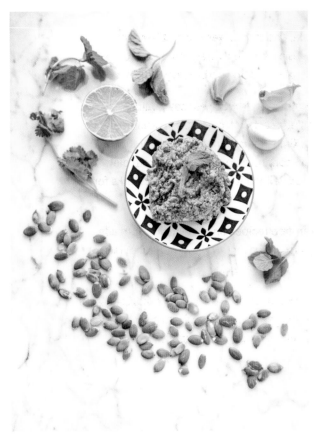

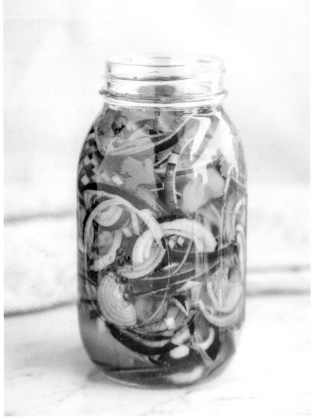

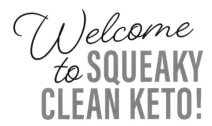
Welcome to SQUEAKY CLEAN KETO!

Not just another run-of-the-mill keto cookbook, *Squeaky Clean Keto* is a new approach to the ketogenic diet—a method designed to accelerate weight loss, reduce inflammation, increase energy, and so much more!

Before we get into the nuts and bolts of how to do Squeaky Clean Keto, I want to briefly introduce myself and give you a little backstory into how and why I developed the Squeaky Clean Keto Challenge (SCKC) program and this book.

A foodie to the bone, I've been cooking since I was four years old. I've worked in restaurants, done private catering, competed on television cooking contests, and fed hundreds of people at a time. In short, I know my way around a kitchen, and I'm good at food. I tell you this not to brag but to let you know that when it comes to cooking—and more specifically, my ability to help *you* become better at cooking—you're in capable hands.

When sharing my recipes with others, my aim is always to make sure that people can execute the recipes at home to rave reviews and requests for seconds. It's something I work hard at, and if the Amazon feedback and blog comments I've received so far are any indication, then I'm not horrible at it.

Like most people who love to cook, I also love to eat, and therein lies my problem with keeping weight off. Once I realized that limiting carbs was the only way I could consistently maintain my weight, I lamented the idea of missing out on all the carb-heavy foods I loved.

Determined to avoid food boredom, I set out to create low-carb recipes that would be so delicious that I wouldn't miss my old carb-heavy favorites like bread, pasta, pizza, and rice—and I shared those recipes with others on my website, *I Breathe I'm Hungry* (ibreatheimhungry. com). That was more than eight years ago, and IBIH continues to thrive as the keto diet becomes more and more popular with people who have tried it and found that it works for them.

In addition to posting delicious low-carb and gluten-free recipes on my website, I provide free meal plans for basic keto, a five-day keto egg fast, and a five-day keto soup diet (see pages 64 to 67) that have helped tens of thousands of people lose weight.

Since starting my blog, I've learned what works and what doesn't, not just for me but also for a lot of my readers. Their feedback via email and social media has been invaluable for figuring out what the biggest challenges are to starting and maintaining a keto diet.

Although some of those challenges are common to everyone (tracking macros, finding time to meal prep, keeping to a budget, getting enough variety, etc.), others struggle with getting results due to extenuating circumstances like health conditions, medications they take, and food intolerances, just to name a few.

In my first book, *Keto for Life* (my mom says it's awesome; you should totally read it), I compared keto to snorkeling and discussed how keto fins are not one-size-fits-all; you may need different "fins" to fit your age, health problems, medications, gut health, and so on. Some of the "fins," or methods, you might use when regular keto isn't working for you are intermittent fasting, fat fasting, and eliminating specific foods like dairy or sweeteners that you might be reacting to.

As a follow-up to that analogy, I developed the SCK program—the mother of all keto fins! Squeaky Clean Keto marries the elimination diet standards of plans like the Whole30 with a very clean approach to the ketogenic diet. It's definitely more restrictive than a typical keto diet, but the fantastic results are absolutely worth it.

The program was incredibly successful with my readers on the website, so I decided to write this book in the hope that it would reach an even wider audience of people who are under the mistaken impression that their bodies just aren't compatible with keto or even capable of losing weight and feeling good at all.

And of course, the purpose of this book isn't just to provide the SCK guidelines but also to offer you practical tips, suggestions, and, most important, delicious recipes that will help you reach your goals without sacrificing the joy of eating great food!

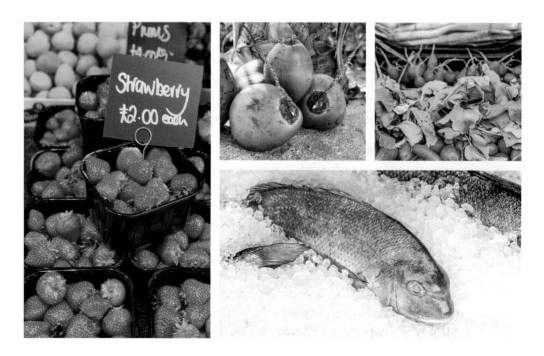

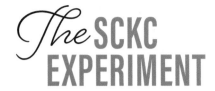

The SCKC EXPERIMENT

Squeaky Clean Keto is an approach that has worked for me without fail time and time again, even when my health and life were at their most challenging. I knew it could work for my readers too, so I fine-tuned the program and shared it free on my website in January 2019. In spite of my own success eating Squeaky Clean Keto, even I am amazed by the incredible results reported by the thousands of people who have tried the program.

It was those inspiring success stories that led me to write this book—and I'm sharing some of them with you to help inspire you to give the SCKC a try and reap the incredible benefits for yourself.

So many people struggled like I did, even on regular keto, but when they "went squeaky," they started seeing immediate and dramatic results. Of course, weight loss is paramount to most people embarking on a keto diet, but many people reported other incredible benefits and improvement of even chronic health issues as well! Here's a short, inexhaustive list of some of the conditions the first round of "squeakers" have reported are improved: inflammation, rosacea and psoriasis, sleep, heartburn, mood stability in those with depression, and joint pain.

The results were so dramatic that even though the program was originally a thirty-day challenge, many of the original members from January 2019 have made Squeaky Clean Keto a permanent way of life.

A lot of us did the program in January and got to know each other through the closed Facebook community I created for support. There was plenty of commiserating about how sad we were to be missing out on cheese, nuts, sweet treats, and the occasional glass of wine. After gutting through the thirty days, everyone was excited to start reintroducing dairy, nuts, sweeteners, and alcohol a little at a time to see how those foods affected them.

Many people felt so awful after adding back those foods—especially dairy and nuts—that they decided the discomfort wasn't worth it, and they went back to the SCK way of eating. Some of these same people had tried every loophole at the beginning of the thirty-day trial—surely just a little cream in their coffee wouldn't hurt anything? Pretty please? But after sticking it out to complete the SCKC, they realized that part of the reason they hadn't been losing weight, were feeling tired, and/or were having joint pain had been their beloved dairy or nuts (or both).

Other people found that sweeteners were the culprit. Or that they were snacking too much on nuts and cheese—or having too many desserts and consuming more calories than they needed. All these things have the potential to slow progress.

Across the board, everyone in the challenge lost weight—some more than 20 pounds in a single month—but all agreed that the big takeaway was how insanely good they felt while eating Squeaky Clean Keto. That feeling of good health is what kept so many of them coming back to the group even after weeks or months away.

So, if you're frustrated with your lack of results, or you aren't feeling your best and want to see if you can improve your overall health and sense of well-being, then I urge you to give Squeaky Clean Keto a try. You can do anything for thirty days—and I can promise that if you stick it out and don't cave in to temptation and cheat, you'll see amazing progress not just on the scale but also in your overall health and energy levels.

But I warn you: once you experience the benefits of Squeaky Clean Keto, you may never be content with regular keto again!

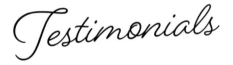 Here are some of the nice things my readers have said about the SCKC and how it has changed their lives. I hope to hear from you about *your* success!

"I had been on keto for four months and had very good results; however, I still felt drained all the time, noticed my face and fingers were always puffy, and although I had lost over 35 pounds at that point, still felt awful. I started SCKC on January 2, 2019, and by no means was it an easy task to give up cheese. I had grown to rely on cheese for my fats; however, with the SCKC, I learned how to rely on other healthier foods such as avocados. I learned different ways to use avocados so I would eat them, began to like both broccoli and cauliflower, and learned how to make homemade mayonnaise, and with Mellissa's recipes I created a whole monthly menu that the family loves! By the end of the challenge, I had not just lost 11 pounds, the most so far in one month, but noticed both my face and fingers had slimmed down. I felt better, I had lost the fogginess, I felt detoxed, and it truly helped my Hashimoto's disease. It's just 30 days—you can do anything for 30 days!"

— Joni L.

"I started my Squeaky Clean Keto journey almost one year ago. I was severely depressed, overweight bordering on obese, and overwhelmed. I thought this would be hard, but I needed to change. I hoped weight loss would help the chronic pain I lived with from severe spinal arthritis. I never imagined that at the end of the first month I'd be down 20 pounds, almost pain free, with amazing, glowing skin. I don't think I can adequately express the change in my pain levels—not only am I able to take part in regular life activities, but I am medication free. No pain meds, no anti-inflammatories, no blood pressure medications, and no medication for my depression and anxiety. This way of living saved my life! The recipes are all delicious and easy to make, and they are also family friendly. The Brazilian Shrimp Stew is a hands-down favorite! Thank you for helping me take back my life, Mellissa!"

— Terri M.

"I started the Squeaky Clean Keto Challenge because I had tried literally every diet there is and was not seeing any results. Even with regular keto, I just wasn't feeling my best. I loved how everything was laid out for me on the website, and the recipes were using ingredients I could find even in my rural town. I prepared all of my meals for the week hoping I liked the food so it wouldn't be wasted and I wouldn't cheat. Well, I LOVED the food. And after a week, I noticed my body did too. I used to be constantly bloated, but that went away. I always had joint pain, and my knees would give out on me from time to time. I'm twenty-five; my knees shouldn't be giving out! Well, I felt like I could sprint miles after a week on the plan. My face cleared up for the first time since before I was diagnosed with PCOS at age eighteen. My eczema, which is normally cracking and bleeding, was almost nonexistent, and my skin was almost its natural color—in just a WEEK! My brain fog was gone—to be honest, I didn't even realize how foggy my brain was before, I just knew how better I felt after it was lifted! I was happier and had a better outlook on everything. I weighed myself after two weeks and found that I had lost 15 pounds! Normally I can't get the scale to budge more than a pound or two. One day, I forgot my lunch at home, and a coworker was ordering from my favorite fast food restaurant and I thought, one day wouldn't hurt. Oh, how I was wrong. The next day, my joints ached so badly, I noticed a bump or two popping up on my face, and my head felt foggy and tired all day. So I jumped right back on plan to finish healing my body and haven't looked back. I haven't officially weighed myself yet, but I have gone from a pants size 24 to 18!"

— *Melissa C.*

"I started with cutting out gluten. Then I heard about keto. Two months in, and with wonderful weight loss results, I stumbled onto the SCKC. I had been dealing with a nasty patch of eczema that varied in intensity but never went away. It struck a chord, and I decided to do it. After the month, made entirely possible by recipes and support from *I Breathe I'm Hungry,* I started adding food back. Turns out in addition to a gluten sensitivity, I am also triggered by dairy and, the biggest shocker, soy. My poor body! I had no idea. I have returned to dirty keto, with occasional non-keto, while avoiding those triggers, and my weight has been stable (and 10 pounds under my goal weight!) for ten months. I cannot thank Mellissa enough for leading me through this journey. And I never felt like I was depriving myself to boot."

— *Katja*

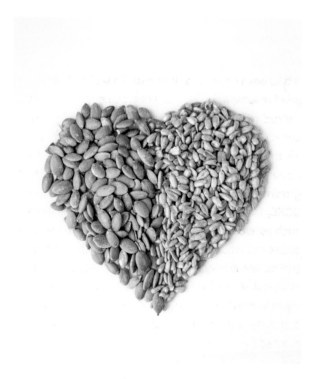

"I always thought giving up foods I'm allergic to would be so overwhelming, but the way you've laid it out it's easy to stay on track without getting frustrated. In two months I dropped 40 pounds. I have so much more energy when I'm eating this way, and my body has never felt so good. With tons of bowel issues, GI problems, plus autoimmune problems, keeping out the dairy, gluten, and sugar has been such a game changer. When eating better I also don't need anxiety, depression, or ADHD meds. Way of eating is so so important!!"

———————————————— *Sarah B.*

"I'm sixty-two years old with a lifetime of dieting. I have more than one autoimmune, and most days my body hurts all over. At the beginning of this year I could not stand myself any longer, and I was desperate to lose weight, feel better, and tie my shoes without huffing and puffing. I had heard about the ketogenic diet but steered away because people were telling me it was not healthy. Out of desperation to lose weight, I searched the internet and found Mellissa Sevigny. I wanted something easy to follow, and I felt I could relate to her easy no-nonsense 30-day SCKC. Within three days, all of my inflammation went down, and I could not believe how good I felt. SCKC is like no other diet I had been on before. I lost 13 pounds the first month. I felt so good I was afraid to go off of her SCKC. When I do decide to add cheese and nuts, I find myself unable to lose weight and then I always end up back on her SCKC. A few months later, I do not hurt all over, I do not use sweeteners, and I can tie my shoes with no problem. I can proudly say, I have lost more weight since my original 13 pounds. I have never felt better, I am so happy to have found Mellissa's SCKC."

———————————————— *Ramona I.*

"Only two more days to go, and I'll have finished my thirty-day challenge. I've adhered to it faithfully, which in truth has really not been difficult at all. Before I started, I had issues with insomnia, extreme morning stiffness, muscle cramps in my sides, feet, calves, and hands, GERD, stomach pain, brain fog, and almost debilitating fatigue. I could sleep ten hours and two hours after I got up, fall asleep on the couch for another hour. Going to the grocery store was starting to feel like a major achievement. This was the reason I decided to do the challenge. The greatest improvement has been in my fatigue—I think I've accomplished more in the past month than I have in the past year. I wake up without stiffness. Muscle cramps are gone, as are stomach pain, GERD, and insomnia. I have definitely lost pounds and inches, which is great, but nothing compares to feeling better."

———————————————— *Janine J.*

"Woot woot, I made it 30 days. I feel so much better. I've discovered that gluten is a major issue for me. I realized that I do need to watch calories, even with keto. I realized that I was eating way too much dairy, specifically cheese. I discovered sunbutter and coconut milk/cream. I wasn't perfect by any means. I almost gave up halfway through because the dang scale wasn't moving. But I stuck with it and I'm down 9 pounds. This is awesome for me since I am challenged with a thyroid issue. I'm going to do the 5-Day Soup Diet again and then head back into squeaky. I have 15 more pounds to goal, and now I feel like I can make it. Don't give up. Focus on the actions and results will come!"

———————————————— *Alisa R.*

THE *Program*
(aka the Nuts and Bolts)

Okay, now that I've hopefully sold you on Squeaky Clean Keto and gotten you excited about giving it a go, let's get down to what it is and how to do it.

The Squeaky Clean Keto Challenge is a thirty-day whole foods, clean eating keto plan that is designed for faster weight loss and better overall health. The focus is less on perfect macros (percentages of fat, carbs, and protein eaten in a day) and more on the quality of food with which you're nourishing yourself.

The basic principles of the Squeaky Clean Keto Challenge are pretty simple—keep to the following guidelines and you're good to go:

1 Keep your net carbs (total carbs – fiber carbs = net carbs) at or below 20 grams per day.

2 Weigh in at the beginning and end of the thirty days and take measurements weekly. (See page 23 for guidelines on taking measurements and a printable chart for tracking.)

3 Don't consume animal-derived dairy products. In other words, no dairy from cows, sheep, goats, water buffalo, unicorns—*nada*. (Butter is the one exception.)

4 Stay away from alcohol. (Flavored extracts like vanilla are the one exception.)

5 Don't consume nuts, nut butters, nut flours, or nut milks made from almonds, cashews, hazelnuts, macadamias, pecans, walnuts, and so on. (Coconut is the one exception.)

6 Don't eat legumes such as peanuts or other starchy beans. (Green beans are the one exception.)

7 Stay away from anything containing gluten or grains—wheat, spelt, bran, oat, quinoa, etc. (Those low-carb tortillas have to go.)

8 Don't use sugar or sweeteners, whether natural or artificial (sugar, honey, maple syrup, agave, stevia, monk fruit, sucralose, aspartame, xylitol, saccharin, erythritol, etc.).

9 Avoid carrageenan, MSG, and food dyes, especially Red 40. (This one isn't strictly required, but you get bonus points if you can do it.)

Boom, you're ready! You can now skip to the recipes and meal plans, right?

Hold on, hold on. The basics are indeed simple, and you could totally follow that list of guidelines and have success, but I've packed a lot of supplemental guidance and tools into this book to help you not only get through the thirty days and see the benefits but do it in a way that takes (most of) the pain out of it.

I want to set you up for success with some additional guidelines, meal plans, meal prep tips, and advice about goal setting and tracking, measuring, journaling, and transitioning. In other words, I want to do everything I can to make sure you're fully equipped to accomplish, and even exceed, your goals on this program.

If you want to skip to the shopping list and get started ASAP, go ahead and do that, but set a goal to get back to this front section soon to go through the other material designed to make the SCKC really work for you and help you change some bad habits and make new healthier ones so that after you've made it through the thirty days of the SCKC, you can continue to make progress toward better health and fitness.

Clean Keto vs. Dirty Keto vs. Lazy Keto vs. Squeaky Clean Keto

If you've been on or looking into the keto diet for any amount of time, you've probably come across the terms *clean keto, dirty keto,* and *lazy keto* and wondered what they mean.

At its core, the phrase *keto diet* simply refers to being in a ketogenic state, which a person typically achieves and maintains by eating 20 grams or less of net carbs per day. Some people can eat a little more than that and maintain ketosis, but 20 grams is what most people aim for.

That's it. If you're doing that, congratulations, you're on the keto diet.

How people approach being on a keto diet can vary wildly. My husband, whom I call Mr. Hungry, would live on cold-cut pickle roll-ups and get all his carbs from cottage cheese if left to his own devices. Other people eat only grass-fed beef and local organic vegetables. Some go "carnivore" and literally live on only meat and fat. If you're like me, well, let's just say that cheese is its own food group and can be used in and on everything.

All these approaches can work if your only aim is to achieve ketosis and drop some extra pounds. You have plenty of options for how to "do" keto; the style you choose depends on your current state of health, your fitness goals, and other factors.

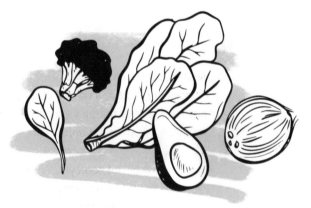

LAZY KETO

Many experts believe that the ideal macronutrient breakdown for a keto diet is to have 70 percent of your calories coming from fats, 25 percent from protein, and 5 percent from carbohydrates. Others say more fat and less protein or vice versa. Most agree that to stay in ketosis, you need to eat no more than 30 grams of net carbs per day—with 20 grams or less being considered optimal.

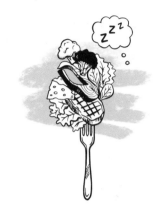

When someone is doing "lazy" keto, it usually means that person is tracking net carbs only (and sometimes only loosely) and isn't worrying about fat or protein intake at all. This approach is good for people who abhor tracking and who are okay with slower results over the long haul.

DIRTY KETO

Dirty keto refers to an approach that follows the typical keto macro ratios, but the components include "dirty" foods like fast food, packaged convenience foods, processed meats, artificially sweetened diet sodas and sports drinks, and unhealthy, highly refined oils like canola and vegetable oils.

Can you lose weight on dirty keto by eating hot dogs, deli meats, excessive amounts of cheese, fast food without the bun, and so on? Yes, absolutely. But you won't be nourishing your body and diminishing your toxic load, thereby reducing inflammation. While you can absolutely get into ketosis and lose weight eating dirty keto, you will definitely not be living your best keto life.

Another term related to dirty keto is *IIFYM*, or "if it fits your macros." That means pretty much anything goes as long as you can fit it into 20 grams of net carbs per day. Four pints of keto-friendly ice cream in one day? Sure, as long as it fits your macros. Protein and fat all day and then four beers with dinner? You betcha. Are you still in ketosis? Probably. Are you reaping the health benefits of lowered inflammation, better digestion, and more energy that can come with a keto diet? I doubt it.

Dirty keto is fine occasionally. Life gets busy, and sometimes your choices are to have a couple of bunless burgers at your local fast food joint or to quit keto altogether because you can't find something clean to eat before you starve to death. Or maybe you're just starting, and you can't bear to give up packaged convenience foods and diet soda yet. Do what you have to do to get in the groove; you can always refine your approach and clean up your diet gradually. Baby steps.

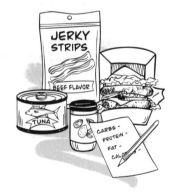

CLEAN KETO

Clean keto is a strict approach to the keto diet that involves diligent macro tracking and eliminating processed foods, artificial sweeteners, unhealthy processed oils, etc. Someone who is eating clean keto may also insist on cage-free eggs, grass-fed and pastured meats and dairy products, and local organic produce. Although that is a nice goal (even if you're not eating keto), not everybody has a budget that allows for that level of clean eating. In my opinion, any time you work with whole foods that are minimally processed and as close to their natural state as possible, you're on the right track.

What one person considers clean keto may not be the same for another. Some people think dairy is fine; others do not. The occasional keto dessert is okay for some; others believe all keto sweeteners are from the devil. Clean keto is open to interpretation, and that interpretation often depends on an individual's ideas of what *healthy* is.

Unfortunately, it's usually the very strict clean keto people who can be incredibly dogmatic about their opinions of what is clean enough. These people are typically the ones on social media who are labeled as the "keto police" because they love to inform you that your bunless burger with a salad isn't keto because the beef isn't from grass-fed cows, your greens aren't organic, and your dressing is made with unhealthy canola oil instead of olive oil. In other words, you are a complete keto failure and "RIDDLED WITH INFLAMMATION, my friend!!!!!" Don't be that guy.

These same people usually identify themselves *as* keto. They don't just eat keto; they *are* keto. You'll often hear them say, "Oh, I can't eat that; I'm keto." In my opinion, this is an unbalanced viewpoint. Keto is nothing more than one of many approaches to healthy eating. It doesn't (or shouldn't) define who you are—it's simply how you're eating right now to reach your goals. Even if you adopt keto as a long-term lifestyle, it shouldn't be how you relate to the world. I'm just saying.

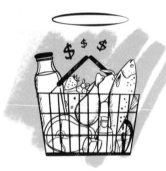

Squeaky Clean Keto

Squeaky Clean Keto (SCK) is an approach that aims for sweeping improvements in your overall eating, removing the main culprits to inflammation and food intolerances, and cutting out foods that lead to overeating and compulsive snacking—primarily dairy, grains, alcohol, sweeteners, and nuts.

Making those changes will drastically improve your health and the speed of your weight loss, but you don't have to go so overboard that you can't realistically sustain these healthier habits long-term. You don't have to be overly dogmatic or buy only ridiculously high-priced "clean" ingredients that aren't affordable or are hard to find.

So many people give up on eating "healthy" because it seems exceedingly complicated and too much work to maintain. Although it's true that convenience foods are called that for a reason, eating healthy whole foods can also be convenient (and delicious) when you do a little advance planning and use recipes that don't require you to spend hours in the kitchen. That said, purchasing condiments like mayonnaise, salad dressings, and other popular seasonings can make daily life easier and the overall plan more sustainable.

The SCK plan isn't quite as restrictive as some people would consider necessary to be "clean" because it doesn't require you to avoid every gram of sugar in condiments or even bacon like the Whole30 plan does. A gram or two of sugar in a salad dressing or some Sriracha isn't going to affect you long-term (as long as you're counting those carbs in your daily allowance), and it makes shopping for food easier and cheaper because you don't have to be so restrictive.

SCK also makes allowances for the occasional use of deli cold cuts for convenience and allows butter as the one exception to the no-dairy rule.

A "Healthier" Way to Keto

People throw around the term *healthy* with regard to recipes and eating plans, but what does it even mean? The term is subjective or dependent on a person's ideals. Someone who eats vegan would categorize a recipe as healthy if it contains no animal products. Others would consider a recipe healthy if it is low-fat or even fat-free. Those on a keto diet consider something healthy if it is high in fat, contains no sugar, and has very few carbohydrates.

I think most people will agree, though—even when at odds about meat versus veg, low-fat versus low-carb, etc.—that a healthy diet consists of whole foods or mostly unprocessed ingredients. In other words, foods that are as close to their natural state as possible.

When it comes to the different ways to approach keto, a good analogy is to view your body like a car engine and the various keto styles like different types of fuel. If you're filling up on premium fuel, your engine will run cleaner and more efficiently—possibly extending the overall life of the car—i.e., you. If you're putting in low-grade sludge, that fuel will still get you where you're going (at least for a while), but eventually it's going to clog you up and leave you sputtering and possibly broken down on the side of the road.

Now that I'm in my mid-forties, my approach to eating and weight loss is less about vanity or reaching a perfect ideal and more about balance and how I feel. I'm more interested in getting the most out of my body so that I can have the energy and stamina to live a satisfying life in my fifties, sixties, and beyond. That requires more than simply restricting carbohydrates and calories as I did back in my twenties.

As with an older car you love, you baby your body a little more as it ages to keep it running smoothly—and premium fuel is one of the ways to ensure that you get the most life out of an engine or yourself. When you're putting only good stuff in and limiting or omitting altogether the unhealthy and inflammation-causing alcohol, grains, dairy, sweeteners, and, yes, for some people even nuts, you will see rapid and tangible results not just on the scale but in other areas as well.

The human body is amazing. Because our cells regenerate constantly, almost any damage can be undone or mitigated when we adopt better eating habits and improve our fuel intake—resulting in good health and boundless energy, even later in life. Although I wish I'd known about the benefits of Squeaky Clean Keto sooner so I could have built a strong foundation from the get-go, it's never too late to start.

In a nutshell, doing Squeaky Clean Keto even 80 percent of the time will both make a big difference in how you feel and affect your weight-loss speed. But you'll never know if you don't try it!

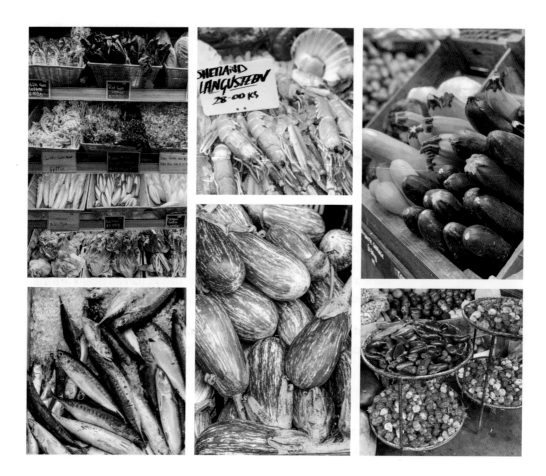

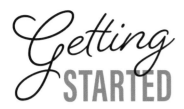

Getting STARTED

This section outlines the basics of how to get started eating Squeaky Clean Keto. I provide a chart (or cheat sheet, if you will) that gives you the program guidelines at a glance. You can photocopy it to keep handy on your fridge or download it from my website to print or save for future reference.

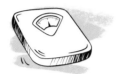

1 NET CARBS 20G OR LESS PER DAY

Keep your net carbs at or below 20 grams per day (total carbs – fiber carbs = net carbs). Weigh at the beginning and end of the challenge.

2 NO DAIRY PRODUCTS

No animal-derived dairy products—cow, sheep, goat, water buffalo, unicorn—*nada.* (Butter is the one exception.)

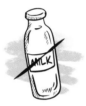

3 NO SUGAR OR SWEETENERS

No added sugar or sweeteners (sugar, honey, maple syrup, agave, aspartame, erythritol, monk fruit, saccharin, stevia, sucralose, xylitol, etc.).

4 NO GRAINS, LEGUMES, OR NUTS

No gluten or grains—wheat, bran, oats, quinoa, spelt, etc.

No legumes—peanuts or other starchy beans. (Green beans are the one exception.)

No nuts, nut milks, or nut flours—almonds, cashews, hazelnuts, macadamias, pecans, walnuts, etc. (Coconut is the one exception.)

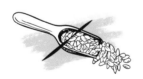

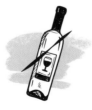

5 NO ALCOHOL

Small amounts of alcohol are fine in extracts like vanilla; no drinking or flavoring recipes with wine or spirits is the goal this month.

Detox: What to Expect

It's going to be hard. Suck it up. Don't quit. The end.

The Mental Game: Coping with Cravings and Emotional Triggers

Weight loss is all about the mental game. We quit diets because we're frustrated, bored, angry about what we're missing out on, or looking for comfort in food. Nobody's hand has an involuntary reflex that makes it start stuffing cookies into one's mouth. That behavior starts in your brain—and a choice to eat off-plan.

Obviously, if the process were as simple as deciding to lose weight and not to eat the bad stuff (or even too much of the good stuff), nobody would be fat. I know what I need to do to lose weight and keep it off, but it's still an ongoing struggle. Why? If I knew the answer to that question, or rather, if I had an easy and foolproof solution to the problem, I'd be a gajillionaire and a size two for the rest of my life.

Unfortunately, there's no way for me, or anyone else, to make you lose weight. Eating keto can help you, and eating Squeaky Clean Keto can speed up the weight-loss process and make you feel healthier and more energetic to boot. But not without a price. And that price isn't in dollars, but in discipline and self-sacrifice.

You have to do the work and make the decision to eat right (or, more importantly, not to eat wrong) every minute of every day. Sometimes it's going to be hard. But it can be done, and the results are worth it. If you believe that and work the program, you'll eventually get where you want to be.

One of the things I've noticed about starting keto again after I've been off for a while (which inevitably leads to weight gain for me because my body's legit superpower is turning carbs into fat) is that for the first few days I feel a little depressed—sometimes I even get irrationally mad about it.

After talking to others, I found that many struggle with the same thing on keto—especially initially. I spent some time thinking about why I'd get so angry and frustrated when starting keto, and I realized that it wasn't actual hunger—I mean, I'm not starving or anything. I, even more than most people, can cook up lots of delicious keto-friendly food like it's my job—because it literally is.

What it boils down to is that I just miss the normalcy of eating what I want to eat and drinking what I want to drink—especially when having dinner with friends, or relaxing, or treating myself after a long, hard day.

So what is really at the core of my frustration is that it just doesn't seem fair that to lose weight and thus be happy with how I look, I have to deprive myself of eating and drinking what I enjoy. I can't just go with the flow and have it be easy. I have to plan, say no to things, and work harder than everyone else who is just ordering what they like off the menu or making a quick sandwich to take for lunch. Now everything is more complicated—even going to a friend's house for dinner becomes rife with anxiety and wondering if I should bring my own food or maybe not go at all so I'm not tempted to cheat and go off-plan.

Cue massive pity party.

Inevitably, though, if I hang in there and don't quit, I get in the groove within a few days, and the scale starts moving in the right direction. Within a couple of weeks, it feels easy peasy. I remember why I love eating keto, and until the next time a vacation or traveling has me going off-plan for a bit, it feels like I could do it forever and never miss the carbs.

Maybe if you've done keto before, you know the initial struggle I'm talking about—and I hope you also know from experience that if you just stick it out for a week or two, it will be pretty effortless from then on.

But now we're talking Squeaky Clean Keto. That means, in the already (initially, at least) challenging keto construct, you're also giving up dairy, nuts, sweeteners, and alcohol. That means saying bye-bye to keto ice cream, dark chocolate, whiskey nightcaps, and rum and Diet Cokes with friends—at least for thirty days.

If you're thinking, "No problem, I've got this," then I admire your optimism. But—I'm just keeping it real here—it's going to be hard at times. Don't delude yourself into thinking that you won't face some challenges. Otherwise, you won't be mentally prepared for them, and you might just give up before you start to benefit from the positive effects.

The five stages of squeaky (even if you've already been keto for a while) are typically as follows:

1. **Optimism:** I'm going to lose so much weight! I'm going to look amazing and feel better than I ever have! I'm going to fit into those goal jeans (or dress or bathing suit) by the end of the month!

2. **Grief:** I miss cream in my coffee. Why do I even get out of bed in the morning? All my friends are going out this weekend, and I can't even have a drink or eat nachos; maybe I should just stay home alone. I walked by the cheese aisle while grocery shopping today and had to choke back a sob.

3. **Anger** (for me the most dangerous stage): This is stupid! I can lose just as much weight on regular keto; why am I doing this to myself?! I miss my nightly wasabi almonds. The internet says nuts are anti-inflammatory, and this plan says I can't eat nuts. Who does this chick think she is? I hate her and everything she stands for. I would rather be fat than live without joy! I WANT TO QUIT!

4. **Acceptance:** I'm glad I didn't quit. This isn't easy, but I feel good, and my clothes fit better. My skin is clearer, and I'm getting a solid eight hours of sleep for the first time in years. Coffee without cream isn't as bad as I thought it would be; I actually like it with cocoa butter. Who knew?

5. **Determination:** I am killing it. I'm down a dress size, my skinny jeans will zip up again, and I took the stairs today just because I could. I can easily eat squeaky for another couple of months—and if I actually start using that gym membership I bought, I might have visible abs by the summer.

There's no set timeline for the five stages of SCK. You might experience them all in one week, have some overlap, or even repeat them throughout the month—especially if you're a woman with active monthly hormonal cycles. But if you stay the course, the grief and anger stages will eventually give way to the acceptance and determination stages—and once you're there, it's usually pretty smooth sailing.

TIPS FOR GETTING THROUGH THE FRUSTRATING MOMENTS

Stop using food as entertainment. Enjoy what you're eating, but put meals in their place—your entire source of joy and comfort should not be tied to food. Replace that crutch, or you'll go right back to old habits when the challenge is finished.

When you're eating with friends, focus on the conversation rather than the food. You can still eat, but that shouldn't be the highlight of the evening. If it is, then you probably need to start looking for new friends.

If you enjoy the occasional evening tipple like I do, instead of having that glass of wine or vodka martini, make a cup of tea. I know that might sound crazy, but it works. I recommend investing in a cute mug and tea infuser that will make it more fun. You can order some really delicious and relatively inexpensive craft teas online—Amazon carries tons of them. Do whatever it takes to make tea drinking an event you enjoy and even look forward to at the end of the day. Bonus points that tea is pretty much calorie-free, so even if you decide to reintroduce alcohol after the challenge, tea drinking is a healthy habit that you can hold onto.

If you tend to use food as a reward at the end of a long day, or if you're a habitual nighttime snacker, find other ways to treat yourself and keep your hands busy.

Give yourself a home facial or pedicure. Groom your pet or play a game with your kids—do anything to break those old evening habits of sitting and eating. For me, staying busy and avoiding the couch and Netflix is a good way to keep my mind off snacking. When I do catch up on my shows, a cup of tea helps keep my hands and face busy. If you're good at multitasking, you can take up crocheting or knitting, and that will keep your hands busy while you watch TV.

Finally, if you're going to do the thirty-day Squeaky Clean Keto Challenge, commit fully. Don't look for loopholes and ways to keep your old habits in place while you're supposed to be squeaky—that's a slippery slope that can lead to giving up. Instead, use the challenge as an opportunity not just to lose weight faster but to change old habits that were hindering your progress to begin with.

Then, when the challenge is over, you can carry on with those healthier habits firmly in place, hopefully for life.

SNACKING

Speaking of ditching old habits, let's talk about snacking. I'm a world-class snacker. I mean, I can snack like nobody's business. It doesn't matter if I'm technically hungry or not—when the sun goes down and the TV goes on, I'm like one of Pavlov's dogs, and my fingers are itching to feed my face. Back in the day, it was popcorn, chips, crackers—you name it, and I will snack it straight to the bottom of the bag. True story.

Many people are under the misconception that calories don't matter on keto, and as long as you're under your carb budget for the day, you can snack your little heart out. That's simply not true. There are plenty of keto-friendly snack options out there—crackers, cheese, nuts, pepperoni chips, Whisps, etc. They're all calorie-dense and will inhibit your progress if you eat them with wild abandon—the same as their carb-heavy counterparts.

The fact is, most people (myself included) use snacking as entertainment. Like, why even bother relaxing if I can't eat while doing it? It all goes together—especially when watching TV or movies. They sell popcorn at the movies for a reason, right? And people pay eight dollars for that bucket for a reason. Without it, the whole movie-theater experience doesn't feel complete.

Snacking behavior is a mindset. To be successful at losing weight and keeping it off, you need to change your mindset. It's that simple.

Stop snacking for entertainment. Find something else to do with your hands until you can turn on the TV without reaching for the chips—even if they are keto-friendly ones. Once you stop eating mindlessly, you'll see the weight drop off, and you'll be able to keep it off, even with the occasional weekend movie marathon indulgence.

That said, if you find yourself needing a little somethin'-somethin' between lunch and dinner to keep you going, then eating SCK-friendly whole foods like half an avocado, a few pickles, or some hard-boiled eggs with mayo won't hurt you. Just be sure you're eating because you're hungry and not because you're bored.

Tracking Your Progress: Measuring vs. Weighing

Inches are the real holy grail—they're what people see with their eyes and what determine how your clothes fit. That number on the scale and whether it's up or down by a few ounces every morning is not really important. It's the long game that matters, and I encourage you not to weigh yourself at all during the first thirty days.

If you can stand to hold out for the whole challenge, you'll be thrilled with the big drop at the end rather than being stressed that it doesn't go down every day or even goes up slightly some days due to water weight from hormone fluctuations and other temporary factors.

The biggest problem with weighing is that after a few days of no visible drop on the scale, people tend to get frustrated at their perceived lack of progress and give up—which helps nothing.

So I'm providing you with a measurement chart and a tutorial on how to measure yourself properly to help you track how many inches you lose each week. I recommend that you weigh yourself only once a month; remember, the scale is a big fat lying liar and not an accurate barometer of your progress. Measurements are where it's at.

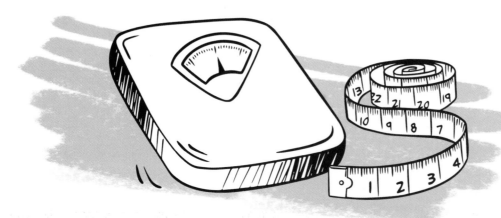

TIPS ON TAKING YOUR MEASUREMENTS:

1. Use a soft measuring tape or string that can be measured

2. Always measure in the same place with the same tightness

3. Relax, try not to suck in or puff out!

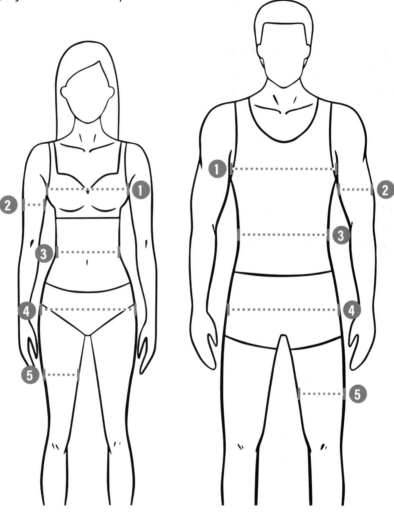

1 CHEST

Measure around your fullest part, under your armpits and around your shoulder blades.

2 ARMS

Measure around the largest part of your arm—don't flex.

3 WAIST

Measure around the smallest part of your waist—above your belly button and below your ribcage.

4 HIPS

Measure the widest part of your hips—around your buttocks.

5 THIGHS

Measure around the fullest part of your thigh—upper middle leg.

Journaling for Success

Journal your progress. Journaling can feel weird if you're not used to it, but we're not talking about writing *War and Peace* here. Just keep track daily of anything important.

Here's an example of how easy and brief your journal can be while still being effective at reminding you of how the month went and where you might want to tighten up or do some more experimenting.

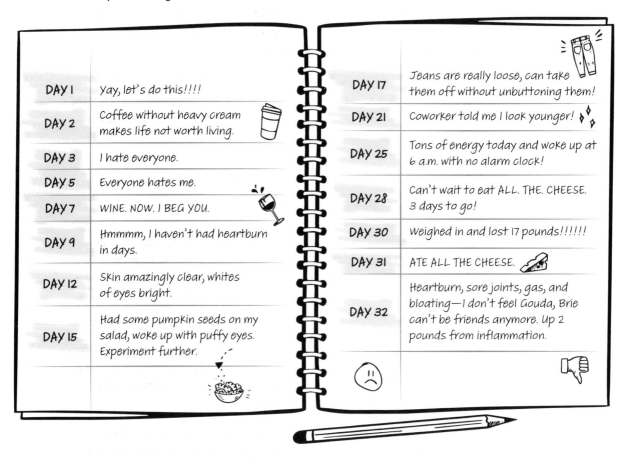

DAY 1	Yay, let's do this!!!!
DAY 2	Coffee without heavy cream makes life not worth living.
DAY 3	I hate everyone.
DAY 5	Everyone hates me.
DAY 7	WINE. NOW. I BEG YOU.
DAY 9	Hmmmm, I haven't had heartburn in days.
DAY 12	Skin amazingly clear, whites of eyes bright.
DAY 15	Had some pumpkin seeds on my salad, woke up with puffy eyes. Experiment further.
DAY 17	Jeans are really loose, can take them off without unbuttoning them!
DAY 21	Coworker told me I look younger!
DAY 25	Tons of energy today and woke up at 6 a.m. with no alarm clock!
DAY 28	Can't wait to eat ALL. THE. CHEESE. 3 days to go!
DAY 30	Weighed in and lost 17 pounds!!!!!!
DAY 31	ATE ALL THE CHEESE.
DAY 32	Heartburn, sore joints, gas, and bloating—I don't feel Gouda, Brie can't be friends anymore. Up 2 pounds from inflammation.

Now don't go panicking and saying, "I'm not doing the SCKC if it's going to make me allergic to dairy!!!" This is a fictional example of how it might go and how you could discover that you have always had an underlying issue with some ingredients but just didn't realize it. Or maybe you suspected it but have been ignoring it because it's easier to delude yourself without the facts staring you in the face.

It's up to you to decide whether to indulge in those foods occasionally. Just make sure it's worth it when you do!

Best gelato of my life in Italy? Worth it every time, even if I'm doubled over the next day. Cheese on my bunless burger on an average Wednesday night? Probably going to skip it and not take the chance. Extra bacon for me, please, and I won't even be sad about it.

Take "Before" Photos

If you're not happy with the way you look right now, I know you probably don't want photo proof of it, but trust me, photos are a great way to see your progress in a tangible form, and you don't have to share them with anyone. When you're looking at yourself in the mirror daily, it's easy to miss the changes that take place over time.

Ideally, you want face shots from both the front and the side (I'm looking at you, double chin) and full-body shots (clothed is fine) from the front, sides, and back if you have someone who can take them for you. At the very least, plan to take one face photo per week. You'll be glad you did, even if no one but you ever lays eyes on them!

You may find it hard to believe now that you'll ever show anyone those photos, but once you're rocking that brand-new body, you'll want everyone to know how far you've come! And even if you decide never to share them, you'll have those photos to help keep you from sinking back into old unhealthy habits and gaining the weight again.

After the Challenge/Transitioning

Once you've completed your first thirty days of Squeaky Clean Keto, it's time to start reintroducing some of the foods that you've been avoiding to see if they have been negatively affecting you. The best way to do so is one food at a time; if you start eating dairy, nuts, and alcohol all at once and then feel bloated or experience other symptoms, how will you isolate the culprit?

I recommend reintroducing one item per week; the order doesn't matter. After a week, evaluate whether you're experiencing any negative impact from that food. If so, cut it out again. If not, continue eating it and reintroduce another item. Repeat until you've added back in whatever foods you wanted to and then evaluate any that caused issues.

If you added back all dairy and had problems, try eating only aged hard cheeses that don't contain much lactose, or heavy whipping cream but no milk or yogurt. See if you can drill down to what it is about dairy that bothers you—you might have to cut out some things but not others.

For me, mozzarella causes issues, but Parmesan doesn't. Gelato is a killer, but whipped cream sweetened with erythritol is no problem. You'll have to figure out what it is that causes an issue—and maybe you will find that you are totally fine with all dairy but that almonds make your joints hurt. Or low-carb tortillas made with gluten make your face break out every single time.

The results will be different for everyone. And maybe you'll get away scot-free with no adverse effects from anything—but at least you'll know!

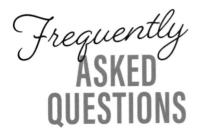

Frequently ASKED QUESTIONS

When I first rolled out the Squeaky Clean Keto Challenge on my website, readers asked some of the same questions over and over again. I've addressed them on the website and in the SCKC Facebook group, but I'm also providing an easy-to-reference list here with answers to some of the most frequently asked questions about the program.

Can Squeaky Clean Keto Help Me Break Through a Plateau?

The short answer is yes; many people have used SCK to break through a stall or plateau. But what is a "plateau," anyway? A real weight-loss plateau is when you haven't lost any weight for four to six weeks or more, even though you are actively trying to. Many people think they are in a "stall" because the scale isn't moving fast enough for them, but that's not a true stall; it's just the unfortunate reality of losing weight at a slow but steady pace.

It's natural for us to gain weight by degrees, so it's easy to ignore or justify as water weight or temporary bloating at first. Then we get complacent about those extra 10 pounds, which turns into 20, or 30, or more over time if we don't make the necessary changes. If it happened really fast and our weight shot up 30 pounds in a month, we would panic, and as a result, we would probably self-arrest and change our habits quickly to fix the problem—but that's typically not how it works.

For most of us, weight loss happens in a similar way to, or even more slowly than, weight gain does. To avoid getting discouraged by how slowly you're losing, especially if you have a lot of weight to lose at first, set smaller goals on the way to the big one. Let your body adjust by tens, and don't expect that you're going to drop 30 to 40 pounds in a month or two.

The majority of people who've done the plan and reported their results have found that they lose weight much faster on Squeaky Clean Keto than on "regular" keto. But you still need to be realistic about how fast your body can shed weight healthily and sustainably.

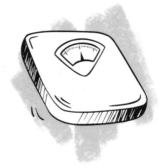

Can I Do Intermittent Fasting with Squeaky Clean Keto?

Absolutely! Intermittent fasting is a great tool to help you reach your health and weight-loss goals on any eating plan, including Squeaky Clean Keto.

Week 4 of the SCKC meal plan (see pages 62 and 63) incorporates a short window of fasting to get your feet wet. If you find it tolerable and feel up to tackling longer periods, I recommend doing some research on the benefits of and different approaches to intermittent fasting before you decide which one is right for you. I highly recommend Dr. Jason Fung's book *The Complete Guide to Fasting* as a starting point.

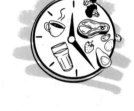

Once you start fasting more often, there are a few apps available that can help you track your fasts and journal your results. I use an app called Zero, and it definitely keeps me accountable and helps me stay the course when I'm tempted to stop short of my fasting goal with just a few hours left.

Can I Work Out While Doing Squeaky Clean Keto?

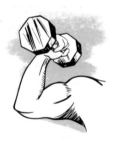

Yes, and you may find that once you get through the detox phase, which could include some temporary fatigue, you'll have more energy than ever to devote to your workouts.

I'm a Vegetarian/Vegan; Can I Still Do Squeaky Clean Keto?

Yes! Following a keto eating plan while not consuming meat or animal products can be a challenge, but it's definitely possible. There are plenty of plant-based SCK-friendly recipes in this book to get you started. (The Sheet Pan Veggie Burgers recipe on page 306 is one of my favorites.) Shelled hemp seeds (aka hemp hearts) are one of the few plant sources that contain all the essential amino acids that make up a complete protein, so you'll want to stock up on those. The most important thing to remember is that plant foods contain more carbs than meat, so you'll have to be diligent with meal planning and tracking to keep your net carbs under 20 grams per day so you can stay in ketosis.

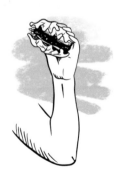

What About My Social Life?

Although you may find it a bit of a test to be around friends who are drinking and eating the things you're avoiding while on the plan, there's no reason to live like a hermit during your SCKC.

The Drinks & Snacks chapter of the book (beginning on page 312) doesn't contain any actual cocktails, but it does feature plenty of tasty beverages that will make you feel like you're getting your sip on without actually imbibing.

When planning get-togethers, try to make eating and drinking less of a focus by having an activity on deck rather than simply sitting around at a restaurant or bar. Start a knitting club, have a pedicure party, play cards or board games, and, when possible, provide plenty of compliant foods that everyone can enjoy.

If you end up going out, at least pick a place with a dart-board or billiards table so you can enjoy time with friends without having your hands free to head toward your face with non-squeaky eats.

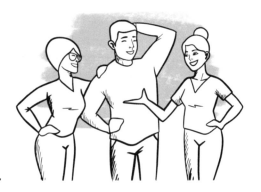

When you do find yourself faced with eating at a restaurant, you can't go wrong with ordering grilled meat or seafood and a side of sautéed vegetables—just ask for any sauce or dressing to be on the side so you can make sure it's not sweetened before your entire plate is drowning in it.

I'm Not Made of Money; Won't Eating This Way Be Super Expensive?

Lots of people are under the misconception that eating keto, let alone Squeaky Clean Keto, is more expensive than their typical diet, and that is simply not always the case.

Although it's true that many expensive supplements and other keto products are being promoted on blogs and social media these days, there are very few "extras" that are essential to a successful keto diet—and most of them aren't expensive at all.

The few specialty ingredients recommended in this book can be purchased in bulk from Amazon, Thrive Market, and other websites at very reasonable prices.

Here are some examples of how eating Squeaky Clean Keto compares in cost to the standard American diet (SAD) and regular keto. All these prices are based on what I found on Amazon or Walmart at the time I was writing this manuscript. Obviously, prices can vary based on timing and location—but this chart gives you a general idea.

SAD	16 ounces brand-name peanut butter	$2.48
KETO	16 ounces unsweetened almond butter	$10.99
SCK	16 ounces homemade sunflower seed butter	$3.37
SAD	64 ounces whole milk from cows	$1.79
KETO	64 ounces unsweetened almond milk	$2.97
SCK	64 ounces homemade hemp milk	$2.76
SAD	16 ounces all-purpose wheat flour	$0.86
KETO	16 ounces almond flour	$7.38
SCK	16 ounces homemade sunflower seed flour	$3.00

So, as you can see from these few examples, eating SCK isn't the least expensive option, but it's not significantly more expensive than the SAD, and it's actually cheaper than regular keto in some cases.

Take into account all the money you won't be spending on beer, wine, spirits, heavy cream, cheese, and nuts, and you might find that you're actually saving money in the long run.

Do I Have to Track My Macros?

Although it's crucial that you track your net carbs to maintain a ketogenic state (20 grams or less being optimal), I don't think it's necessary to track every gram of fat or protein that passes your lips. If you're the type of person who enjoys the process of tracking everything you eat, then by all means, you can continue to do so while eating SCK. However, if the thought of tracking and entering every morsel into an app or journal makes you want to give up before you even start, then don't despair! Simply follow the meal plans beginning on page 54, and you'll see results with no tracking required.

Once you get the basics down, you'll find that keeping track of your carb intake becomes easier and easier. Should your weight loss slow or stop as you get closer to your goal weight, you can start looking at fat and protein to see if you can make further adjustments to those macros to lose those last few pounds.

There are so many apps available for macro tracking that it can be hard to decide which one to use. Because apps come and go, whatever I recommend at the time of writing may no longer be relevant by the time you're reading this book. Currently, Carb Manager and Cronometer are the two that seem most popular with the SCK Facebook group, so you can check them out if you like. I don't recommend MyFitnessPal because the database is full of errors and the carb counts of ingredients are often way off as a result.

Do I Need to Take Supplements?

If the internet is to be believed, you can't be successful on any keto diet without a pantry full of pricey MCT powders, protein shakes, exogenous ketones, electrolyte replacement drinks, and the like. No wonder people think keto is expensive!

In spite of all the hype surrounding the supplements and gadgets that so many popular keto "influencers" are hawking on blogs and social media these days, you don't need all that stuff to get results. There are, however, a few legitimate (and inexpensive) additions to your keto diet that you may want to consider:

- **Sugar-free daily multivitamin:** You may want to consider one to fill in any nutritional gaps and ensure you're getting enough vitamins—especially vitamin C.

- **Calcium:** Since you're eliminating dairy products for at least the first thirty days of SCK, you need to make sure you're getting enough calcium. Sardines, spinach, kale, and sunflower seeds are all high in calcium, but you can also supplement with a pill if necessary.

- **Potassium:** Potassium is an important electrolyte that you'll need to replenish often because you don't retain fluids on keto. Salmon, avocados, spinach, and tomato sauce are all rich natural sources of potassium that are SCK friendly. The easiest way to replenish potassium, though, is a product called lite salt, which you can find in the spice aisle of almost any grocery store. A few shakes a day is all you'll need to ensure you're getting enough potassium. Be sure not to overdo it, because too much potassium is even worse than not enough.

- **Magnesium citrate:** You can get magnesium citrate, which is inexpensive and effective at replenishing magnesium, in liquid, pill, or powder form at most pharmacies. Beware of powders like Natural Calm that contain sweeteners, which are a no-no on Squeaky Clean Keto. You can also get magnesium from SCK-approved natural sources like sardines, hemp seeds, pumpkin seeds, and sunflower seeds.

- **Moringa:** Although it's not necessary for success, moringa, especially in tea form, is excellent for reducing appetite and inflammation in the body. As moringa has grown in popularity for its many health benefits, moringa tea has become available in most grocery stores—even Lipton has several flavors to choose from.

- **Sauerkraut:** Whether homemade or store-bought (live and unpasteurized), immunity-boosting sauerkraut is a healthy addition to your keto diet. Sauerkraut is loaded with vitamins, fiber, and, most important, beneficial probiotic bacteria, making it good for your gut and your overall health. Just a tablespoon or two a day can work wonders, and there are many delicious flavors to be had. You can usually find them in the refrigerated area of your grocery store's produce section.

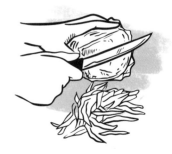

What Fruits and Veggies Can I Eat on the SCKC?

I am not going to give you a list of foods to eat on the SCKC because people tend to see a list of approved foods and think that as long as they eat from that list, they will succeed. Unfortunately, it's not that simple. Keto is about chemistry—you can't simply work off of a list of foods that are deemed "keto-friendly" or even "SCK-friendly" without also counting the carbohydrates.

If you eat too many carbohydrates, you'll get kicked out of ketosis—it doesn't matter if those carbs come from chocolate, bananas, potatoes, or spinach. You have to track what you eat if you want to stay in ketosis and reap the benefits of a ketogenic diet. There are no loopholes, potions, or supplements that will allow you to cheat the system and stay in ketosis while overeating carbohydrates—no matter how healthy the source of those carbs might be.

With that caveat in mind, there are some fruits and vegetables that are lower in carbs and easier to fit into your keto lifestyle than others. I've made a list of my favorites, along with their carb counts per cup for your reference. Please keep in mind that this is not an exhaustive list; there are plenty of other low-carb greens and veggies that fit very well into the SCK program. Just be sure to calculate the net carbs and count them toward your daily budget of 20 grams.

SCK-Friendly Fruits and Vegetables

INGREDIENTS	NET CARBS IN 1 CUP RAW	INGREDIENTS	NET CARBS IN 1 CUP RAW
Blackberries	7g	Red radishes	2.4g
Raspberries	7g	Asparagus	2.5g
Strawberries	8g	Avocado	3g
Blueberries	17g	Cauliflower florets	3g
Spinach	0.4g	Yellow summer squash, sliced	3g
Romaine lettuce	0.5g	Zucchini, sliced	3g
Spring greens	0.7g	Green cabbage, shredded	3.2g
Swiss chard (aka Silverbeet)	0.7g	Broccoli florets	3.5g
Cucumbers, sliced	1.8g	Green beans, sliced	4g
Celery, sliced	1.9g	Brussels sprouts	4.7g
Eggplant, cubed	2g	Turnips, chopped	6g
White mushrooms	2g	Spaghetti squash	7.5g

Note: Blueberries are the highest in carbs by volume. For that reason, I recommend keeping your serving size to ⅓ cup or less.

How Come I Can Have Butter but Not Heavy Whipping Cream? Aren't They Basically the Same Thing?

I get this question a lot, and often people ask because they want to justify having cream in their coffee—and I get it; I do (see "But First, Coffee" on page 34). But the sad fact is, although butter is an almost pure fat containing only trace amounts, if any, of the common allergens lactose, whey, and casein, heavy whipping cream is usually only about 36 percent fat—the rest is essentially milk.

If you churn heavy whipping cream, you'll end up with a chunk of butter and a large amount of liquid by-product called buttermilk. One cup of buttermilk contains about 12 grams of sugar and 8 grams of protein. Those by-products are what you're trying to avoid while on Squeaky Clean Keto—at least until you can determine if they're inflammation triggers for you.

Why Can't I Have Nuts? Aren't They Healthy and Anti-Inflammatory?

Nuts are a common allergen that can raise inflammation if you have even a slight intolerance. Just because your throat doesn't close up when you eat nuts as it would in someone with a life-threatening allergy doesn't necessarily mean that your body tolerates nuts well. You can't really know whether they are affecting you unless you cut them out for a while.

Even if you aren't sensitive to nuts from an inflammation standpoint, they are incredibly calorie-dense and far too easy to overeat, which inhibits weight loss.

How Can I Combat Keto Breath Without Sugar-Free Gum or Mints?

Keto breath is real, and it's not pleasant—especially for the people close to you. While many people rely on sugar-free gum and mints to mask keto breath, they are a no-no on SCK because of the sweeteners they contain.

If you're an introvert who prefers to avoid people anyway, then this isn't a problem—but the rest of you may want to employ a few of the following strategies to keep from losing your friends along with the weight.

- **Brush your teeth.** Seriously, there's no substitute for a clean mouth—it's the foundation of fresh breath.

- **Drink more water.** Because you excrete ketones (the source of keto breath) in both urine and exhalations, the more water you drink to flush and dilute them, the less you are going to be exhaling onto others.

- **Keep your distance.** Nobody likes a "close talker," but it's especially awkward if your breath leaves something to be desired. When in doubt, keep a minimum of 2 feet between you and your victim.

- **Chew mint leaves.** You can simply chew a few mint leaves throughout the day to keep your breath fresh—easy and cheap (especially if you have a garden). Parsley and cilantro also work wonders!

- **Use peppermint oil.** Keep a vial of peppermint oil handy in your purse or car and apply a drop of it to your tongue as needed.

- **Chew cardamom pods.** You can find cardamom pods in the spice aisle, and they're very effective at freshening breath—just be sure to discreetly spit out the woody remains rather than swallowing them.

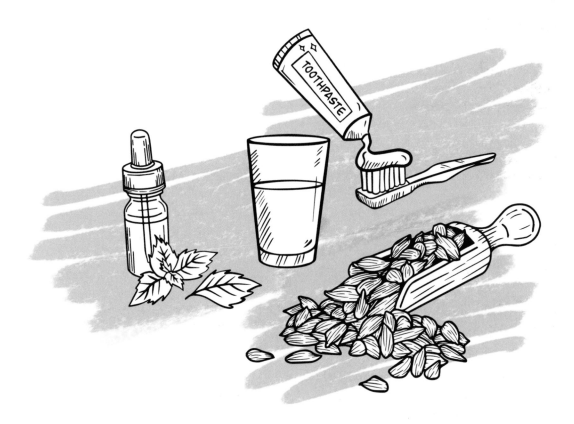

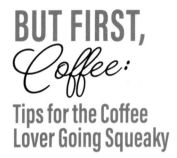

BUT FIRST, *Coffee:*
Tips for the Coffee Lover Going Squeaky

The number one question I get about taking on the Squeaky Clean Keto Challenge is, "But what about my coffee? I can't possibly drink it black/unsweetened/etc."

If you're like me, coffee is one of the highlights of your day. Sometimes I go to sleep smiling, already anticipating that first cup of steaming cappuccino or light and sweet cold brew. Because yes, my dream coffee does usually include copious amounts of dairy—and occasionally sweeteners too.

So what's a latte-loving girl (or guy) to do when staring down thirty days of dairy-free, sweetener-free, almond milk–free coffee? Don't give up just yet, because I've got some tips to shore up your squeaky coffee game.

Buy Better Coffee

Now, I'm not saying you have to pony up for the best beans out there (who wants to drink something harvested out of jungle cat poop, anyway?), but paying a couple of dollars more per pound is completely worth it if you're a coffee lover.

Contrary to popular belief, those famous chain coffeehouse beans they sell at your local grocery store for $12 a pound aren't actually the best you can do. Lots of small craft roasters out there are making incredible (and sustainable) coffee and selling it relatively cheap on sites like Amazon. You can even join a coffee club that will send you 2 pounds of different coffees from all over the world every month—for less than the price of four pretentiously named, carb-laden lattes from your favorite coffee shop.

Like anything else you plan to eat or drink, you don't need a lot of extras to make it taste good when you start with high-quality fresh ingredients—it's going to be delicious right out of the gate. So start shopping around for better coffee; with all that money you'll be saving on heavy whipping cream, you can afford to. Hopefully, it will make your morning coffee experience more pleasurable even if you go back to cream and sweeteners when the challenge is over.

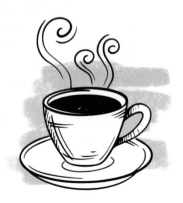

Coping Without Cream

No matter how good the quality of the coffee you're starting with, black coffee just doesn't have the luscious, creamy mouthfeel of coffee with heavy cream added to it. If you just can't even with black coffee, don't despair; you have plenty of delicious and creamy options to choose from while keeping it squeaky.

COCOA BUTTER

I'm going to start with my favorite nondairy coffee additive, and that's cocoa butter, which is the pure fat extracted from cocoa beans. You can purchase cocoa butter (or cacao butter— same thing) from health food stores or online in bulk from sites like Amazon, and it usually comes in a resealable bag. I store mine in the fridge to keep it from melting. I just throw a few chunks (about 2 tablespoons' worth) into the blender along with my hot coffee, which gives me an ultra-creamy coffee topped with a delicate foam. The cocoa butter imparts a subtle chocolate flavor to the coffee that is simply delicious.

COCONUT MILK

Canned coconut milk or coconut cream (which is a little thicker) is an easy and inexpensive addition to your morning cup of joe. Canned coconut milk is shelf-stable, and you can store the unused portion in the refrigerator for up to a week. You can also purchase packets of coconut milk powder, which stays fresh for a long time and gives coffee an even thicker consistency because no water has been added. Or try my Vanilla Mocha Coconut Creamer on page 322, which works great hot or iced!

MCT OIL

Extracted from coconut oil, MCT (medium-chain triglyceride) oil has none of the coconut flavor that some people find off-putting, particularly in coffee. (MCT oil or coconut oil is a key ingredient in the famous bulletproof coffee.) A pure fat and an excellent source of energy, MCT oil has antifungal properties that make it a healthy addition to your keto diet. Some people find that MCT oil has a laxative effect, so start small (no more than 1 tablespoon per day) and work your way up to several tablespoons or more if desired. This will ensure that you don't get blindsided by the potential unpleasant side effects.

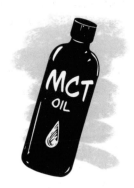

HEMP MILK

Hemp milk works very well as a coffee creamer. I especially love to whip it into a foam in my blender and use it for a Hemp Milk Cappuccino (page 330), which tastes surprisingly legit!

UNSALTED BUTTER

Blending butter into your coffee may sound weird, but it's quite delicious! When you add unrefined coconut oil or MCT oil in addition to butter, you've got a Basic Bulletproof Coffee (page 324).

Emulsify

Emulsi-what? If you've never heard of emulsifying, it's simply the process of blending two liquids of different consistencies so thoroughly that they appear to be one. It's most commonly used when referring to salad dressing—typically a blend of oil and vinegar, which everyone knows can't truly be mixed. You can shake them together, but after a few minutes they will quickly separate again. When you blend them at high speed, however, you get an emulsification that allows the fatty oil to thicken the watery vinegar, and the flavors are fully combined when consumed.

You can do the same thing with the fats you add to your coffee. It's important to emulsify butter or oil into your coffee with a blender or frother to turn the whole cup creamy rather than simply having the fat sit on top like an oil slick. Even when you start with a fully emulsified beverage, if you don't drink it within a few minutes, the fat will begin to separate.

However, you can slow down how quickly the fat separates, and increase the creaminess of your coffee, by adding a tablespoon of powdered collagen peptides (aka hydrolysate) to the mix. The collagen stabilizes the emulsification and keeps the coffee and oil from separating after a few minutes.

Sweet Nothings

You can (almost) fool your face into thinking there's sweetener in your coffee by using flavored extracts—not syrups, which contain sweetener, but actual extracts and flavorings that you find in the baking aisle. I like vanilla, chocolate, and, surprisingly, maple extracts best, but you can use whatever works for you. Again, there is no substitute for starting with a good-quality coffee—if you usually sweeten because you find coffee bitter, then look for a mellower roast with overtones of chocolate or caramel.

MEAL PREP
Tips

As mentioned in the introduction, my goal with this book isn't just to provide you with a diet plan and some recipes but also to help you become a better cook overall. Part of that training involves acquiring some skills at doing some easy prep work at home that will save you money on grocery shopping.

One of the easiest ways to save money on groceries is to purchase foods in their whole form and cut them up, or "break them down," at home. The more hands that touch your food to get it ready to consume before you buy it, the more money you will pay for that item.

Sometimes it's worth paying extra for the sake of convenience, or if the preparation requires some skill that you don't have, such as trimming meat. But cutting a head of broccoli into florets or trimming boneless chicken breasts is a simple matter of a sharp knife, a cutting board, and a few minutes of time. If you're willing to put in that time, you can save potentially hundreds of dollars a month on groceries.

If you have a large freezer, you can purchase larger quantities from bulk retailers like Costco and pay less per pound for most meats and vegetables. But even if you don't have a large freezer, breaking down your own meats from the grocery store and freezing them until you need them will save you a significant amount of money. You can invest in a vacuum sealer if you like, but honestly, a sturdy plastic zip-top freezer bag will do the trick almost as well without a big payout upfront.

The following are some basic techniques for breaking down whole ingredients. If you're not feeling confident the first time, there are plenty of YouTube videos that will walk you through these techniques step by step until you've got them down pat.

Chicken

BREASTS

Buy chicken breasts in large packages—they're cheaper by the pound when you buy in bulk. Then spend a few minutes trimming the gristle from the edges, and they're ready to use.

There's no need to pay extra for chicken "tenders" when you can simply cut a breast into strips. The same applies to chicken "cutlets," which are thinner pieces that have been cut from the breast. You can make chicken cutlets yourself by cutting a breast in half or thirds horizontally, with your knife parallel to the cutting board. For even thinner cutlets, place a cutlet in a large plastic freezer bag (unsealed) and pound it with a meat mallet to your desired thickness. Keeping it in the bag while pounding prevents juice and bits of raw chicken from showering both you and your kitchen as you work. Discard the bag when finished.

Refrigerate (or freeze, if well in advance) your chicken pieces in 1-pound portions so that you have them ready to throw into recipes like Tuscan Chicken with Zoodles (page 170), Sesame Chicken Fingers (page 180), or Crispy Lemon Chicken (page 192).

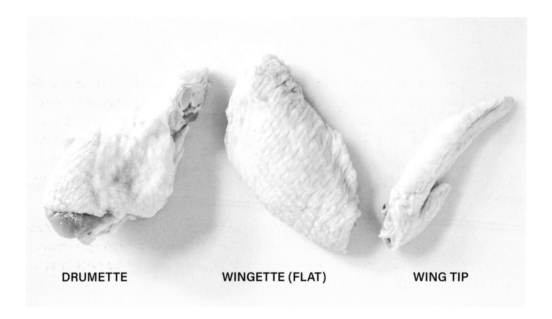

DRUMETTE   **WINGETTE (FLAT)**   **WING TIP**

WINGS

Stop spending money on precut chicken wings! You will spend as much as $2 per pound or more for chicken wing "drumettes" that are already cut and frozen—and they won't taste nearly as good as fresh. Purchase large packages of whole chicken wings and use a large sharp knife to cut through the joint at the wing tip and the joint between the drumette and "armpit." (See the photo above.) You will be left with three pieces. Reserve the drumette and wingette (aka flat) for making my Everything Chicken Wings (page 178) and freeze the collagen-rich wing tips to add to your next batch of bone broth (page 72).

Beef

CHUCK ROAST

You can often find chuck roast on sale at very reasonable prices. Stock up when it's cheap, and cut it into 1½-inch pieces to use in stews, curries, and chili instead of buying lean and often tough "stew beef." It will cost you less and give you a much more tender and luscious end result.

RIB-EYE

If you have room in your freezer, you can purchase a whole boneless or bone-in rib-eye for $5 less per pound than you can purchase rib-eye steaks. Portioning a rib-eye is even easier than trimming a tenderloin (see below); you literally remove the rib-eye from the bag and slice it into steaks. If I'm planning a party, I sometimes purchase a whole rib-eye, cut half of it into steaks for the freezer, and roast the rest of it whole to serve as prime rib to my guests.

TENDERLOIN

I've purchased a whole beef tenderloin on sale for as little as $6.99 a pound, and I've seen the same grocery store sell filet mignon steaks for $18.99 a pound. The only difference between the two is that the steaks have been trimmed and sliced. For this reason, I always purchase beef tenderloin whole when it's on sale. I take it home, trim off the inedible membrane (commonly referred to as "silver skin"), and then slice the meaty center piece into 1½-inch steaks. Finally, I cut the thin ends into bite-sized pieces for stir-fries, stews, or curries. Nothing goes to waste, and it costs about the same per pound as premium ground beef.

If you search "how to break down a beef tenderloin" on YouTube, you'll find lots of easy tutorials to teach you how to do it. Anyone can master this basic technique, but a sharp, somewhat flexible knife is the key to getting off the silver skin without wasting a lot of the meat. I freeze the trimmings to add to bone broth (page 72).

Pork

BACON

This is more of a time-saver than a money-saver, but there's no need to cook bacon to order every day! You can cook 1 to 2 pounds in a single layer on a sheet pan in the oven. (Bake it at 400 degrees Fahrenheit for about 18 minutes, until the desired crispness is reached.) Then transfer the cooked bacon to a paper towel–lined plate to drain any extra grease. Store the leftovers in a covered container in the refrigerator for up to a week and use them in a Chicken Club Wrap (page 164) or Cobb Salad (page 150) or heat them up for breakfast. Don't forget to strain the grease from the pan into a clean glass jar and store it in the fridge to use for frying eggs, mushrooms, or anything else to which you'd like to add a bit of bacon flavor.

CHOPS

Most boneless pork chops are cut from the loin, which you can purchase whole and cut into chops yourself for a fraction of the price. The added benefit is that you can cut them to the thickness you want—thicker for stuffing or thinner for grilling. You can also cut a few chops into bite-sized pieces to use in stir-fries and curries, like my Vindaloo on page 232.

Vegetables

MUSHROOMS

Purchase mushrooms whole instead of sliced. Often you see pretty slices at the top of the package, but underneath will be some extra stems and inedible pieces thrown in to make weight. In most cases, you get more usable mushroom out of a package of whole ones than from a package of slices.

Never wash your mushrooms with water or they will become slimy. Simply brush them clean with a soft brush or a piece of paper towel.

RICED CAULIFLOWER

Stop buying riced cauliflower at the store at a 300 percent markup! Buy a few heads when cauliflower is on sale and make large batches of riced cauliflower in just minutes using your blender. Simply trim off any leaves and then cut each head into about six pieces. Place the pieces in the blender and fill the jar with water to about 3 inches from the top. Pulse for about 10 seconds, or until the cauliflower is riced but not liquefied. Pour it through a strainer to drain and then put 1 or 2 cups of "rice" in each freezer bag with a little bit of water. Keep frozen for up to three months, then thaw, drain, and use as needed.

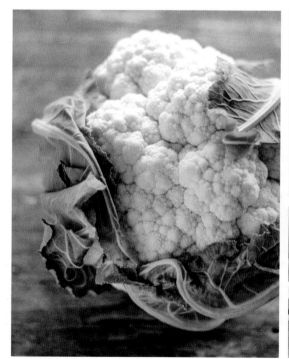
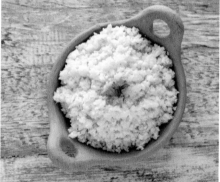
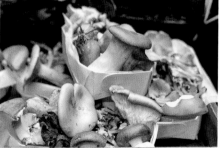

KITCHEN Safety

When you rely on packaged foods, you don't have to worry much about contaminants because those foods contain so many chemicals and preservatives that few bacteria can survive. Working with whole foods—raw meats, fresh vegetables, eggs, and so on—requires that you take a few basic precautions to keep everyone healthy and free from food-borne illnesses.

Meat and Seafood

Never cut raw meat (including poultry and seafood) near exposed clean dishes that can become contaminated. Be sure to sanitize your cutting board, knife, and counter (even after washing them with dish soap) with a solution of one part bleach to four parts water to ensure that they are fully clean and that any lingering bacteria has been eradicated after use.

Even then, it's a good idea to have a dedicated meat cutting board that you replace every six months or so, because cuts in the board can harbor bacteria. Wood and bamboo cutting boards are permeable, so avoid using them for preparing meat.

Chicken

I've done a lot of cooking on construction projects with volunteer crews of home cooks, and I'm always surprised at how few people are aware of basic kitchen safety. This is especially true when it comes to prepping and cooking chicken, arguably one of the more dangerous sources of bacteria that can cause food-borne illness.

When I lived in South Carolina, a common practice was to rinse raw chicken in the sink to get off any bacteria before cooking. Please don't do this—it actually *increases* your chances of getting sick from bacteria! Washing raw meat can spread bacteria via splashing and dripping onto counters, sinks, faucets, towels, and any clean dishes or utensils that might be nearby.

Any bacteria on or in the chicken (as long as it's fresh and unspoiled) will be destroyed by cooking it to an internal temperature of 165 degrees Fahrenheit. You can test it with a meat thermometer to be sure, but if there is no pinkness left in the meat, you can be pretty confident that it's reached a safe temperature for consumption.

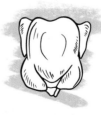

Eggs

Eggs are a staple of the keto diet, and you want to be sure you're handling them safely. When we lived in Belize, where eggs are stacked in crates on the floor in stores without air-conditioning and the temperature can rise to more than 100 degrees Fahrenheit, I became sick several times and thus became a lot more cautious about egg safety.

When living in the United States, I took for granted that the eggs I was buying from the grocery store were always fresh and safe to eat. Since I started testing all the eggs I eat, I have found that this isn't true in every case, even when purchasing eggs from reputable grocery stores.

The best way to check your eggs for freshness (always right before eating) is the float test. Fill a bowl with water and place an egg in it. If it sinks like a stone, it's fresh; if it floats to the top, it's no good; and if it kind of hovers just above the bottom, you probably shouldn't risk eating it. Even if your eggs pass the float test, if you crack them into a pan or bowl and the yolks disintegrate into a watery mess, discard them immediately.

If you're getting your eggs fresh from a farm and they've never been refrigerated, you don't need to refrigerate them, either. They'll keep for months in a cool, dry place. Once an egg has been refrigerated, though, it must remain refrigerated until eaten.

Never wash your eggs until right before you use them, or you'll rinse off the coating that prevents air from permeating the shell and keeps your eggs from spoiling. Dry the rinsed eggs thoroughly before cracking them to prevent the spread of any bacteria.

If you're consuming eggs raw for mayonnaise or in other applications, be sure to purchase pasteurized eggs so that any salmonella or other bacteria has been killed.

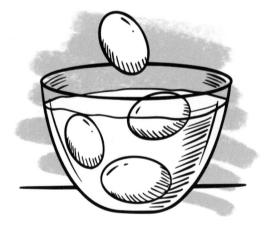

Vegetables

Just because something looks clean doesn't mean that it is. This is especially true of produce from the grocery store. It may be shiny and look perfect when you purchase it, but it's been handled by multiple people, traveled by truck (and possibly even boat or plane), been sneezed on, and maybe even fallen onto the dirty store floor multiple times before you buy it.

I'll be honest: When I lived in the United States, I wasn't especially diligent about washing my produce before eating it. I'd give it a quick rinse under water, but I rarely used anything to sanitize it.

Living in Central America has opened my eyes to the bacteria and chemicals that my produce comes in contact with before it arrives in my kitchen. My local grocery stores spray their produce with Raid to keep the bugs off. Before it even gets to the store, it travels in open pickup trucks in which boxes of lettuce, squash, and loose cabbages are snuggled up to uncovered freshly butchered pigs. It's horrific.

Now, I'm fanatical about washing *allllll* my produce, even the stuff that gets cooked before we eat it. You can purchase vegetable washes at the store, but honestly there's no need to spend that kind of money to get your produce clean. A simple and inexpensive solution of one part white vinegar to four parts water will remove most chemical residue and kill bacteria—even E. coli. Soak your veggies in a large bowl of this solution for five minutes and then air-dry it on paper towels before storing it. If you have a lot of vegetables to wash, you can sanitize your kitchen sink with bleach, rinse it well, and then fill the sink with the vinegar-and-water solution to clean a large number of vegetables at once.

I'm not a fan of soaking raspberries and strawberries for a long time because they will absorb the liquid and become waterlogged. For berries, I recommend a one-minute soak, which should be long enough to sanitize them for fresh eating. Be sure they're fully dry before you put them in the refrigerator; if you put them away while they're soaking wet, they will spoil much faster.

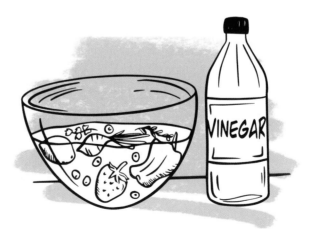

Essential SQUEAKY CLEAN KETO PANTRY

I created the recipes in this book to be as simple to prepare and as budget-friendly as possible. Still, because you're eliminating some mainstream keto foods, you may want to stock up on certain ingredients that will make your Squeaky Clean Keto life easier and tastier. You can do without them, but not having these ingredients on hand will limit your already restricted options quite a bit. Stocking up online using sites like Amazon and Thrive Market will save you money and time.

Hemp Seeds, Shelled (Hemp Hearts)

Rich in vitamins, minerals, fiber, antioxidants, and essential fatty acids, hemp seeds are known to be anti-inflammatory, making them an excellent addition to your SCKC. Hemp seeds are also one of the few plant sources that provide all nine essential amino acids of a complete protein, so if you're looking to reduce your meat consumption, hemp seeds will be instrumental to getting the protein and nutrients you need to function at optimum levels.

At about 50 cents per ounce of hemp hearts when bought in bulk, you can make the delicious and easy homemade hemp milk on page 328 for much less than you can buy any nut milk at the grocery store.

Oh, and in case you're worried, no, you can't get high from hemp seeds, and they won't make you fail a drug test, either.

Pumpkin Seeds, Shelled (Raw)

Pumpkin seeds, the flat and oval-shaped green seeds that are also known as pepitas, are high in omega-3s as well as magnesium, iron, zinc, selenium, and beta-carotene, which our bodies convert to vitamin A. They make a great addition to salads and work well as a garnish for curries and soups for texture. Don't get too free with them when snacking, though, because ½ cup contains about 11 grams of net carbs.

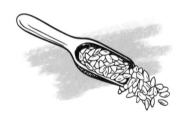

Sunflower Seeds, Shelled (Raw & Roasted)

Sunflower seeds can be turned into butter (see page 78) or flour (see page 74), making them a versatile staple on your nut-free SCKC. They are also high in vitamins and minerals like magnesium, potassium, iron, B6, and (most notably) calcium—which is important since you'll be getting less of it while you're not eating dairy.

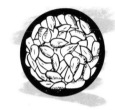

Coconut Flour

Coconut (which is not technically a nut, despite the name) and all products made from it, including flour, are acceptable for SCK. Coconut flour is high in fiber and healthy fats and relatively low in net carbs. Slightly gritty and very absorbent, coconut flour works well when combined with sunflower seed flour in baked goods and also makes a great breading for baking or frying.

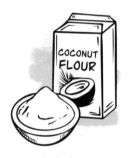

Coconut Milk & Coconut Cream

Canned full-fat, unsweetened coconut milk is a great nondairy alternative to heavy cream in soups, sauces, and curries. Coconut cream, a thicker version, is a tasty alternative to non-squeaky heavy cream for coffee. Not all coconut milk is created equal, and the carb amounts can vary widely, so make sure to read the labels and purchase the one with the least net carbs per serving.

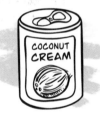

Coconut Milk Powder

A couple of recipes in this book call for coconut milk powder, which is pretty inexpensive and can be purchased online or in the international food aisles of some grocery stores. If you can find it, buy a bunch because it keeps for a long time and you can make instant coconut milk or cream just by adding it to water. (Instructions are usually included on the packaging.) This is especially helpful when you need only a small amount and don't want to open an entire can of coconut milk or cream.

As an added benefit, coconut milk powder is even more effective than canned coconut milk for thickening soups, sauces, curries, and even smoothies.

Psyllium Husk Powder

I've only recently started using psyllium husk powder in recipes, and I'm totally in love with it. High in fiber, psyllium helps you stay regular and is a prebiotic that nourishes good gut bacteria, improving overall digestive health. The high fiber content can also increase your feeling of fullness, which can reduce your appetite and help you cut back on calorie consumption almost effortlessly. While those are all great benefits, what I love most about psyllium husk powder is how it improves the texture of baked goods and bready recipes like my Spinach Wraps (page 112). It also helps batters and breadings stick during frying—like in the Fried Calamari on page 254. At only about 50 cents an ounce, it's inexpensive and, in my opinion, a critical addition to any keto pantry.

Tip: Some brands of psyllium husk powder have been known to turn purple during cooking, so read the reviews before you purchase. I use Healthworks brand, which I buy on Amazon, and I haven't had any issues with it.

Unsweetened Shredded Coconut

Unsweetened shredded coconut, also sold as desiccated (which just means dried out) coconut, can be blended to make the Coconut Butter on page 76. It also bulks up the Sheet Pan Veggie Burgers on page 306.

Avocado Oil

Avocado oil is my go-to cooking oil because of its high smoke point and neutral flavor. While it's a little more expensive than other oils, it's rich in essential fatty acids and antioxidants that make it a healthy keto option, and it performs better than olive oil in most recipes.

Coconut Oil

High in medium-chain triglycerides (MCTs), coconut oil is a great addition to your keto diet when your body relies on fat rather than carbohydrates for energy. The fat in coconut oil is converted to energy much quicker than the fats in other oils. The high concentration of lauric acid found in coconut oil gives it antiviral and antifungal properties that can kill harmful pathogens in the gut. It's especially effective against Candida albicans, a yeast that feeds on sugar and can overrun your body and cause a variety of health problems.

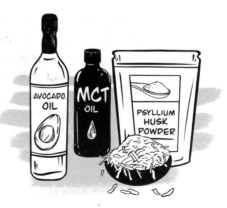

Cocoa Butter

Extracted from cocoa beans, cocoa butter is a pure fat with a milk chocolate flavor that stays solid at room temperature. While I don't call for it in any of the recipes in this book, it's a great staple for a Squeaky Clean Keto kitchen, primarily because it is incredibly delicious when blended into coffee (see "Coping Without Cream" on page 35) and is loaded with powerful phytosterols, antioxidants, and essential fatty acids that boost heart health and lower inflammation.

Coconut Aminos

Boasting a complex sweet and salty flavor, coconut aminos is an excellent gluten-free and squeaky-compliant substitute for soy sauce and Worcestershire sauce. You can find coconut aminos in many grocery stores (I can even get it here in Honduras) or purchase it online for around $8 per bottle. The flavor is intense, and a little goes a long way, so while you'll find it used often in my recipes, it's usually only in small amounts. Also, it does contain some carbs, so be sure to count them if you're using coconut aminos as a condiment.

Xanthan Gum

A neutrally flavored thickener that is commonly used in soups, sauces, gravies, and dressings, xanthan gum also gives gluten-free baked goods a chewy texture and keeps them from being too crumbly. It is inexpensive and has a long shelf life, so just a few ounces will last the average cook an entire year.

Collagen Peptides

While not strictly essential for Squeaky Clean Keto, powdered collagen peptides (aka collagen hydrolysate) is beneficial for skin, hair, nails, bones, joints, and gut health. It dissolves easily into hot or cold liquids and is a great addition to smoothies, gravies, sauces, and soups. Be sure to purchase an unflavored and unsweetened version while squeaky—you will find the lowest prices online in most cases.

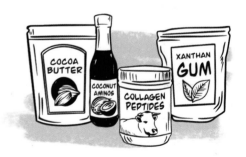

Salt

While salt may seem like a no-brainer, not all salt is created equal, and the type you use can affect the outcome of a recipe. My go-to salt for most recipes is Morton's coarse kosher salt. I mention the brand Morton's specifically because the same type of coarse kosher salt from Diamond Crystal has a lot less sodium by volume because the grains are larger and take up more room when measured. Because a fine salt like table salt or finely ground sea salt has very small grains, more salt fits into a teaspoon, making a recipe seasoned with 1 teaspoon of fine salt a lot saltier than a recipe seasoned with 1 teaspoon of coarse salt (kosher or otherwise). For best results when following my recipes that call for kosher salt (and most of them do), use coarse kosher salt and then taste and adjust the seasoning to your preference when the dish is finished. If you prefer to use sea salt or Himalayan salt for the higher mineral content, look for a converter online and adjust the amount of salt you use accordingly. In most cases, you can season sparingly at first and then finish the dish to taste with your preferred salt.

Butter

Butter (the one exception to the dairy-free rule on the Squeaky Clean Keto program) is a basic ingredient that you'll want to have on hand for a lot of my recipes. I use salted butter in nearly all of my cooking; the exception is when the neutral flavor of unsalted butter is preferred, as is the case for the Basic Bulletproof Coffee and Bulletproof Chai Latte recipes on pages 324 and 326, or when the other ingredients in a recipe add plenty of salt, as in the Bagna Cauda recipe on page 288. You can use unsalted butter in these recipes if you want; just remember that I based the seasoning on using salted butter, so you will likely need to increase the quantity of salt or add some salt if none is called for in the recipe. *Note:* A conservative ratio to use when replacing salted butter with unsalted butter is to add ¼ teaspoon salt (fine or coarse) for every stick (4 ounces) of butter.

For a richer flavor (and supposedly more nutrients), purchase grass-fed butter if you can get it at a reasonable price. If you choose not to use butter at all during your SCKC, you can substitute coconut oil or lard in most of the recipes that call for butter.

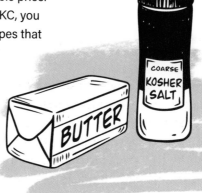

KITCHEN *Arsenal*

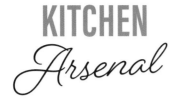

Your kitchen doesn't need to be stocked like a Williams Sonoma store for you to be a good cook. You need very little equipment to churn out restaurant-quality meals at home. Primarily, you should have a sharp knife, a cutting board, and a few decent pots and pans. Although many of the items I've listed in this section are not absolutely necessary to execute the recipes in this book, they will make your prep work go much faster. These are my key recommendations for equipping your kitchen with everything you need to prepare delicious squeaky meals at home easily.

Immersion Blender

A handheld blender, also known as an immersion or stick blender, is relatively inexpensive (about $40 for a basic model), so it's a budget-friendly upgrade to your kitchen tool drawer. This versatile appliance is easy to store and clean and can be used to blend soups and sauces right in the pot, but I use it most frequently to blend bulletproof coffee or tea to a delightfully creamy and foamy consistency.

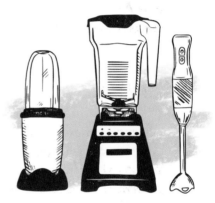

Personal-Sized Blender

A lot of the sauce and dressing recipes in this book make less than 2 cups, which isn't very much to put in a typical large blender. I love a personal-sized blender (common brands include Magic Bullet and NutriBullet) for working with smaller quantities that make a large blender overkill. A personal-sized blender is easy to use and quick to clean, and it'll run you as little as $30.

High-Powered Blender

A high-powered blender makes short work of even low-liquid recipes like the Coconut Butter on page 76 and the Sunflower Seed Butter on page 78. Although these blenders are typically a bit of an investment—with a price tag of $200 to $400 or more—most will last for years and come with an excellent warranty. If you're a serious cook, you might want to consider investing in a high-powered blender, which has many uses beyond the recipes in this book. I have both a Vitamix and a Blendtec, and I highly recommend both brands. Amazon often has sales on these brands and others, especially around the holidays.

Handheld Frother

This gadget is not a necessity, but if you're a coffee lover like I am, you may want to consider a battery-powered handheld frother. You can purchase one for as little as $10, and it's great to keep around in case your coffee begins to separate from the oil, butter, or cocoa butter that you've blended into it. You can't stick an immersion blender into a cup of coffee after you've served it, but a frother can re-emulsify your coffee right in the cup and is small enough to bring with you pretty much anywhere.

Food Processor

I have two food processors, but to be honest, I hardly ever use them. That said, they do come in handy for dealing with thick or chunky items that may not pulse uniformly in a blender, like the Pumpkin Seed Pesto on page 82. If you don't have a high-powered blender and don't want to invest in one, a food processor is a much cheaper way to get a similar result—even when making coconut butter or sunflower seed butter—though it may take longer, and the final consistency won't be quite as creamy as if you had used a high-powered blender.

Spiral Slicer

A spiral slicer is an inexpensive gadget (expect to spend about $40 for a good one) that turns zucchini or daikon radish into tasty noodles that you can serve in a variety of delicious ways. Cases in point: the Tuscan Chicken with Zoodles on page 170 and the Shrimp Piccata with Zoodles on page 240.

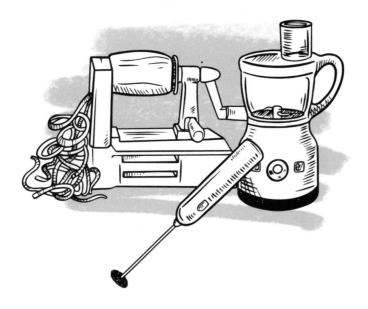

High-Quality Knives

A good sharp knife is a cook's best friend and can replace almost any fancy kitchen gadget if you've got the time and skill to use it. A dull knife is dangerous because it can slip or roll instead of slicing through, leaving you with a nasty cut that could require a trip to the emergency room. Better to invest that money in at least one decent knife, though I recommend two: a paring knife for trimming and a chef's knife for slicing and chopping. If you decide to add to your collection over time, a fillet knife and a vegetable knife are two others to consider.

Silicone Kitchen Utensils

Silicone rubber spatulas, flipping spatulas, serving spoons, and ladles are inexpensive, are easy to clean, and won't scratch your cookware or melt because of high heat. You can find them in fun colors in most department stores and online, and they will last for years if you care for them properly.

Cutting Boards

No kitchen is complete without at least a few cutting boards, both small and large. Small ones are great for chopping just one or two items in petite quantities, and large ones are good for big cuts of meat or large quantities of vegetables.

Never purchase glass cutting boards; they will dull your knives, and the smooth, hard surface can cause the blade to slip, potentially resulting in serious injury. Wood and bamboo cutting boards look cool and are easy on your knives, but they're porous and can harbor bacteria. Plastic cutting boards are my preference because they are nonslip, easy on knives, nonpermeable, and pretty inexpensive. No matter which material you choose, you should replace cutting boards when they start showing a lot of wear; all those cuts and scratches in the surface can harbor bacteria.

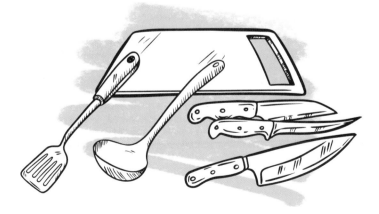

Cookware and Bakeware

The basic cookware you need to execute the recipes in this book includes a large (12- to 14-inch) heavy-bottomed nonstick skillet (a heavy bottom distributes heat evenly and prevents scorching) and a large (4-quart) saucepan with a lid. A 10-inch skillet is the best size to use for making the Prosciutto & Tomato Omelette on page 128, but you could use a slightly smaller or larger skillet if need be. Also useful but not necessarily imperative (because you can often use a larger pan when a smaller one is called for) are a medium-sized (1- to 2-quart) saucepan, a small (2- to 3-cup) saucepan, a medium-sized (9- or 10-inch) skillet, and a small (7- or 8-inch) skillet. If you'd like to make the Chorizo & Turnip Hash on page 120, you will need a skillet that can go from stovetop to oven, such as cast iron or stainless steel.

You also need a standard-sized and a jumbo muffin tin and one or two standard-sized sheet pans. You can purchase these items very reasonably on Amazon, at Target or Walmart, or at discount home stores like HomeGoods, Marshalls, and T.J. Maxx.

Storage Containers

Storage containers are ideal for both meal prep and storing leftovers. You need small (2-cup or less) to medium-sized (4-cup) containers, and it's a good idea to have at least a few large ones (6 to 8 cups) as well. I have transitioned away from plastic containers and now primarily use glass storage containers (with plastic lids). I recommend doing so if your budget allows because glass is easy to clean, doesn't scratch, doesn't retain odors or stains, and—unlike plastic—can be used for reheating food in the microwave or oven, which saves you the step of transferring the food to another container.

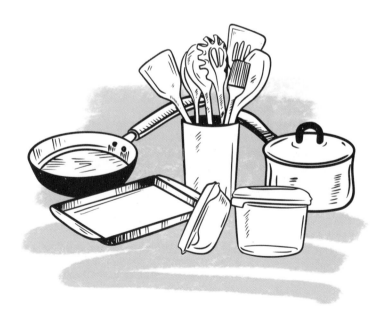

Microplane Grater

When I'm not eating squeaky, I use my Microplane grater to grate everything from dark chocolate to Parmesan cheese. Even when I am eating squeaky, this small but useful tool gets a workout grating garlic, ginger, and, most often, citrus zest. A Microplane grater costs only around $10, and it's definitely worth the price.

Parchment Paper

Although it's not strictly necessary, parchment paper is handy for making the Everything Hemp Crackers on page 342 and for lining a sheet pan to make cleanup easy when cooking bacon or chicken wings. You can typically find parchment paper in the same grocery aisle as the aluminum foil, but if your store doesn't carry it, you can purchase it on Amazon in rolls or even in precut sheets.

Multicooker

Multicookers are all the rage, with the most popular brands being the Instant Pot and the Ninja Foodi. Boasting the capabilities of a slow cooker and a pressure cooker—and in the case of the Foodi, also an air fryer and a dehydrator—these versatile appliances can save you a lot of time and produce consistently delicious results. You can purchase one for as little as $79, though the more functions it has, the pricier the appliance will be. An added benefit of a multicooker is that it can save space in the kitchen because it eliminates the need for separate appliances (slow cooker, pressure cooker, air fryer, dehydrator) that do the same jobs.

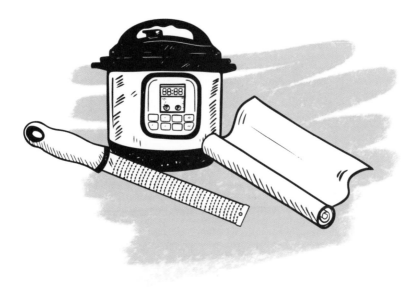

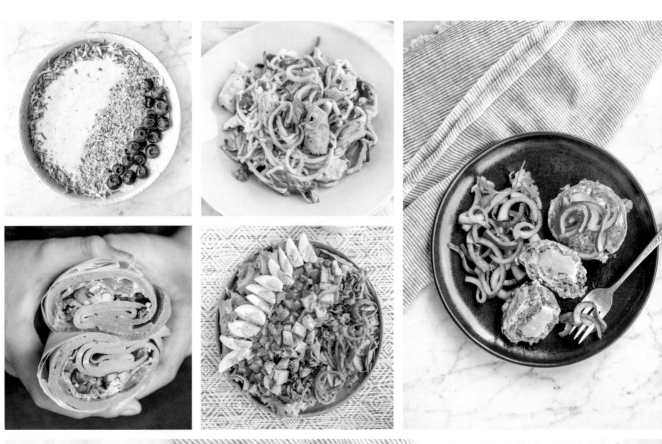
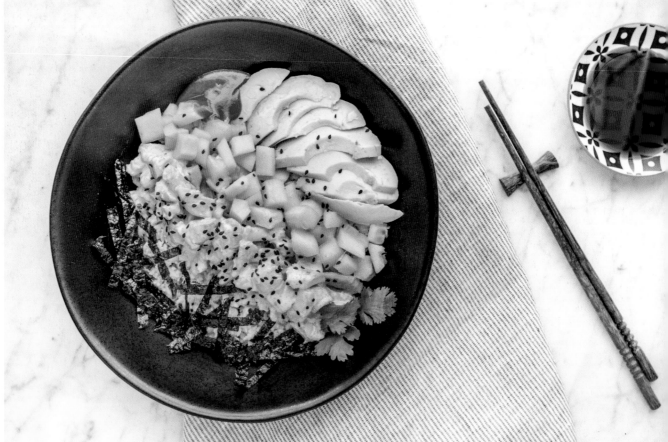

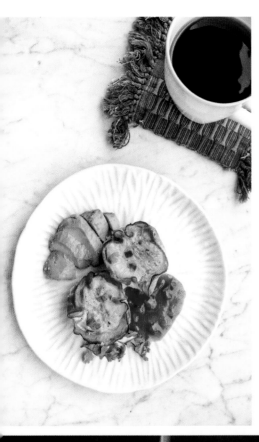

MEAL PLANS

These meal plans are meant to feed one person, so if you're doing Squeaky Clean Keto for two, plan to double everything. The daily nutrition information assumes one serving as defined in each recipe. A weekly shopping list follows each week's plan.

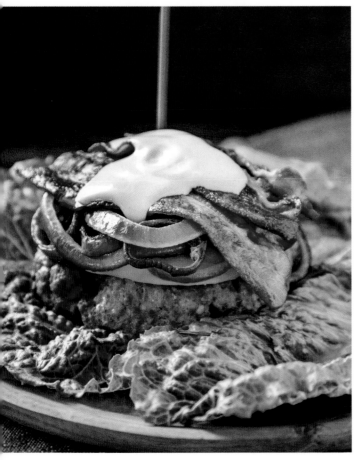

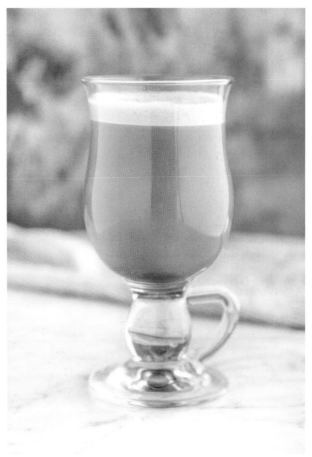

SQUEAKY CLEAN KETO MEAL PLAN

Week 1

	BREAKFAST	LUNCH	DINNER	NUTRITION INFO	
DAY 1	Basic Bulletproof Coffee 2 Fiesta Egg Cups (324 / 116)	Cobb Salad with Warm Bacon Vinaigrette (150)	Crispy Lemon Chicken 1 cup cauliflower rice (192)	CALORIES	1,376
				FAT	98g
				NET CARBS	13g
				PROTEIN	87g
DAY 2	Basic Bulletproof Coffee 2 Fiesta Egg Cups (324 / leftover)	Crispy Lemon Chicken 1 cup cauliflower rice (leftover)	Spanish Rice Hamburger Skillet ½ Hass avocado (198)	CALORIES	1,304
				FAT	92g
				NET CARBS	10g
				PROTEIN	87g
DAY 3	Basic Bulletproof Coffee 2 Fiesta Egg Cups (324 / leftover)	Spanish Rice Hamburger Skillet ½ Hass avocado (leftover)	Crispy Lemon Chicken 1 cup cauliflower rice (leftover)	CALORIES	1,304
				FAT	92g
				NET CARBS	10g
				PROTEIN	87g
DAY 4	Basic Bulletproof Coffee Blueberry Bliss Smoothie Bowl (324 / 118)	Easy Tuna Salad (148)	Crispy Lemon Chicken 1 cup cauliflower rice (leftover)	CALORIES	1,334
				FAT	97g
				NET CARBS	13g
				PROTEIN	79g
DAY 5	Basic Bulletproof Coffee 2 Fiesta Egg Cups (324 / leftover)	Cobb Salad with Warm Bacon Vinaigrette (leftover)	Crispy Lemon Chicken 1 cup cauliflower rice (leftover)	CALORIES	1,376
				FAT	98g
				NET CARBS	11g
				PROTEIN	87g
DAY 6	Basic Bulletproof Coffee 2 Fiesta Egg Cups (324 / leftover)	Crispy Lemon Chicken 1 cup cauliflower rice (leftover)	Spanish Rice Hamburger Skillet ½ Hass avocado (leftover)	CALORIES	1,304
				FAT	92g
				NET CARBS	10g
				PROTEIN	87g
DAY 7	Basic Bulletproof Coffee Blueberry Bliss Smoothie Bowl (324 / 118)	Easy Tuna Salad (leftover)	Spanish Rice Hamburger Skillet ½ Hass avocado (leftover)	CALORIES	1,395
				FAT	120g
				NET CARBS	15g
				PROTEIN	56g

Prep Notes

✓ *Make the Fiesta Egg Cups at the start of the week. Reheat in the microwave for 30 seconds.*

✓ *Make the Crispy Lemon Chicken on Day 1. Store the cauliflower rice in a separate container. Reheat the chicken, sauce, and rice together on a plate in the microwave for 2 minutes or until hot.*

✓ *Make the Spanish Rice Hamburger Skillet on Day 2. Reheat in the microwave for 2 minutes or until hot.*

✓ *Make the Easy Tuna Salad on Day 4. Serve leftovers cold.*

Shopping List

PRODUCE

blueberries or raspberries, ½ pint

cauliflower, 2 large heads, or 9 cups riced cauliflower

garlic, 1 bulb

Hass avocados, 4

lemons, 2

parsley, 1 bunch

spring mix salad greens, 8 ounces

tomato, 1

PROTEIN

bacon, 1 pound

chicken, 6 (6-ounce) cutlets, or 2½ pounds boneless, skinless chicken breasts

deli ham, 10 slices

eggs, large, 1 dozen

ground beef (80/20), 1 pound

DAIRY

butter, 1 stick salted and 1 stick unsalted

PANTRY

chicken broth, 1 (10-ounce) can

chopped green chilis, 1 (4-ounce) can

diced tomatoes, 1 (14-ounce) can

tuna, 2 (5-ounce) cans

unsweetened coconut milk, 1 (14-ounce) can

unsweetened shredded coconut, 1 (8-ounce) bag

CHECK YOUR KITCHEN FOR THESE ITEMS:

coconut flour

coconut oil

coffee

collagen peptides (if using)

Dijon mustard

dried onion flakes

dried oregano leaves

extra-virgin olive oil

garlic powder

ground cumin

hemp seeds (aka hemp hearts)

mayonnaise

salsa

Sun-Flour (page 74), ⅓ cup

white balsamic vinegar

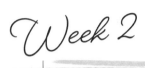

Week 2

	BREAKFAST	LUNCH	DINNER	NUTRITION INFO	
DAY 1	324 / 130 Basic Bulletproof Coffee 2 Baked Scotch Eggs	166 1 Pastrami Roll-Up	216 Sheet Pan Bacon Burger	CALORIES	1,407
				FAT	108g
				NET CARBS	6g
				PROTEIN	80g
DAY 2	324 / leftover Basic Bulletproof Coffee 1 Baked Scotch Egg	leftover 2 Pastrami Roll-Ups	leftover Sheet Pan Bacon Burger	CALORIES	1,343
				FAT	106g
				NET CARBS	6g
				PROTEIN	76g
DAY 3	324 / leftover Basic Bulletproof Coffee 1 Baked Scotch Egg	152 Simple Egg Salad 4 romaine lettuce leaves	224 Bangers & Mash	CALORIES	1,211
				FAT	104g
				NET CARBS	11g
				PROTEIN	46g
DAY 4	324 / 118 Basic Bulletproof Coffee Blueberry Bliss Smoothie Bowl	leftover 1 Pastrami Roll-Up	leftover Sheet Pan Bacon Burger	CALORIES	1,355
				FAT	113g
				NET CARBS	12g
				PROTEIN	62g
DAY 5	324 / leftover Basic Bulletproof Coffee 1 Baked Scotch Egg	leftover Bangers & Mash	leftover Sheet Pan Bacon Burger	CALORIES	1,495
				FAT	124g
				NET CARBS	12g
				PROTEIN	69g
DAY 6	324 / leftover Basic Bulletproof Coffee 1 Baked Scotch Egg	leftover Simple Egg Salad 4 romaine lettuce leaves	leftover Bangers & Mash	CALORIES	1,211
				FAT	104g
				NET CARBS	11g
				PROTEIN	46g
DAY 7	324 / 118 Basic Bulletproof Coffee Blueberry Bliss Smoothie Bowl	leftover Simple Egg Salad 4 romaine lettuce leaves	leftover Bangers & Mash	CALORIES	1,402
				FAT	124g
				NET CARBS	18g
				PROTEIN	44g

Prep Notes

(✓) *Make the Baked Scotch Eggs on Day 1. Serve leftovers cold, or reheat in the microwave for 30 seconds or until hot.*

(✓) *Make the Pastrami Roll-Ups on Day 1. Serve leftovers cold.*

(✓) *Make the Sheet Pan Bacon Burgers on Day 1. Serve leftovers cold, salad style, over romaine lettuce leaves, or reheat in the microwave for 2 minutes or until hot.*

(✓) *Make the Bangers & Mash on Day 3. Reheat in the microwave for 2 minutes or until hot.*

(✓) *Make the Simple Egg Salad on Day 3. Serve leftovers cold.*

Shopping List

PRODUCE

blueberries or raspberries, ½ pint

cauliflower, 1 large head

chives, 1 tablespoon chopped (can substitute dried chives)

jalapeño peppers, 2

lemon, 1

lime, 1

red onion, 1 small

romaine lettuce, 2 heads

yellow onion, 1 large

PROTEIN

bacon, 6 slices

breakfast sausage, 1 pound

eggs, 6 medium and 6 large

ground beef (80/20), 1½ pounds

pastrami, 8 slices (about 8 ounces)

pork sausages, 4 (about 6 ounces each)

DAIRY

butter, unsalted, 1 stick

PANTRY

kosher dill pickles, whole, 1 (16-ounce) jar

unsweetened coconut milk, 1 (14-ounce) can

CHECK YOUR KITCHEN FOR THESE ITEMS:

caraway seeds

chicken broth

coconut aminos

coconut oil

coffee

collagen peptides (if using)

Dijon mustard

extra-virgin olive oil

garlic powder

hemp seeds (aka hemp hearts)

mayonnaise

red wine vinegar

spicy brown mustard

Sriracha sauce

Week 3

	BREAKFAST	LUNCH	DINNER	NUTRITION INFO	
DAY 1	Basic Bulletproof Coffee **324** / Crispy Radish Corned Beef Hash 2 eggs fried in 1 tsp butter **126**	Curried Chicken Salad 4 romaine lettuce leaves **146**	Tuscan Chicken with Zoodles **170**	CALORIES	1,179
				FAT	87g
				NET CARBS	11g
				PROTEIN	84g
DAY 2	Basic Bulletproof Coffee **324** / Crispy Radish Corned Beef Hash 2 eggs fried in 1 tsp butter *leftover*	Curried Chicken Salad 4 romaine lettuce leaves *leftover*	Tuscan Chicken with Zoodles *leftover*	CALORIES	1,179
				FAT	87g
				NET CARBS	11g
				PROTEIN	84g
DAY 3	Basic Bulletproof Coffee **324** / Blueberry Bliss Smoothie Bowl **118**	Curried Chicken Salad 4 romaine lettuce leaves *leftover*	Ginger Beef Stir-Fry 1 cup cauliflower rice **214**	CALORIES	1,225
				FAT	94g
				NET CARBS	17g
				PROTEIN	70g
DAY 4	Basic Bulletproof Coffee **324** / Crispy Radish Corned Beef Hash 2 eggs fried in 1 tsp butter *leftover*	Muffuletta Wrap **162**	Tuscan Chicken with Zoodles *leftover*	CALORIES	1,473
				FAT	113g
				NET CARBS	10g
				PROTEIN	91g
DAY 5	Basic Bulletproof Coffee **324** / Crispy Radish Corned Beef Hash 1 egg fried in ½ tsp butter *leftover*	Muffuletta Wrap **162**	Ginger Beef Stir-Fry 1 cup cauliflower rice *leftover*	CALORIES	1,429
				FAT	108g
				NET CARBS	10g
				PROTEIN	92g
DAY 6	Basic Bulletproof Coffee **324** / Breakfast Burrito **132**	Tuscan Chicken with Zoodles *leftover*	Ginger Beef Stir-Fry 1 cup cauliflower rice *leftover*	CALORIES	1,299
				FAT	88g
				NET CARBS	17g
				PROTEIN	97g
DAY 7	Basic Bulletproof Coffee **324** / Breakfast Burrito **132**	Curried Chicken Salad 4 romaine lettuce leaves *leftover*	Ginger Beef Stir-Fry 1 cup cauliflower rice *leftover*	CALORIES	1,289
				FAT	95g
				NET CARBS	15g
				PROTEIN	87g

Prep Notes

- ✓ Make the Crispy Radish Corned Beef Hash on Day 1. Reheat in the microwave for 2 minutes or until hot. Fry eggs to order each day to serve with the hash.

- ✓ Make the Curried Chicken Salad on Day 1. Serve leftovers cold.

- ✓ Make the Tuscan Chicken with Zoodles on Day 1. Reheat in the microwave for 2 minutes or until hot.

- ✓ Make the Ginger Beef Stir-Fry on Day 3. Reheat in the microwave for 2 minutes or until hot.

- ✓ Make the Spinach Wraps (you'll need 4 for the week) on Day 3. Store them in an airtight container in the refrigerator until you need them.

- ✓ Make the Olive Salad for the wraps on Day 3 so it's ready for meals later in the week.

Shopping List

PRODUCE

basil, 1 (½-ounce) package

blueberries or raspberries, ½ pint

broccoli florets, 8 ounces (can substitute frozen)

cauliflower, 1 large head, or 4 cups riced cauliflower

cilantro, 1 bunch

garlic, 4 cloves

ginger, 1 small knob

Granny Smith apple, 1 small

Hass avocado, 1

mint, 1 bunch

radishes, 8 ounces

red bell pepper, 1 large

red onion, 1 small

scallions, 1 bunch

spinach, 8 ounces (can substitute frozen)

yellow onion, 1 small

zucchini, 3 medium

PROTEIN

beef steak, boneless, such as sirloin or flank, 1 pound

breakfast sausage, 8 ounces

chicken breasts, boneless, skinless, 2 pounds

eggs, 17 large

Genoa salami, sliced, 2 ounces

mortadella or bologna, sliced, 2 ounces

prosciutto or other ham, 2 ounces

DAIRY

butter, unsalted, 1 stick

PANTRY

black olives, sliced, 1 (4-ounce) can

capers, in brine, 1 (4-ounce) jar

cocktail onions, 1 (4-ounce) jar

corned beef, 1 (12-ounce) can

olives, pimento-stuffed, 1 (10-ounce) jar

pepperoncini, sliced, 1 (10-ounce) jar

sun-dried tomatoes, 1 (8-ounce) jar

CHECK YOUR KITCHEN FOR THESE ITEMS:

avocado oil or other light-tasting oil

coconut aminos

coconut flour

coconut oil

coffee

collagen peptides (if using)

curry powder

dried oregano leaves

extra-virgin olive oil

fish sauce

garlic powder

ground nutmeg

hemp seeds (aka hemp hearts)

mayonnaise

parsley, fresh

psyllium husk powder

pumpkin seeds (pepitas)

red pepper flakes

red wine vinegar

salsa

toasted sesame oil

unsweetened shredded coconut

white vinegar

xanthan gum

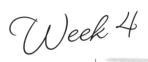

Week 4

	MEAL 1	MEAL 2	NUTRITION INFO	
DAY 1	Basic Bulletproof Coffee **324** Chorizo & Turnip Hash **120**	Spicy Shrimp Sushi Bowl **154**	CALORIES	1,071
			FAT	96g
			NET CARBS	13g
			PROTEIN	42g
DAY 2	Basic Bulletproof Coffee **324** Spicy Shrimp Sushi Bowl *leftover*	Chorizo & Turnip Hash *leftover*	CALORIES	1,071
			FAT	96g
			NET CARBS	13g
			PROTEIN	42g
DAY 3	Basic Bulletproof Coffee **324** Spicy Shrimp Sushi Bowl *leftover*	Sheet Pan Meatballs with Zoodles **208**	CALORIES	1,140
			FAT	100g
			NET CARBS	11g
			PROTEIN	42g
DAY 4	Basic Bulletproof Coffee **324** Chorizo & Turnip Hash *leftover*	Spicy Shrimp Sushi Bowl *leftover*	CALORIES	1,071
			FAT	96g
			NET CARBS	13g
			PROTEIN	42g
DAY 5	Basic Bulletproof Coffee **324** Sheet Pan Meatballs with Zoodles *leftover*	Chorizo & Turnip Hash *leftover*	CALORIES	1,165
			FAT	102g
			NET CARBS	12g
			PROTEIN	50g
DAY 6	Basic Bulletproof Coffee **324** Chorizo & Turnip Hash *leftover*	Sheet Pan Meatballs with Zoodles *leftover*	CALORIES	1,165
			FAT	102g
			NET CARBS	12g
			PROTEIN	50g
DAY 7	Basic Bulletproof Coffee **324** Chorizo & Turnip Hash *leftover*	Sheet Pan Meatballs with Zoodles *leftover*	CALORIES	1,165
			FAT	102g
			NET CARBS	12g
			PROTEIN	50g

Prep Notes

 Incorporate intermittent fasting this week; have black coffee every morning until your first meal.

 Make the Chorizo & Turnip Hash on Day 1. Reheat in the microwave for 2 minutes or until hot.

 Prep the cauliflower rice and make the shrimp salad for the Spicy Shrimp Salad Sushi Bowl on Day 1. Assemble the bowls throughout the week from the prepped ingredients.

 Make the No-Cook Marinara Sauce and the Sheet Pan Meatballs with Zoodles on Day 3. Reheat in the microwave for 2 minutes or until hot.

Shopping List

PRODUCE

cauliflower, 1 medium head, or 2 cups riced cauliflower
cucumber, 1 large
garlic, 1 clove
Hass avocados, 2
lime, 1
red bell pepper, 1 small
turnips, 6 medium
yellow onion, 1 small
zucchini, 4 medium

PROTEIN

chorizo, Mexican-style fresh (raw), 1 pound
eggs, 6 large
ground beef (80/20), 1 pound
shrimp, large, 1 pound

PANTRY

nori (dried seaweed sheets), 1 package
San Marzano tomatoes, 1 (28-ounce) can

CHECK YOUR KITCHEN FOR THESE ITEMS:

chipotle powder
cilantro, fresh
coconut aminos
coconut oil
coffee
dried basil
dried oregano leaves
dried parsley
extra-virgin olive oil
garlic powder
hemp seeds (aka hemp hearts)
mayonnaise
onion powder
parsley, fresh
red pepper flakes
red wine vinegar
rice wine vinegar (no sugar added)
sesame seeds
Sriracha sauce
toasted sesame oil

5-Day
KETO SOUP DIET PLAN

Thousands of people have had success losing up to 10 pounds (and more!) on my keto soup diet. One reason it's so effective is that it gives you the necessary nutrients, antioxidants, and electrolytes to feel your best on keto when losing weight and detoxing. It does that with plenty of healthy fats, but also provides lots of fiber, sodium, potassium, magnesium, B vitamins, vitamin C, vitamin K, and even choline—which nourishes your liver so it can burn more fat.

Most of my other meal plans are luxurious compared to this one. They are designed to help you lose weight in a way that is maintainable longer term so you don't go crazy from deprivation. This five-day keto soup diet plan is different. It's not meant to be adopted as a lifestyle change or to keep you going on keto forever—it's too restrictive for that. That being said, there is no reason you couldn't repeat this plan over and over if it works for you.

If variety in your diet isn't an issue, then you will have zero issues with this plan. It's a no-frills means to an end—tasty, but not fancy by any means.

The meals are simple and require almost no effort to reheat once the initial prep work is done. If you don't enjoy cooking or you just don't have a lot of time, this plan is perfect for you because you make three things and they last all five days.

HOW MUCH SOUP WILL I NEED TO MAKE?

The Chicken & Vegetable Soup recipe (page 144) used for this plan yields 20 cups of soup if you follow the recipe correctly and simmer it covered to avoid excessive evaporation. The keto soup diet calls for 4 cups per day over five days. The math works.

Still, some people have reported they were a little short on the soup by the end of the week. If that happens, stretch it with extra broth or a little more protein (or make another batch), but don't add extra veggies to the existing soup or it will change the carb count.

For best results, I recommend portioning out the soup for the week (even if it's just into five containers, each containing your total soup for each day) all at once if possible. That way, you can make sure you're getting an equal amount of broth and veggies/chicken every day—otherwise, you may find that you have mostly broth and nothing else by day five.

WHAT SHOULD I DO IF I CAN'T FIND SOME OF THE INGREDIENTS CALLED FOR IN THE SOUP RECIPE?

If you can't find celery root where you live, you may substitute an equal amount of cauliflower, turnips, jicama, or rutabaga for roughly the same amount of carbs. Do not use parsnips—they are much too high in carbs and could skew your results.

If you can't find Swiss chard, collards are an excellent substitute for about the same amount of carbs. Do not substitute kale for the Swiss chard—it's too high in carbs and could impede your weight loss.

The following are some carb counts of possible substitutes for celery root and Swiss chard. Note that parsnips and kale are quite a bit higher in carbs than the others, so, as mentioned above, I don't recommend using them.

Root veggies (approx. weight 5 ounces)	Greens (approx. weight 1.3 ounces)
1 cup celery root = 11g net carbs	1 cup Swiss chard = 0.7g net carbs
1 cup cauliflower = 3.5g net carbs	1 cup fresh spinach = 0.6g net carbs
1 cup jicama = 5g net carbs	1 cup collards = 0.7g net carbs
1 cup turnips = 6g net carbs	1 cup kale = 5.5g net carbs
1 cup parsnips = 18g net carbs	

CAN I DO THE KETO SOUP DIET IF I AM A VEGETARIAN?

Yes! While the keto soup diet plan is more limiting without meat, it can absolutely be tailored to be vegetarian.

If you are fine with seafood, you can substitute fish or shrimp in the soup.

If you don't eat any animal flesh, simply omit the chicken or replace it with tofu or another non-meat protein of your choice. If you are fine with eggs, simply increase the eggs to three, omit the bacon from your breakfast, and eat an entire avocado.

Instead of tuna salad, have egg salad for all the snacks.

5-DAY KETO SOUP DIET PLAN

	BREAKFAST	LUNCH	SNACK	DINNER
DAY 1	2 eggs cooked in 1 tbsp butter, 2 slices bacon, ½ avocado, Basic Bulletproof Coffee or tea using 2 tbsp fat (324)	2 cups Chicken & Vegetable Soup (144)	½ cup Simple Egg Salad, 2 large romaine leaves (152)	2 cups Chicken & Vegetable Soup (leftover)
	CALORIES 1,216	**FAT** 83g	**PROTEIN** 84g	**NET CARBS** 17g
DAY 2	2 eggs cooked in 1 tbsp butter, 2 slices bacon, ½ avocado, Basic Bulletproof Coffee or tea using 2 tbsp fat (324)	2 cups Chicken & Vegetable Soup (leftover)	½ cup Easy Tuna Salad, four 5-inch pieces of celery (148)	2 cups Chicken & Vegetable Soup (leftover)
	CALORIES 1,236	**FAT** 83g	**PROTEIN** 91g	**NET CARBS** 18g
DAY 3	2 eggs cooked in 1 tbsp butter, 2 slices bacon, ½ avocado, Basic Bulletproof Coffee or tea using 2 tbsp fat (324)	2 cups Chicken & Vegetable Soup (leftover)	½ cup Simple Egg Salad, 2 large romaine leaves (leftover)	2 cups Chicken & Vegetable Soup (leftover)
	CALORIES 1,216	**FAT** 83g	**PROTEIN** 84g	**NET CARBS** 17g
DAY 4	2 eggs cooked in 1 tbsp butter, 2 slices bacon, ½ avocado, Basic Bulletproof Coffee or tea using 2 tbsp fat (324)	2 cups Chicken & Vegetable Soup (leftover)	½ cup Easy Tuna Salad, four 5-inch pieces of celery (leftover)	2 cups Chicken & Vegetable Soup (leftover)
	CALORIES 1,236	**FAT** 83g	**PROTEIN** 91g	**NET CARBS** 18g
DAY 5	2 eggs cooked in 1 tbsp butter, 2 slices bacon, ½ avocado, Basic Bulletproof Coffee or tea using 2 tbsp fat (324)	2 cups Chicken & Vegetable Soup (leftover)	½ cup Simple Egg Salad, 2 large romaine leaves (leftover)	2 cups Chicken & Vegetable Soup (leftover)
	CALORIES 1,216	**FAT** 83g	**PROTEIN** 84g	**NET CARBS** 17g

Notes

 I've included a daily snack, though if you find you don't need it, then don't force yourself. But because the soup is low in calories, you will likely need the snack to get through the day. You can have this snack between breakfast and lunch or between lunch and dinner, depending on your preference and schedule. Feel free to mix and match the snacks or eat the same snack every day if that's easier for you. As a side note, you can substitute an extra bulletproof coffee or tea for the snack—the calories are around the same.

If you are a man or are working out frequently, you may find that you need more calories to be satisfied. Still, it's important to keep your carbs under 20g per day, even if you do increase your calories. The best way to increase your calories on this plan is to add extra bacon, tuna or egg salad, or bulletproof coffee to your day. Those items are high in fat and have almost zero carbs. Don't increase the amount of soup, because that is where the bulk of your carbs are coming from—eating more soup could kick you out of ketosis.

Shopping List

PRODUCE

avocados, 3
basil, 1 bunch
celery hearts, 1 package
celery root, 1 large
garlic, 1 bulb
green beans, 8 ounces
onion, 1 small
romaine lettuce, 1 head
Swiss chard or collards, 1 large bunch
white mushrooms, 8 ounces
yellow squash, 2 medium

PROTEIN

bacon, 1 package
chicken breasts, boneless, skinless, 2 pounds (you'll need 4 cups of cooked chicken for the soup)
eggs, 16 large

DAIRY

butter, unsalted, 1 stick

PANTRY

chicken broth or stock, 2 quarts (home-made is best, but store-bought is fine)
sun-dried tomatoes, small package (you'll need ¼ cup chopped)
tuna in water, 2 (5-ounce) cans

CHECK YOUR KITCHEN FOR THESE ITEMS:

Dijon mustard
dried onion flakes
lemon juice
mayonnaise
olive oil
red wine vinegar

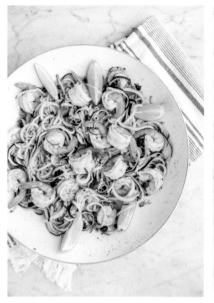
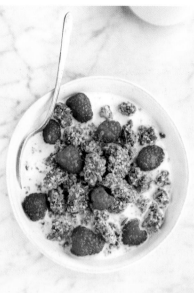
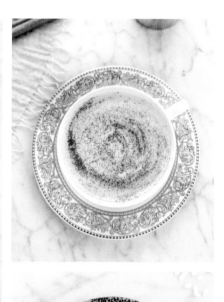

THE RECIPES

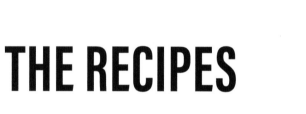
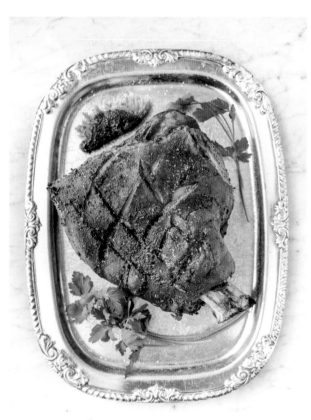
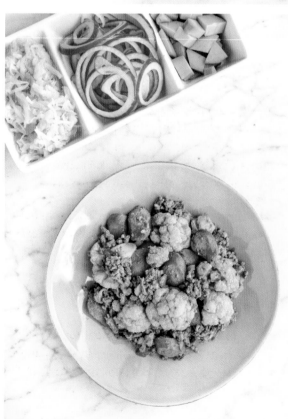

I created the recipes in this book to work within the Squeaky Clean Keto guidelines but also to be delicious enough to appeal to people doing "regular" keto or not eating keto at all. So if you're cooking for family or friends using recipes from this book, you can be confident that—keto or not—they'll enjoy what you're serving. Whether you decide to share with anyone is up to you!

Another of my goals in creating these recipes was to keep the execution easy enough that they simplify rather than complicate your cooking routine. You'll find lots of recipes for sheet pan meals and other meals that you can make in thirty minutes or less. I've also included icons that identify recipes that are coconut-free, egg-free, nightshade-free, and vegetarian. There is also an icon for dairy-free, which may seem strange because dairy other than butter isn't allowed on SCK; however, I realize that some people are intolerant to all forms of dairy. If that describes you, look for recipes with the dairy-free icon or, as I mentioned earlier, where a recipe does call for butter, you can substitute coconut oil or lard with good results.

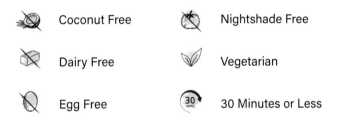

	Coconut Free		Nightshade Free
	Dairy Free		Vegetarian
	Egg Free		30 Minutes or Less

Most of these recipes make four servings because I find that it's easier to double a recipe for big families than to halve it if you're cooking for one or two people. I also include instructions for storing and reheating leftovers where applicable.

This book contains tasty recipes from a range of different cuisines, and if some of these flavor profiles aren't familiar to you, I encourage you to go outside your comfort zone and try them out! Some of my favorite dishes in this book that have an international flair are the Beef Kofta Meatballs on page 206 (Middle Eastern), the Chicken Jalfrezi on page 190 (Indian), and the Inside-Out Egg Rolls on page 226 (Asian).

If your tastes run more toward dishes commonly found in the U.S., not to worry—you'll find SCK-friendly classics like the Meatloaf Cupcakes on page 210, the Sheet Pan Bacon Burgers on page 216, the Simply Roasted Chicken Breasts on page 182, and the Crab Cakes on page 262.

My sincere hope is that you'll discover some new favorite recipes in this book and continue enjoying them for years to come.

Finally, I'd love to see photos and/or videos of you and your family making these recipes! You can post on Instagram or Facebook and tag me (@ibreatheimhungry) or use the #squeakycleanketocookbook hashtag so I'll be sure to see your post and maybe even share it.

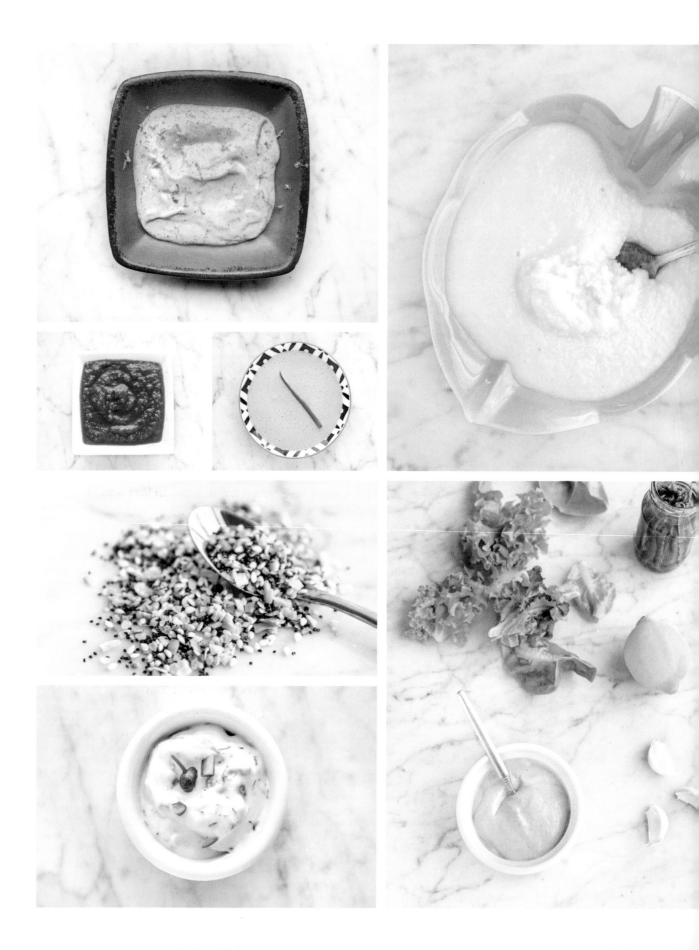

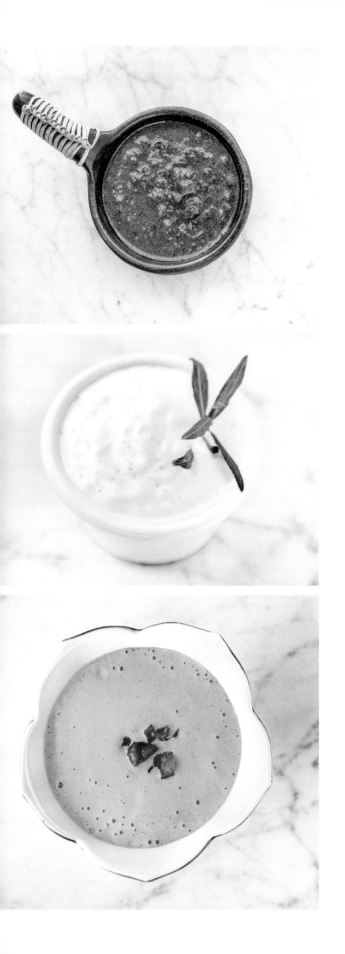

Basics

Easy Chicken Bone Broth / 72

Sun-Flour (Sunflower Seed Flour) / 74

Coconut Butter / 76

Roasted Sunflower Seed Butter / 78

Everything Bagel Seasoning / 80

Pumpkin Seed Pesto / 82

No-Cook Marinara Sauce / 84

Easy Balsamic Glaze / 86

Charmoula Sauce / 87

Easy Salsa Verde / 88

Dairy-Free Caesar Dressing / 89

Sesame Ginger Dressing / 90

Garlicky Lemon & Tarragon Dressing / 91

Tahini Dressing / 92

Creamy Sriracha Dipping Sauce / 93

Roasted Red Pepper Sauce / 94

Dairy-Free Tzatziki / 96

All-Purpose Green Sauce / 98

Chili-Lime Mayo / 100

Sun-Dried Tomato Sauce / 102

Dill Caper Tartar Sauce / 104

Creamy Garlic Sauce / 106

Quick-Pickled Red Onions / 108

Olive Salad / 110

Spinach Wraps / 112

EASY CHICKEN BONE BROTH

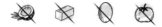

| YIELD: 12 cups | SERVING SIZE: 1 cup | PREP TIME: 5 minutes | COOK TIME: 8 hours in a slow cooker |

Bone broth is a Squeaky Clean Keto staple because it not only improves the flavor of soups and sauces but also is incredibly good for you due to its high concentration of minerals and collagen. It is inexpensive to make at home, and you can freeze it to have handy whenever the need arises. If making your own bone broth isn't something you have time for, there are many quality brands you can purchase online or in stores. I've included some of my favorite SCK-friendly bone broth brands in the Resource Guide on page 344.

1 cooked chicken carcass (most of the meat removed), and any pan drippings

1 (1-inch) piece fresh ginger, rinsed and sliced

1 small onion, quartered

1 cup chopped celery tops with leaves

2 cloves garlic, peeled

2 tablespoons apple cider vinegar

4 quarts filtered water

1. Combine all the ingredients in a 6-quart or larger slow cooker. Cook on high for 8 hours (or longer).

2. Let cool for 1 hour, then strain the solids from the broth and place the broth in the refrigerator to chill overnight.

3. Skim the solidified fat from the top of the broth. Portion the broth into containers as needed and store in the refrigerator for up to 1 week or in the freezer for up to 3 months.

Variation: **Easy Beef Bone Broth.** *You can easily use this same basic method to make beef bone broth. Simply replace the chicken carcass and drippings with about 4 pounds of beef bones and cook as directed above. For the best flavor, use short ribs, oxtail, or marrow bones if you can get them.*

Alternative Method: *Combine all the ingredients in a 6-quart or larger Instant Pot. Seal the lid according to the manufacturer's instructions. Turn on the cooker and set it to manual, high pressure, for 1 hour. When finished cooking, release the pressure according to the manufacturer's instructions. Then follow Steps 2 and 3 above to cool, strain, and store the bone broth.*

| CALORIES: 38 | FAT: 2g | PROTEIN: 3g | CARBS: 1.5g | FIBER: 0g | NET CARBS: 1.5g |

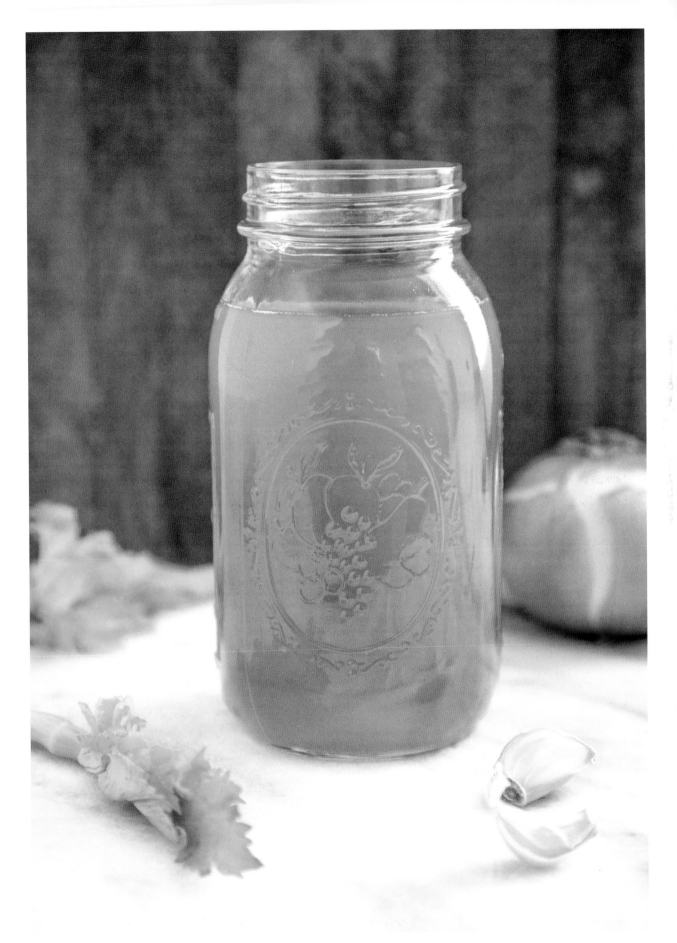

SUN-FLOUR (SUNFLOWER SEED FLOUR)

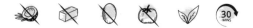

YIELD: 2½ cups | SERVING SIZE: ¼ cup | PREP TIME: 5 minutes

If you've got a blender or food processor and about two minutes of time, you can make this versatile sunflower seed flour, or "sun-flour," as it's also called, for pennies on the dollar compared to store-bought. This is an excellent alternative to almond flour for those with nut allergies.

2 cups shelled raw sunflower seeds

Put the sunflower seeds in a blender and pulse for 20 seconds. Stir. Pulse for another 20 seconds. Pour the mixture into a large-mesh sieve and shake over a large bowl until only the unblended pieces are left. Return the seed pieces from the sieve to the blender and pulse for 20 seconds. Sift and repeat until all the seeds have been turned into a fine flour. Store in an airtight container or plastic bag in the refrigerator for up to 3 months.

CALORIES: 160   FAT: 14g   PROTEIN: 6g   CARBS: 4g   FIBER: 2g   NET CARBS: 2g

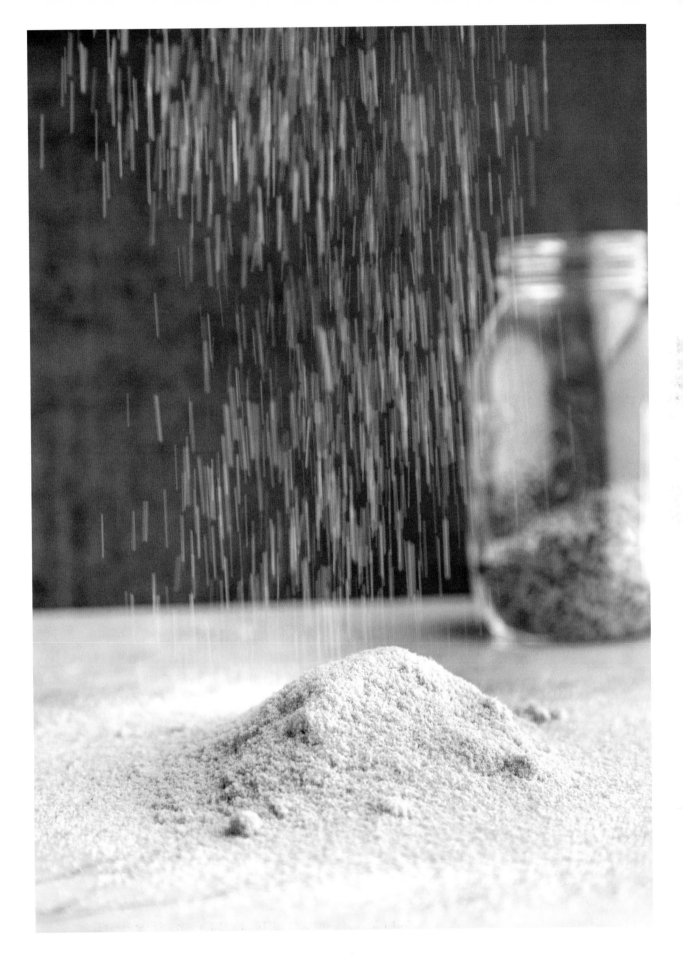

COCONUT BUTTER

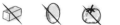

YIELD: 1¼ cups | **SERVING SIZE:** 2 tablespoons | **PREP TIME:** 5 minutes

This homemade coconut butter, which is basically just blended coconut, makes for a rich and naturally sweet snack. It is delicious eaten right out of the jar with a spoon, or you can go a step further and customize the flavors to switch it up a bit (see the note below for some ideas). For easy serving and portion control, you can chill the butter and then roll 2-tablespoon quantities into balls, or freeze the butter in ice cube trays. If you're not squeaky, feel free to sweeten it with a little powdered erythritol.

4 cups unsweetened shredded coconut

3 tablespoons coconut oil

Pinch of kosher salt

Put the ingredients in a blender or food processor and blend until liquefied. The longer you process, the smoother the butter will become. I like a little texture to it, so I usually blend mine for about 5 minutes. Store in an airtight jar in the refrigerator for up to 1 month or in the freezer (as cubes or balls) for up to 3 months.

Note: There are many ways to flavor this butter. Try mixing in vanilla, rum, or mint extract or forming it into balls and rolling them in cocoa powder like truffles. And/or mix cocoa powder directly into the butter.

CALORIES: 260   **FAT:** 26g   **PROTEIN:** 2g   **CARBS:** 8g   **FIBER:** 5g   **NET CARBS:** 3g

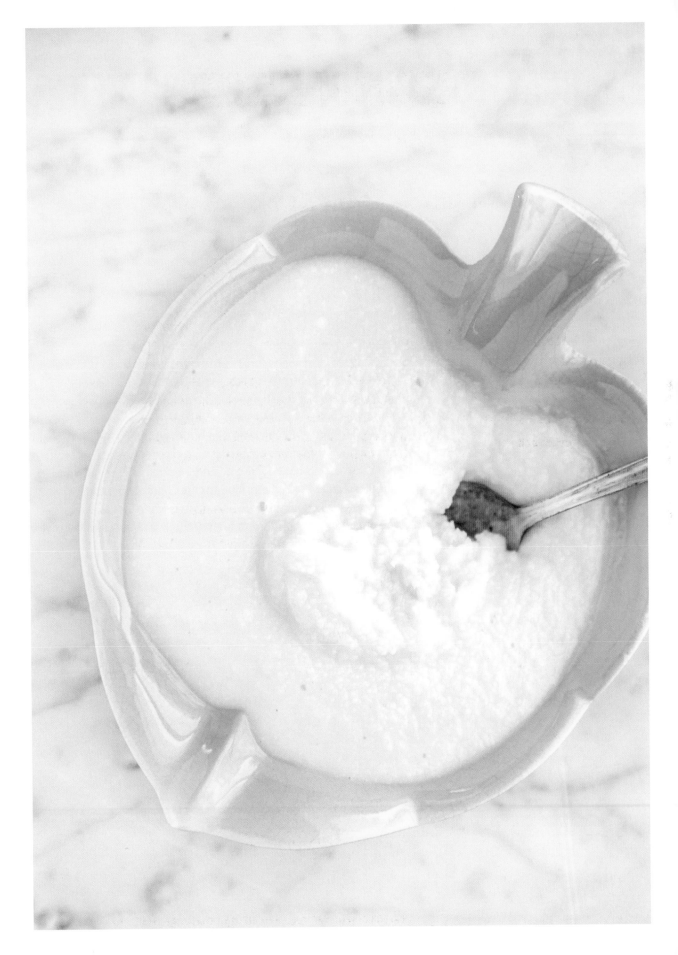

ROASTED SUNFLOWER SEED BUTTER

YIELD: 1⅓ cups | **SERVING SIZE:** 2 tablespoons | **PREP TIME:** 12 minutes

Store-bought sunflower seed butter is often full of added sugar and unhealthy oils—not to mention that it can be really expensive. Making your own sunflower seed butter at home requires a little time and a food processor, but the results are worth it because it's so much cheaper and healthier than store-bought!

3 cups roasted and salted shelled sunflower seeds

2 tablespoons coconut oil

Put the sunflower seeds in a food processor fitted with an "S" blade. Process the seeds for 3 to 5 minutes, until finely ground. Open and scrape the sides of the bowl. Add the coconut oil. Process for another 5 to 8 minutes, scraping the sides occasionally to remove any stuck-on butter. Your mixture will go from powder to a sticky ball, and eventually will thin out to a creamy butter consistency. If you find that it is not smoothing out enough for you, add another tablespoon of coconut oil and blend until creamy. Store in an airtight container in the refrigerator for up to 2 months. While the consistency should remain spreadable when chilled, you may find it easier to spread at room temperature. If necessary, warm it in the microwave for 30 seconds before using.

Notes: *If you can't find roasted and salted sunflower seeds, purchase raw shelled sunflower seeds and roast them for 15 minutes at 325°F. Let cool for 15 minutes before blending. Season the butter with salt to taste.*

The butter can be flavored with cinnamon, cocoa powder, or vanilla extract if desired. Sweeten with powdered erythritol to taste if not squeaky.

CALORIES: 192 | **FAT:** 17g | **PROTEIN:** 5g | **CARBS:** 6g | **FIBER:** 3g | **NET CARBS:** 3g

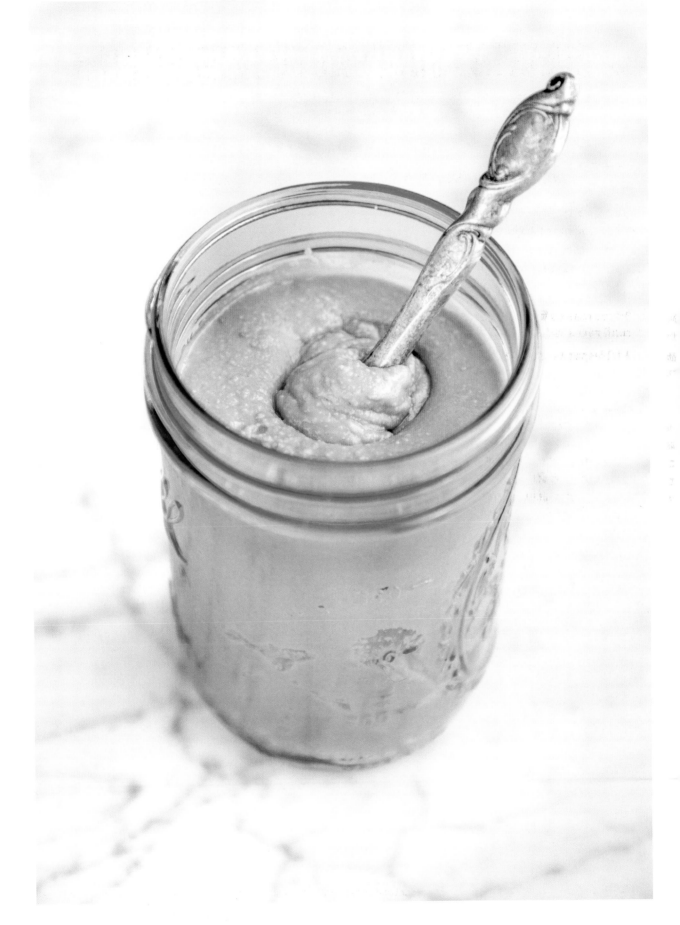

EVERYTHING BAGEL SEASONING

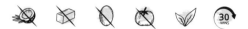

YIELD: ⅓ scant cup | SERVING SIZE: 1 tablespoon | PREP TIME: 5 minutes

Stop paying top dollar at specialty stores for a seasoning that can be made easily and cheaply at home! If you're like us and find yourself putting everything seasoning on, well, everything, then you're going to want to stock up on some basics and start making this addicting seasoning by the quart. We especially love it on the Everything Chicken Wings on page 178 and the Everything Roasted Cauliflower Steaks on page 304.

2 tablespoons poppy seeds

2 tablespoons sesame seeds

1 tablespoon dried onion flakes

2 teaspoons coarse Himalayan pink salt

1 teaspoon dried minced garlic

Put all the ingredients in a small bowl and mix well. Store in an airtight container for up to 3 months.

Note: I prefer the coarse grains of Himalayan pink salt in this recipe because of their crunchy texture and burst of saltiness when you bite them. Their larger size and texture also allow them to incorporate better than coarse kosher salt, which is more of a flake, among the bigger grains of dried minced garlic, poppy seeds, and sesame seeds. If coarse kosher salt is all you have, it will work, just not quite as well in my opinion.

CALORIES: 36 FAT: 3g PROTEIN: 1g CARBS: 2g FIBER: 1g NET CARBS: 1g

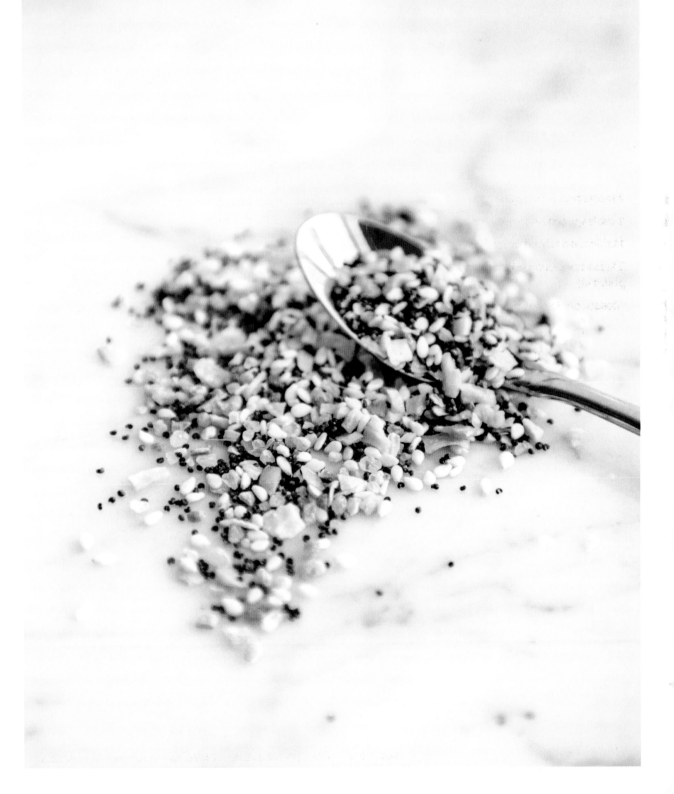

PUMPKIN SEED PESTO

YIELD: 1½ cups | **SERVING SIZE:** 2 tablespoons | **PREP TIME:** 10 minutes

This garlicky pumpkin seed pesto will make everything you eat taste 10000000% percent better, and you won't even miss the dairy! Loaded with cilantro and fresh mint, this zippy pesto will take your grilled or roasted meats, seafood, and veggies to the next level. I particularly love adding a dollop of this pesto to Chicken Korma (page 176) or Easy Vegetable Curry (page 278).

2 cups shelled raw pumpkin seeds (pepitas)

6 cloves garlic, minced

½ cup fresh mint leaves

2 tablespoons fresh cilantro leaves

1 tablespoon seeded and sliced jalapeño peppers

1 tablespoon fresh lime juice

½ cup extra-virgin olive or avocado oil, plus more for the top

2 teaspoons kosher salt

Put all the ingredients in a food processor and blend until a grainy consistency is achieved: it should be not quite smooth, but creamy looking and mostly uniform in color. Taste and adjust the seasoning if desired. Spoon into an airtight container, flatten, and pour an extra tablespoon of oil over the top before storing covered in the fridge for up to a week.

CALORIES: 201 **FAT:** 19g **PROTEIN:** 6g **CARBS:** 2g **FIBER:** 1g **NET CARBS:** 1g

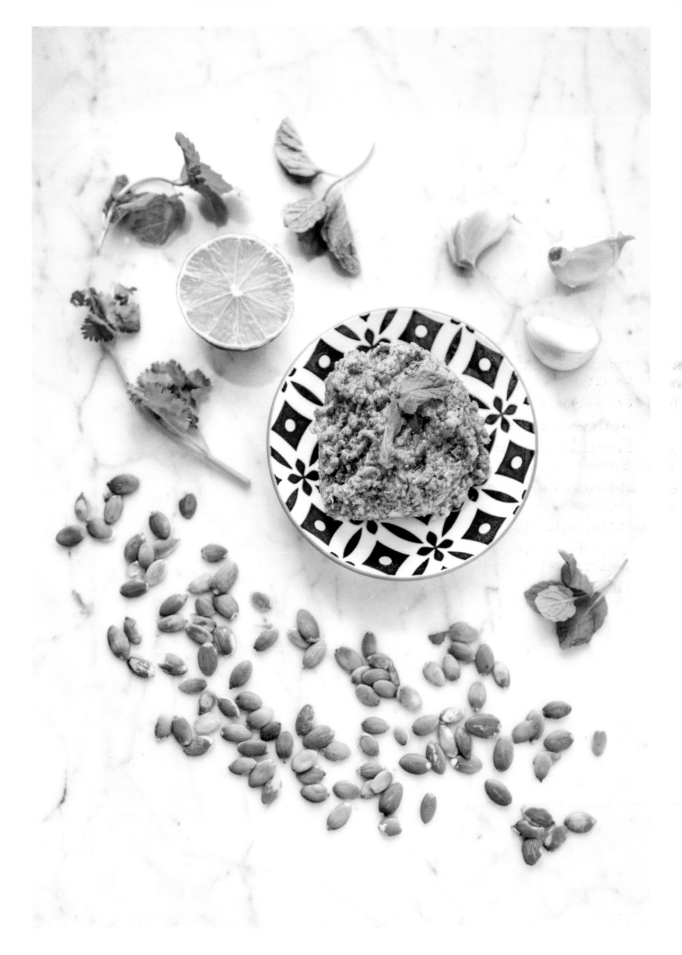

NO-COOK MARINARA SAUCE

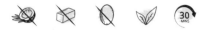

YIELD: 4 cups | **SERVING SIZE:** ½ cup | **PREP TIME:** 5 minutes

A good marinara sauce is a staple not just of Italian cooking but of keto cooking as well, which is why I'm including this essential recipe here even though it's already published on my website and was included in my first book, Keto for Life. Finding a decent-tasting store-bought marinara is possible but is no easy task, and the ones available can be pricey. (See my recommendations for store-bought options on page 345.) Making a delicious keto marinara sauce at home is easy and inexpensive—try it for yourself and see what a difference it makes!

1 (28-ounce) can peeled whole San Marzano tomatoes

¼ cup extra-virgin olive oil

2 tablespoons red wine vinegar

1 teaspoon kosher salt

1 teaspoon dried basil

1 teaspoon dried oregano leaves

1 teaspoon dried parsley

1 teaspoon garlic powder

1 teaspoon onion powder

½ teaspoon red pepper flakes

¼ teaspoon ground black pepper

Put the tomatoes and olive oil in a blender and blend for 30 seconds, or until the desired consistency is reached. If you prefer a chunkier sauce, pulse instead of blend for about 15 seconds. Stir in the remaining ingredients. Store in an airtight container in the refrigerator for up to 1 week or in the freezer for up to 6 months.

Note: If freezing, store this sauce in multiple small containers of 1 cup each so that you don't have to defrost the entire batch when you need a small amount for a recipe.

CALORIES: 84   **FAT:** 7g   **PROTEIN:** 1g   **CARBS:** 5g   **FIBER:** 2g   **NET CARBS:** 3g

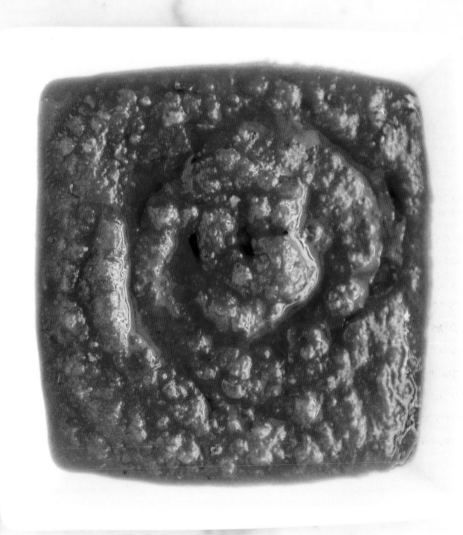

EASY BALSAMIC GLAZE

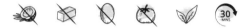

YIELD: 3 tablespoons | SERVING SIZE: 1 teaspoon | PREP TIME: 2 minutes | COOK TIME: 8 minutes

When you're eating Squeaky Clean Keto and forsaking all sweeteners, this glaze made from reducing balsamic vinegar to a syrup can taste as sweet as candy. While those natural sugars do concentrate and add some carbs, a little of this glaze goes a long way, and just a drizzle will elevate the most basic of dishes to restaurant quality. I especially love this glaze on Sausage-Stuffed Onions (page 236).

1 cup balsamic vinegar (no sugar added)

Pour the vinegar into a small saucepan and bring to a boil over medium-high heat. Cook, stirring occasionally, for about 8 minutes, until shiny and thick enough to coat a spoon. Don't let it reduce too long or it will harden like candy, and you'll have to start over with fresh vinegar. Store the glaze in an airtight container in the refrigerator for up to 2 weeks.

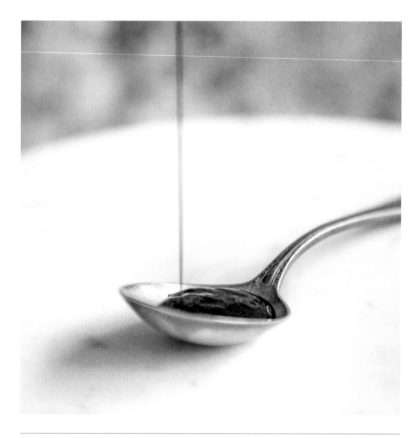

CALORIES: 10 FAT: 0g PROTEIN: 0g CARBS: 3g FIBER: 0g NET CARBS: 3g

CHARMOULA SAUCE

YIELD: ¾ cup | **SERVING SIZE:** 1 tablespoon | **PREP TIME:** 5 minutes

Garlic, lemon, and plenty of fresh herbs give this vibrant green sauce its bold and distinctive flavor. The cumin and smoked paprika add an earthy element that makes it truly delectable when paired with roasted meat and poultry, like my Simply Roasted Chicken Breasts on page 182. If you're trying to include more plant-based options, this charmoula packs so much punch that it will make a simple plate of cooked zucchini, cauliflower, or mushrooms taste like a main course.

½ cup fresh cilantro (leaves and stems)

½ cup fresh parsley (leaves and stems)

1 tablespoon grated lemon zest

1 clove garlic, peeled

1 teaspoon ground cumin

1 teaspoon smoked paprika

⅛ teaspoon cayenne pepper

¼ cup extra-virgin olive oil

Put all the ingredients in a food processor and pulse until blended but not pureed. Store in an airtight container in the refrigerator for up to 1 week or in the freezer for up to 3 months.

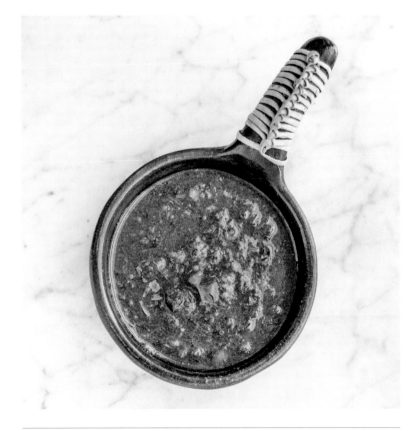

CALORIES: 62   **FAT:** 7g   **PROTEIN:** 0g   **CARBS:** 0g   **FIBER:** 0g   **NET CARBS:** 0g

EASY SALSA VERDE

| YIELD: 2½ cups | SERVING SIZE: ¼ cup | PREP TIME: 5 minutes |

This bright and vibrant salsa verde is tangy, mouth-puckering perfection! In this traditional Mexican salsa, the unique flavor of tomatillos is combined with plenty of garlic, cilantro, and spicy jalapeño. It is a delicious way to dress up grilled meats and veggies or a dairy-free taco salad with plenty of chopped avocado.

1 (28-ounce) can whole tomatillos

2 cloves garlic, peeled

¼ cup fresh cilantro (leaves and stems)

2 jalapeño peppers, seeded

1 tablespoon fresh lime juice

1 teaspoon kosher salt

Put all the ingredients in a small blender or food processor and blend until mostly smooth. Store in an airtight container in the refrigerator for up to 1 week or in the freezer for up to 3 months.

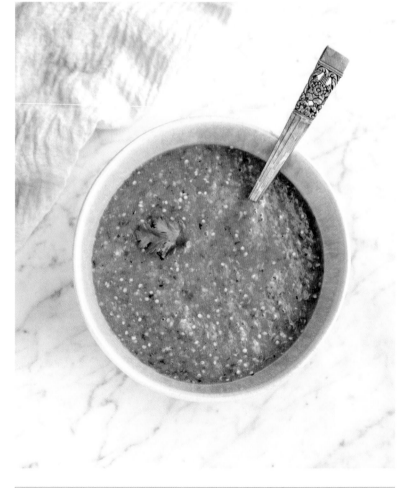

CALORIES: 18 FAT: 1g PROTEIN: 0g CARBS: 3g FIBER: 2g NET CARBS: 1g

DAIRY-FREE CAESAR DRESSING

YIELD: ¾ cup | SERVING SIZE: 2 tablespoons | PREP TIME: 5 minutes

The king of salads, Caesar has always been one of my favorites. While most bottled Caesar salad dressings contain dairy, including Parmesan cheese, this version is so rich from the anchovies, garlic, and lemon juice that you'll never miss it. This dressing also makes a truly delicious marinade for chicken thighs, which you can then bake or grill.

⅓ cup mayonnaise

3 tablespoons avocado oil

2 tablespoons fresh lemon juice

2 teaspoons Dijon mustard

2 cloves garlic, chopped

1 teaspoon grated lemon zest

6 anchovy fillets

¼ teaspoon ground black pepper

Put all the ingredients in a small blender and blend until smooth. Store in an airtight container in the refrigerator for up to 1 week.

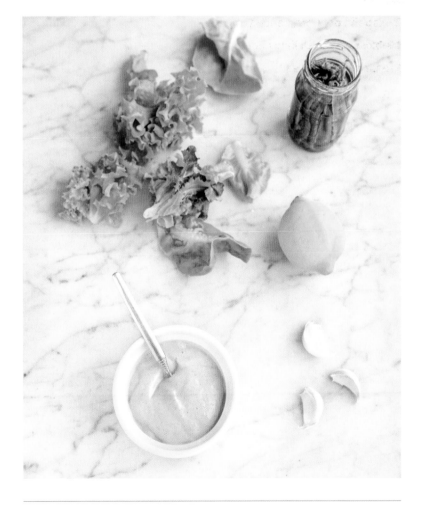

CALORIES: 161 FAT: 17g PROTEIN: 1g CARBS: 1g FIBER: 0g NET CARBS: 1g

SESAME GINGER DRESSING

YIELD: 1 cup | **SERVING SIZE:** 2 tablespoons | **PREP TIME:** 5 minutes

A versatile condiment that can do so much more than just pep up a salad, this dressing can be used as a marinade, a dip, or even a finishing sauce for grilled chicken, shrimp, or fish. The white balsamic vinegar adds a subtle sweetness that perfectly balances the salty fish sauce and sour lime juice. I love this dressing with Coriander & Wasabi–Crusted Tuna (page 248).

3 tablespoons avocado oil or other light-tasting oil

1 teaspoon toasted sesame oil

2 tablespoons filtered water

2 tablespoons fish sauce (no sugar added)

2 tablespoons mayonnaise

1 tablespoon fresh lime juice

1 tablespoon white balsamic vinegar (no sugar added)

⅓ cup chopped scallions, green parts only

2 tablespoons minced fresh ginger

Put all the ingredients in a small blender or food processor and blend until mostly smooth. Store in an airtight container in the refrigerator for up to 1 week. The dressing will separate when stored; shake well before using.

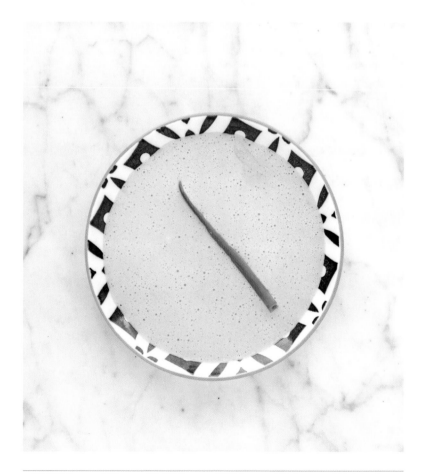

CALORIES: 86 **FAT:** 8g **PROTEIN:** 1g **CARBS:** 2g **FIBER:** 0g **NET CARBS:** 2g

GARLICKY LEMON & TARRAGON DRESSING

  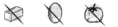

YIELD: ½ cup | **SERVING SIZE:** 2 tablespoons | **PREP TIME:** 5 minutes

Bright and flavorful, this is my go-to salad dressing at home, and it's one of Mr. Hungry's favorites. It is easy to whip up, is made with heart-healthy olive oil, and tastes delicious on everything, especially my Roman Fried Artichokes (page 274).

2 cloves garlic, peeled

1 teaspoon grated lemon zest

¼ cup fresh lemon juice

¼ cup extra-virgin olive oil

1 teaspoon kosher salt

⅛ teaspoon ground black pepper

1 teaspoon chopped fresh tarragon

Put all the ingredients except the tarragon in a small blender or food processor and blend until smooth. Stir in the tarragon. Store in an airtight container in the refrigerator for up to 1 week.

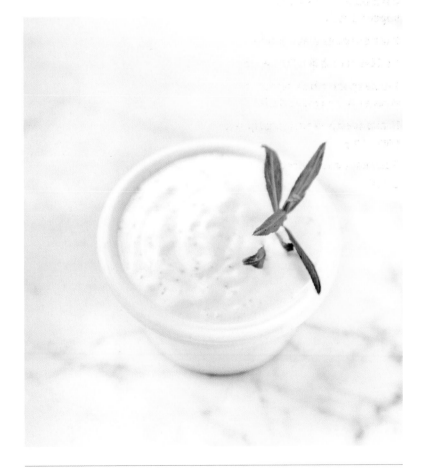

CALORIES: 126 **FAT:** 14g **PROTEIN:** 0g **CARBS:** 2g **FIBER:** 0g **NET CARBS:** 2g

TAHINI DRESSING

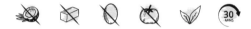

YIELD: ½ cup | **SERVING SIZE:** 2 tablespoons | **PREP TIME:** 5 minutes

---

This rich and nutty tahini dressing works well as a dipping sauce or a salad dressing. It's our go-to whenever we want to add a Mediterranean flair to grilled meats or wraps. It's an absolute must for Beef Kofta Meatballs (page 206).

⅓ cup tahini

2 tablespoons filtered water

1 teaspoon fresh lemon juice

½ teaspoon minced garlic

½ teaspoon kosher salt

Put all the ingredients in a small blender and blend until smooth. Store in an airtight container in the refrigerator for up to 1 week.

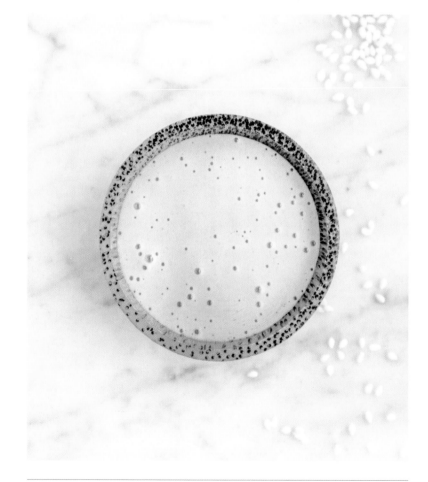

CALORIES: 157   **FAT:** 14g   **PROTEIN:** 1g   **CARBS:** 3g   **FIBER:** 1g   **NET CARBS:** 2g

CREAMY SRIRACHA DIPPING SAUCE

YIELD: ¾ cup | **SERVING SIZE:** 2 tablespoons | **PREP TIME:** 5 minutes

---

A little spicy and slightly sweet from the coconut aminos, this addicting sauce is a great way to dress up the Sheet Pan Veggie Burgers on page 306 or the Sheet Pan Bacon Burgers on page 216. While the Sriracha sauce does contain sugar, it's a negligible amount and won't affect your progress while squeaky. If you're a true purist, though, you can use a chili paste like sambal oelek instead, which has a similar flavor to Sriracha and typically doesn't contain sugar.

½ cup mayonnaise

1½ tablespoons Sriracha sauce

1 tablespoon fresh lime juice

1 teaspoon coconut aminos

Put all the ingredients in a small bowl and stir well until combined. Store in an airtight container in the refrigerator for up to 1 week.

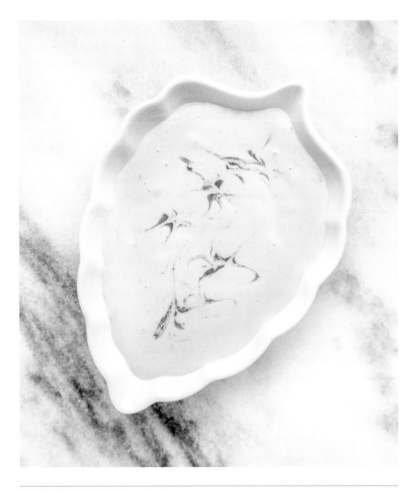

CALORIES: 138 **FAT:** 16g **PROTEIN:** 0g **CARBS:** 2g **FIBER:** 0g **NET CARBS:** 2g

ROASTED RED PEPPER SAUCE

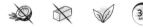

YIELD: ¾ cup | SERVING SIZE: 2 tablespoons | PREP TIME: 5 minutes

I love roasted red peppers, and this tempting sauce makes that flavor even easier to enjoy. Use it as a salad dressing or dipping sauce or to liven up chicken or seafood dishes—there's no end to what you can do with this tasty and versatile condiment. One of my favorite ways to enjoy it is with Crab Cakes (page 262). If I'm feeling extra fancy, I'll drizzle some onto a Chicken Club Wrap (page 164).

⅓ cup mayonnaise

⅓ cup chopped roasted red peppers

1 teaspoon chopped garlic

1 teaspoon fresh lemon juice

½ teaspoon kosher salt

¼ teaspoon ground black pepper

Put all the ingredients in a blender or food processor and blend until smooth. Store in an airtight container in the refrigerator for up to 1 week.

CALORIES: 93   FAT: 10g   PROTEIN: 0g   CARBS: 1g   FIBER: 0g   NET CARBS: 1g

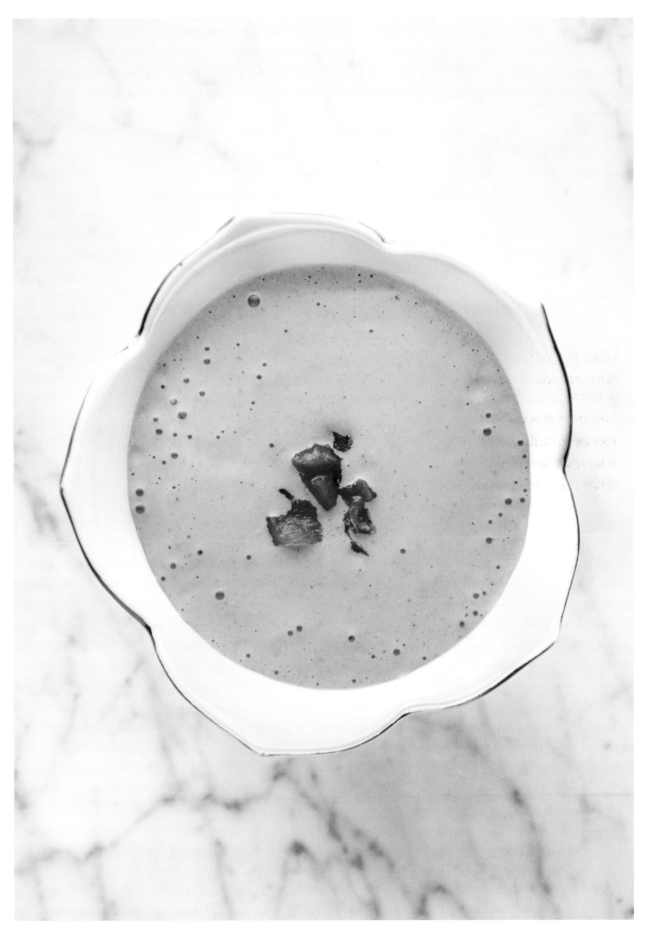

DAIRY-FREE TZATZIKI

YIELD: 1¾ cups | **SERVING SIZE:** 2 tablespoons | **PREP TIME:** 5 minutes

My family became addicted to tzatziki while traveling in Greece, where it is served with almost every traditional Greek meal—especially those featuring grilled meats. In this dairy-free version, vinegar adds the tang that you'd typically get from yogurt, and coconut milk brings the creaminess. The coconut flavor is almost nonexistent and adds just a hint of pleasant sweetness. This is a refreshing and versatile condiment that you'll want to put on everything—especially Beef Kofta Meatballs (page 206) and Greek Zucchini Fritters (page 270).

½ cup canned coconut milk

½ cup mayonnaise

1 teaspoon white vinegar

1 teaspoon grated lemon zest

½ teaspoon kosher salt

¼ teaspoon ground black pepper

¾ cup peeled, seeded, and finely chopped cucumbers

2 tablespoons chopped fresh dill

Put the coconut milk, mayonnaise, vinegar, lemon zest, salt, and pepper in a small bowl and whisk until smooth. Stir in the cucumbers and dill. Store in an airtight container in the refrigerator for up to 1 week.

CALORIES: 67 **FAT:** 7g **PROTEIN:** 0g **CARBS:** 1g **FIBER:** 0g **NET CARBS:** 1g

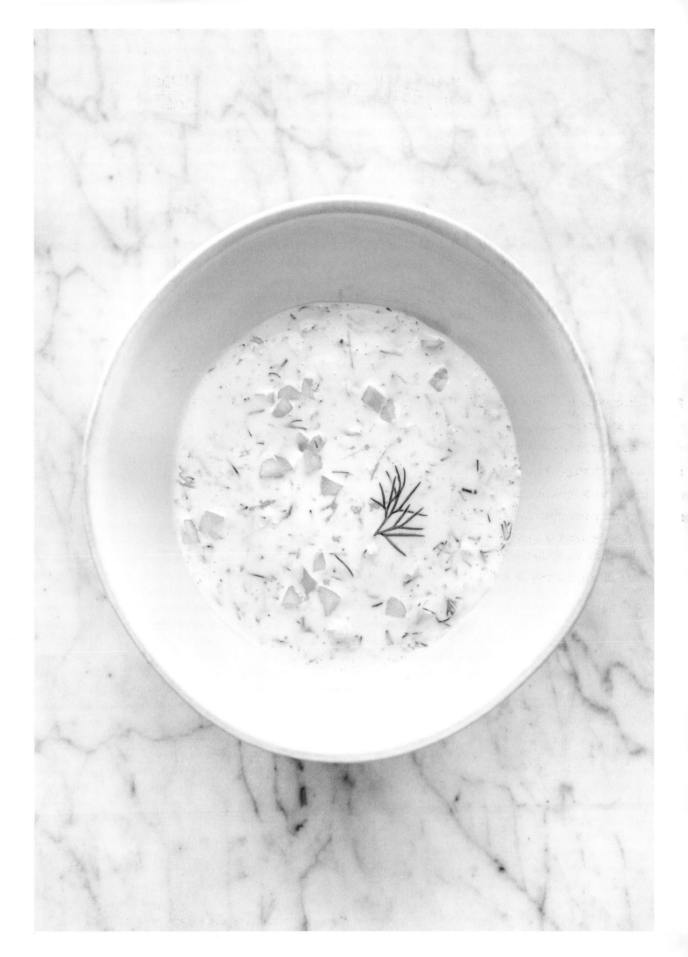

ALL-PURPOSE GREEN SAUCE

YIELD: ¾ cup | **SERVING SIZE:** 2 tablespoons | **PREP TIME:** 5 minutes

This green sauce is my attempt to re-create the addictive green sauce that we always get with our Peruvian chicken order. It quickly became the darling of our Squeaky Clean Keto Facebook group, with fans using it on salads, wraps, veggies, meats, and seafood, and even to dress up their eggs in the morning. There is almost nothing that can't be made more delicious with this tangy, garlicky, and slightly spicy green sauce.

¾ cup fresh cilantro (leaves and stems)

2 jalapeño peppers, seeded and sliced

2 cloves garlic, peeled

1 teaspoon grated lime zest

2 teaspoons fresh lime juice

⅓ cup mayonnaise

2 tablespoons extra-virgin olive oil

1 tablespoon white vinegar

½ teaspoon kosher salt

Put all the ingredients in a blender or food processor and blend until smooth. Store in an airtight container in the refrigerator for up to 1 week.

CALORIES: 133 | **FAT:** 16g | **PROTEIN:** 0g | **CARBS:** 0g | **FIBER:** 0g | **NET CARBS:** 0g

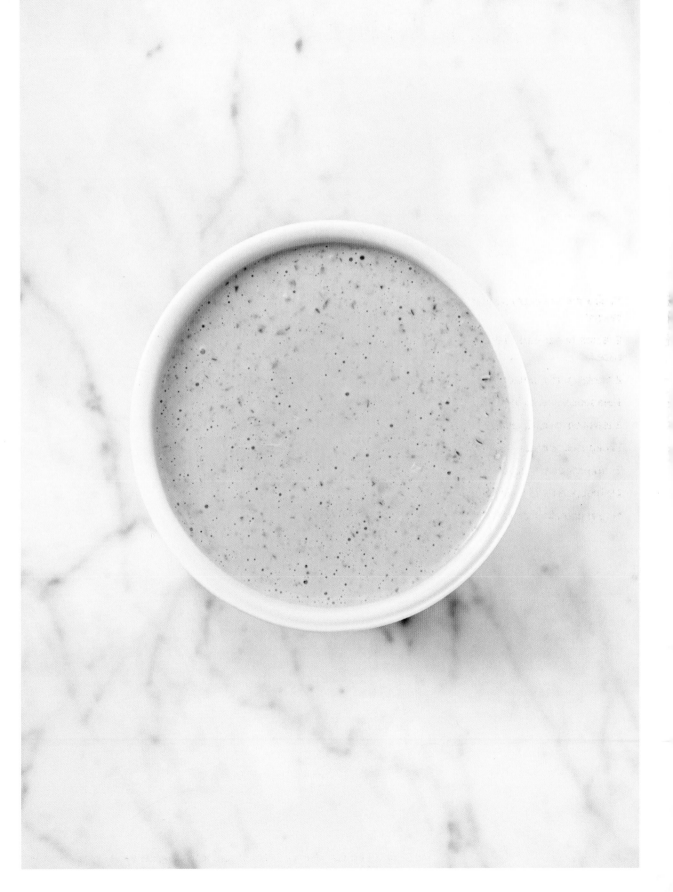

CHILI-LIME MAYO

YIELD: 6 tablespoons | **SERVING SIZE:** 1 tablespoon | **PREP TIME:** 5 minutes

Super easy to throw together, this mayo packs a punch. Spicy, sour, and mildly sweet from the coconut aminos, this sauce is fantastic for dipping and is the perfect accompaniment to my Five-Spice Pork Chops (page 230).

⅓ cup mayonnaise

1 teaspoon coconut aminos

1 teaspoon grated lime zest

1 teaspoon fresh lime juice

½ teaspoon cayenne pepper

Put all the ingredients in a small bowl and whisk until smooth. Store in an airtight container in the refrigerator for up to 1 week.

CALORIES: 91 **FAT:** 10g **PROTEIN:** 0g **CARBS:** 0g **FIBER:** 0g **NET CARBS:** 0g

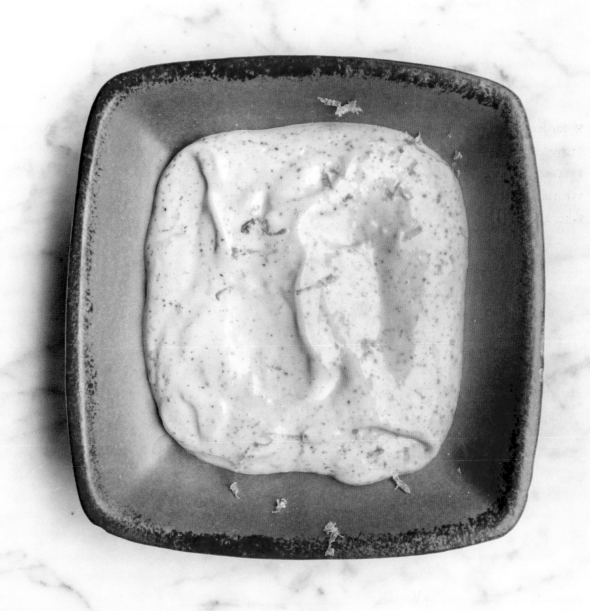

SUN-DRIED TOMATO SAUCE

| YIELD: ⅓ scant cup | SERVING SIZE: 1 tablespoon | PREP TIME: 5 minutes |

Bright and intensely flavored, this sauce is perfect for spreading on wraps or brushing onto grilled chicken or seafood. If you want a thinner sauce for dipping, you can add an extra tablespoon of olive oil. The chicken tenders on page 172 are one of my favorite things to dip into this sauce, with sliced bell peppers and cucumber wedges coming in at a close second!

¼ cup sun-dried tomatoes (see Note)

2 tablespoons extra-virgin olive oil

½ teaspoon minced garlic

½ teaspoon dried oregano leaves

½ teaspoon kosher salt

¼ teaspoon red pepper flakes

Put all the ingredients in a small blender or food processor and blend for 1 minute, or until mostly smooth. Store in an airtight container in the refrigerator for up to 1 week or in the freezer for up to 3 months.

Note: Use sun-dried tomatoes packed in oil for the silkiest consistency. If you can find only dried tomatoes, soak them in hot water for 10 minutes to reconstitute them before using.

| CALORIES: 55 | FAT: 6g | PROTEIN: 0g | CARBS: 1g | FIBER: 0g | NET CARBS: 1g |

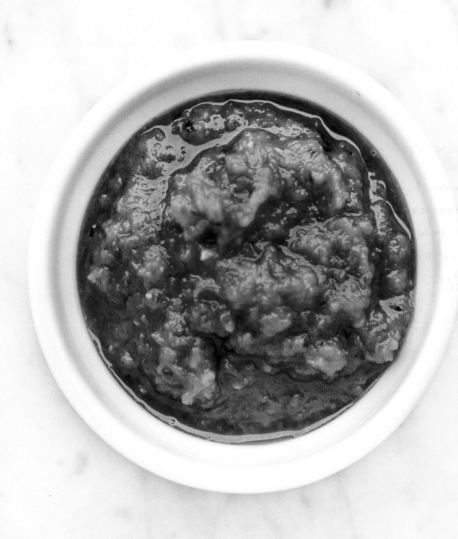

DILL CAPER TARTAR SAUCE

YIELD: ¾ cup | **SERVING SIZE:** 2 tablespoons | **PREP TIME:** 8 minutes

The addition of capers and fresh dill takes this tartar sauce from basic to overachieving. Delish when paired with Salmon Burgers (page 246), it's also a tasty dip for Oven-Roasted Cajun Shrimp (page 242). But it's not just for seafood; you'll want to try this tartar sauce with grilled chicken or even slathered on hard-boiled eggs for a squeaky-friendly lunch or snack.

⅓ cup mayonnaise

2 tablespoons canned coconut milk

2 tablespoons chopped dill pickles

1 tablespoon capers, drained and chopped

1 tablespoon chopped fresh dill

½ teaspoon caper brine (from the jar of capers)

½ teaspoon ground black pepper

Put all the ingredients in a small bowl and whisk until mostly smooth. Store in an airtight container in the refrigerator for up to 1 week.

CALORIES: 93 **FAT:** 11g **PROTEIN:** 0g **CARBS:** 0g **FIBER:** 0g **NET CARBS:** 0g

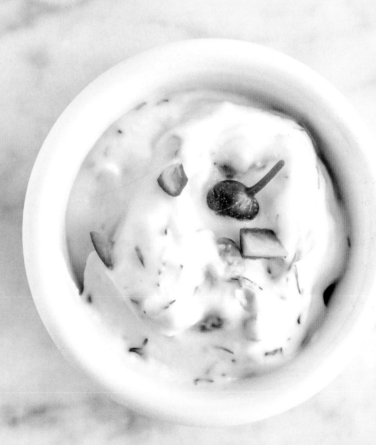

CREAMY GARLIC SAUCE

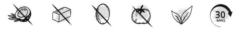

YIELD: 1 cup | **SERVING SIZE:** 1 tablespoon | **PREP TIME:** 10 minutes

Via the magic of emulsification, this simple and tasty garlic sauce has a texture similar to mayonnaise in spite of being egg-free. It was inspired by a classic Lebanese garlic sauce, and you're going to want to slather this luscious potion on meats, veggies, your fingers—I'm not judging, and you won't either once you taste it! My family particularly enjoys this sauce with Prosciutto-Wrapped Chicken Tenders (page 172) and Oven-Roasted Cajun Shrimp (page 242).

⅓ cup chopped garlic

1 teaspoon kosher salt

3 teaspoons fresh lemon juice, divided

¾ cup avocado oil

Put the garlic, salt, and 1 teaspoon of the lemon juice in a 1-quart jar with an opening wide enough to insert an immersion blender. Insert an immersion blender into the jar and blend until smooth. Add ¼ cup of the oil and blend for 1 minute, or until smooth. Add 1 teaspoon of the lemon juice and blend for 1 minute. Slowly pour another ¼ cup of oil into the jar while blending for about 1 minute, or until thickened slightly. Add the remaining teaspoon of lemon juice and blend for 1 minute. Slowly pour the remaining ¼ cup of oil into the jar while blending for about 1 minute, or until thickened, white, and creamy. Store in an airtight container in the refrigerator for up to 1 week.

Note: If the sauce breaks, it will still taste amazing, and it works well as a dressing when liquid. You can also try blending in ¼ teaspoon of xanthan gum to thicken and re-emulsify it if you want a thicker consistency.

CALORIES: 94 **FAT:** 11g **PROTEIN:** 0g **CARBS:** 2g **FIBER:** 0g **NET CARBS:** 2g

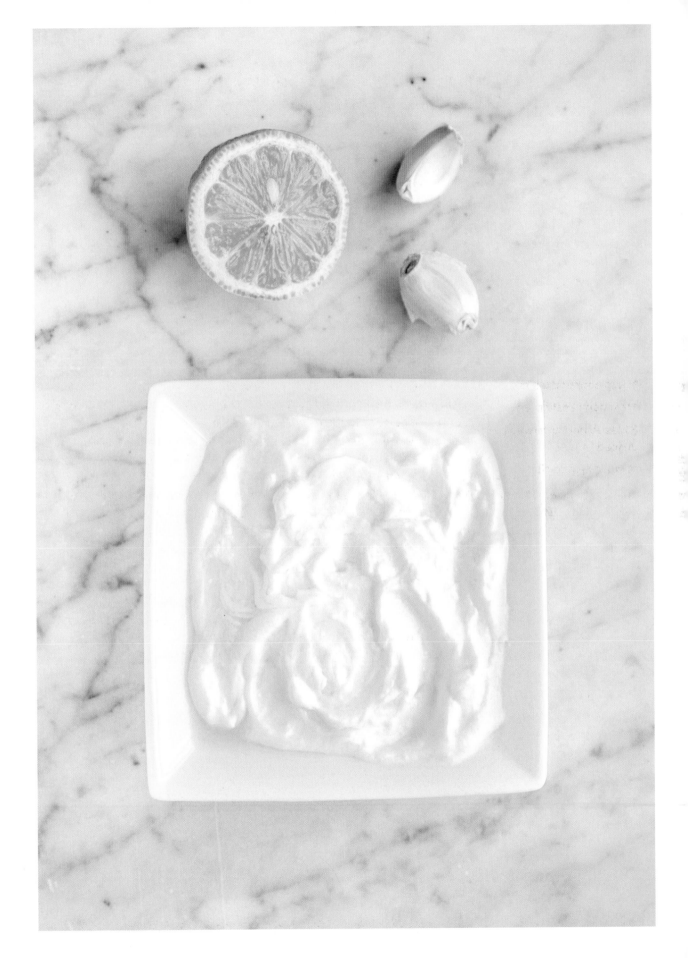

QUICK-PICKLED RED ONIONS

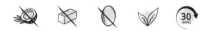

| YIELD: 1 quart | SERVING SIZE: 2 tablespoons | PREP TIME: 10 minutes | COOK TIME: 5 minutes |

A few strands of pungent pickled red onions can elevate almost any dish, bringing another layer of bright flavor and crunchy texture—not to mention that vibrant pink color! Since moving to Central America a few years ago, we've fallen in love with the spicy chilis and sour orange juice that are common in the pickled onions here. This version contains habanero peppers, lime juice, and orange extract, which creates a spicy, sour citrus situation that you won't be able to get enough of!

4 cups thinly sliced red onions

2 whole habanero peppers (any color)

5 sprigs fresh cilantro

1½ cups filtered water

1 cup white vinegar

2 tablespoons fresh lime juice

1 teaspoon orange extract

1 teaspoon kosher salt

Layer the onions, peppers, and cilantro in a clean 32-ounce mason jar. Put the water, vinegar, lime juice, orange extract, and salt in a small saucepan. Bring to a boil, then remove the pan from the heat. Carefully pour the liquid into the jar until the onions are covered. Leave 1 inch of air space between the liquid and the top of the jar. Cover and leave on the counter for 4 hours, or until the liquid has cooled to room temperature. While you can eat these pickled onions immediately, they taste even better after a day or two in the refrigerator, where they will keep for up to 1 month.

Note: To make these pickled onions even spicier, slice the peppers thinly instead of leaving them whole.

| CALORIES: 8 | FAT: 0g | PROTEIN: 0g | CARBS: 2g | FIBER: 0g | NET CARBS: 2g |

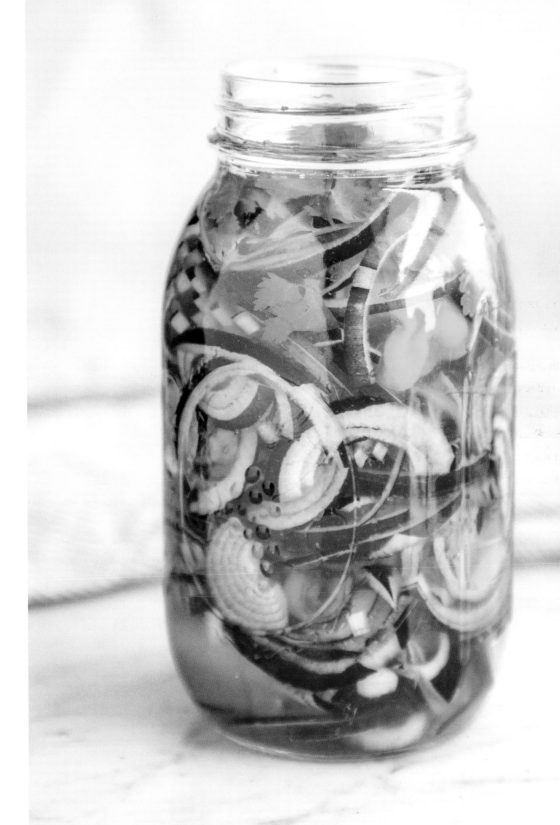

OLIVE SALAD

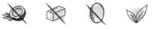

YIELD: 1½ cups | SERVING SIZE: ¼ cup | PREP TIME: 10 minutes, plus 1 hour to chill

Traditionally used as a condiment for the famous muffuletta sandwich (see page 162 for my wrap version), this briny concoction can brighten up any salad or wrap, not to mention grilled meats, seafood, or even your breakfast eggs. Once you make it, you'll want to put it on everything!

8 cocktail onions, cut into quarters

½ cup roughly chopped black olives

½ cup sliced pimento-stuffed olives

¼ cup sliced pepperoncini

3 tablespoons extra-virgin olive oil

2 tablespoons red wine vinegar

2 tablespoons finely chopped red onions

1 tablespoon capers, drained

1 tablespoon chopped fresh parsley

1 teaspoon minced garlic

1 teaspoon dried oregano leaves

¼ teaspoon ground black pepper

Put all the ingredients in a medium-sized bowl and stir well. Cover and refrigerate for at least 1 hour before serving. Store in an airtight container in the refrigerator for up to 1 week.

CALORIES: 95   FAT: 10g   PROTEIN: 0g   CARBS: 2g   FIBER: 1g   NET CARBS: 1g

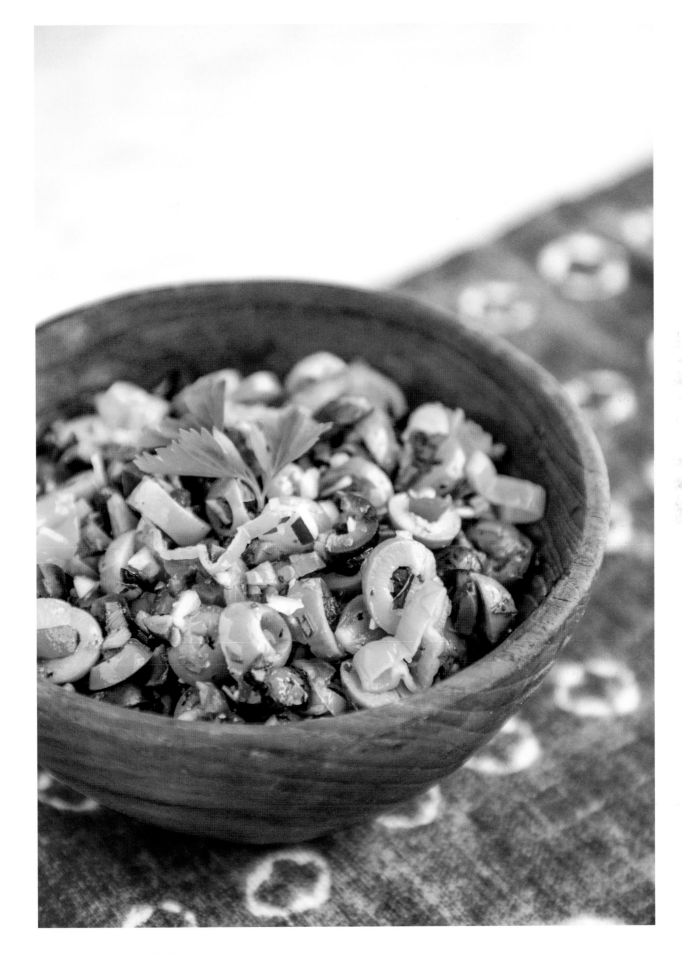

SPINACH WRAPS

YIELD: four 8-inch wraps | **SERVING SIZE:** 1 wrap | **PREP TIME:** 5 minutes | **COOK TIME:** 8 minutes

These versatile spinach wraps are my new favorite because they have no eggy taste and a fantastic texture. The addition of psyllium powder makes them super pliable, and the coconut flour bulks them up just enough to give them an authentically "bready" mouthfeel. I recommend making a bunch and freezing them so you have them on hand whenever a craving for a Muffuletta Wrap (page 162) or Breakfast Burrito (page 132) strikes!

6 large eggs

1 teaspoon white vinegar

½ cup spinach leaves

2 tablespoons coconut flour

½ teaspoon psyllium husk powder

¼ teaspoon kosher salt

⅛ teaspoon garlic powder

⅛ teaspoon ground nutmeg

1 tablespoon avocado oil or other light-tasting oil, for the pan

1. Put all the ingredients except the oil in a blender and blend until smooth and uniform in color.

2. Heat the oil in a large nonstick skillet over medium heat. Pour in one-quarter of the batter and tilt the pan in a circular motion to spread the batter into a circle about 8 inches in diameter. Cook for 1 minute. Flip the wrap with a thin spatula. Cook for an additional 30 seconds, or until firm. Remove and repeat with the rest of the batter, making a total of 4 wraps. Store in an airtight container in the refrigerator for up to 1 week or freeze for up to 3 months. Bring to room temperature before using.

CALORIES: 125 **FAT:** 8g **PROTEIN:** 10g **CARBS:** 3g **FIBER:** 2g **NET CARBS:** 1g

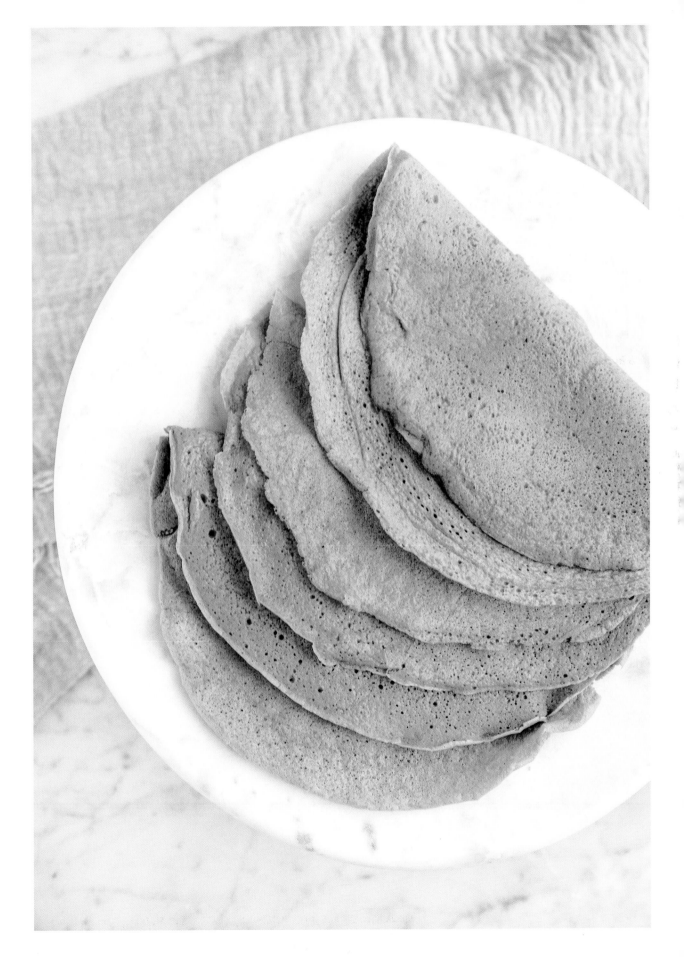

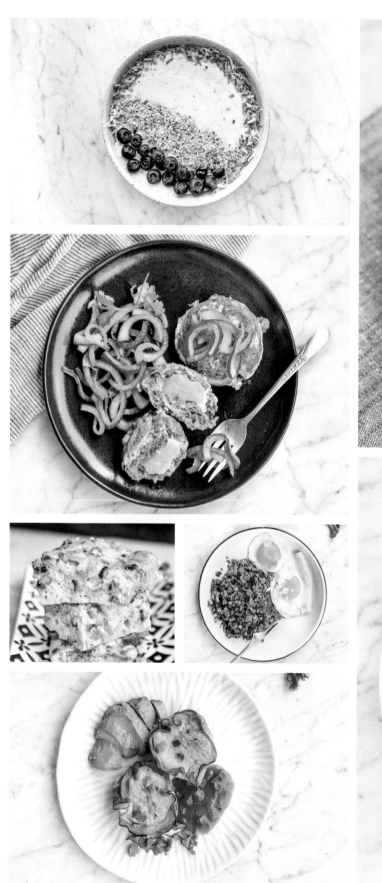
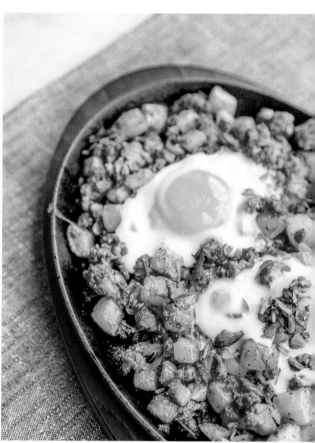
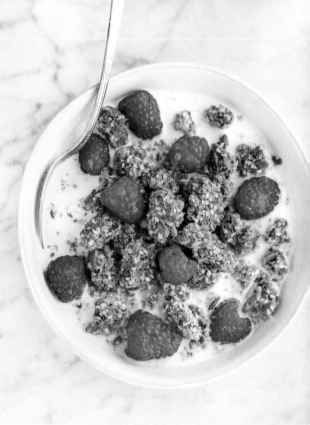

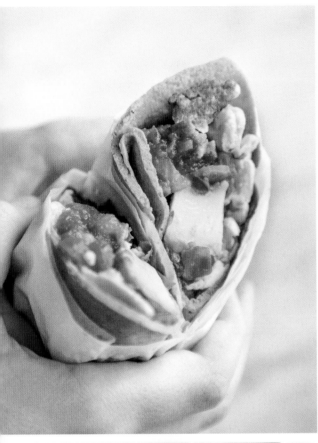

Breakfast

Fiesta Egg Cups / 116

Blueberry Bliss Smoothie Bowl / 118

Chorizo & Turnip Hash / 120

Bacon & Caramelized Onion Breakfast Bake / 122

Cinnamon Maple Granola / 124

Crispy Radish Corned Beef Hash / 126

Prosciutto & Tomato Omelette / 128

Baked Scotch Eggs / 130

Breakfast Burrito / 132

Eggs in Purgatory / 134

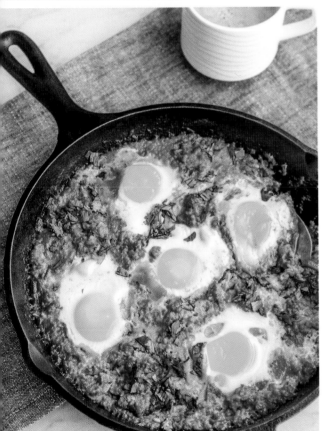

FIESTA EGG CUPS

YIELD: 10 egg cups | SERVING SIZE: 2 egg cups | PREP TIME: 10 minutes | COOK TIME: 18 minutes

Easy to make and perfect for breakfast on the go, these tasty egg cups are a great option to bake in advance and keep on hand for super busy mornings. Using a store-bought salsa means that no chopping is required to get plenty of flavor baked into these protein-packed gems. I like to garnish these cups with chopped fresh cilantro and serve them with extra salsa and some sliced avocado on the side.

10 slices deli ham

8 large eggs, beaten

⅓ cup prepared salsa

½ teaspoon kosher salt

¼ teaspoon ground black pepper

Preheat the oven to 375°F. Line 10 standard-size muffin cups with the ham slices. Mix the beaten eggs, salsa, salt, and pepper in a medium-sized bowl until well combined. Ladle about ¼ cup of the egg mixture into each ham-lined muffin cup. Bake for 18 minutes, or until set. Store leftovers in an airtight container in the refrigerator for up to 5 days or in the freezer for up to 3 months. Reheat in the microwave for 1 to 2 minutes, until hot.

Note: You can add ½ cup shredded cheese to the egg mixture if not squeaky.

CALORIES: 171   FAT: 9g   PROTEIN: 20g   CARBS: 2g   FIBER: 0g   NET CARBS: 2g

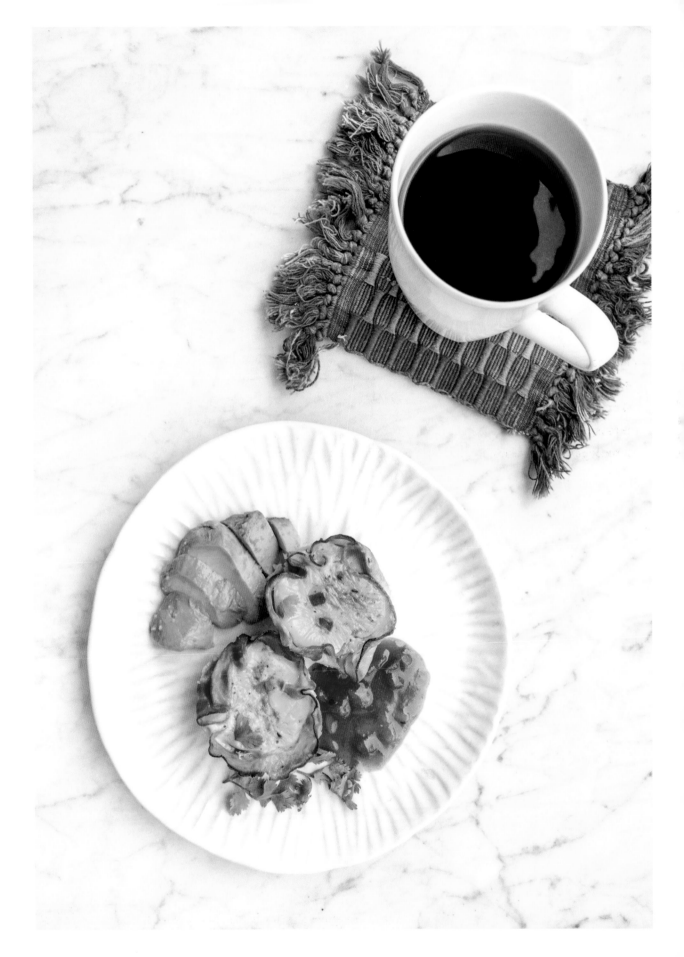

BLUEBERRY BLISS SMOOTHIE BOWL

  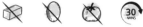

YIELD: 1 serving | **PREP TIME:** 5 minutes

When you're sick of eggs and craving something fresh and a little sweet, this blueberry smoothie bowl will hit the spot! High in fiber and healthy fats, this pretty breakfast bowl will keep you going all morning long.

½ cup chilled canned coconut milk

⅓ cup fresh blueberries or other berries, divided

2 tablespoons collagen peptides (aka hydrolysate)

3 tablespoons unsweetened shredded coconut, toasted

1 tablespoon shelled hemp seeds (hemp hearts)

Put the coconut milk, 2 tablespoons of the blueberries, and the collagen in a small blender or food processor and blend until smooth. Pour the mixture into a cereal bowl and chill for 5 minutes to thicken. Top with the remaining blueberries, toasted coconut, and shelled hemp seeds. Serve immediately.

Notes: You can blend the smoothie portion up to 3 days in advance and assemble the bowl when ready to eat. Feel free to double or triple the recipe if you want to have this bowl more than once a week.

Using raspberries instead of blueberries will reduce the net carbs to 4g.

CALORIES: 434 **FAT:** 35g **PROTEIN:** 14g **CARBS:** 14g **FIBER:** 6g **NET CARBS:** 8g

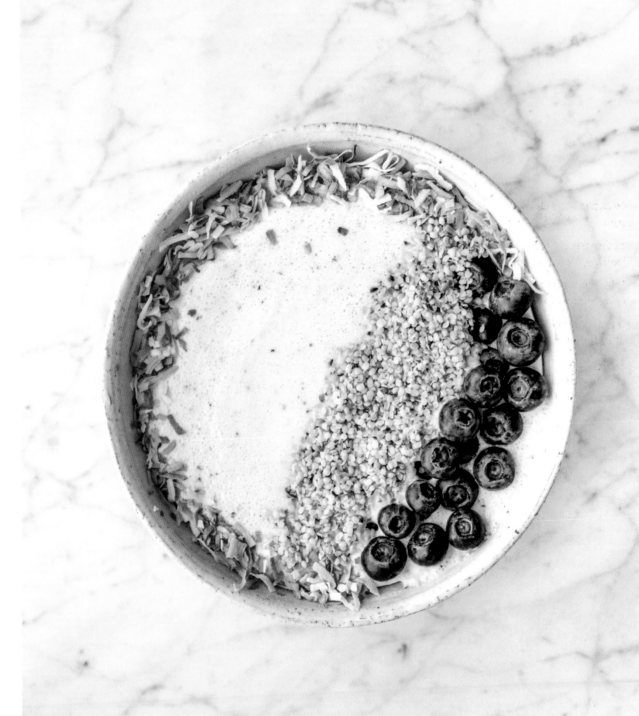

CHORIZO & TURNIP HASH

YIELD: 6 servings	SERVING SIZE: 1 cup hash + 1 egg	PREP TIME: 10 minutes	COOK TIME: 35 minutes

This spicy breakfast skillet is so hearty and flavorful that your family will be begging you to make it on the regular! Turnips stand in for potatoes, and other than a slight natural sweetness, it will be close to impossible to tell the difference. I highly recommend the cilantro garnish to complement the chorizo, but if you aren't a fan, you can use chopped fresh parsley instead. If you're a hash lover like I am, also try my Crispy Radish Corned Beef Hash on page 126 for a more traditional flavor profile.

1 tablespoon extra-virgin olive oil

4 cups peeled and diced turnips

1 pound Mexican-style fresh (raw) chorizo, casings removed

½ cup chopped onions

2 tablespoons chopped red bell peppers

1 teaspoon minced garlic

1 teaspoon kosher salt

½ teaspoon chipotle powder

¼ teaspoon ground black pepper

6 large eggs

2 tablespoons chopped fresh cilantro, for garnish

1. Preheat the oven to 375°F.

2. Heat the oil in a large ovenproof skillet over medium heat until shimmering. Add the diced turnips and cook, stirring occasionally, for 5 minutes, or until they are beginning to brown and soften. Add the chorizo and cook for 5 minutes, stirring to break it up into crumbles. Add the onions, red peppers, garlic, salt, chipotle powder, and pepper and stir well. Cook for 5 more minutes, or until the onions have softened and the turnips are fork-tender.

3. Press 6 depressions into the hash with the back of a large spoon and carefully break an egg into each depression. Transfer the skillet to the oven and bake for 18 minutes for a firm white with a runny yolk; if you prefer a solid yolk, bake for 20 minutes or longer. Remove from the oven and garnish with the cilantro. Serve immediately. Store any leftovers in an airtight container in the refrigerator for up to 5 days.

Note: For easy meal prep during the week, you can make the hash ahead and bake individual portions with an egg in a small ovenproof skillet or ramekin as needed. Or, if you're pressed for time, you can reheat the hash in a skillet (2 to 3 minutes over medium heat) and then plate it and fry your egg in the same skillet for a hot breakfast ready in 5 minutes or less.

CALORIES: 432	FAT: 36g	PROTEIN: 25g	CARBS: 9g	FIBER: 2g	NET CARBS: 7g

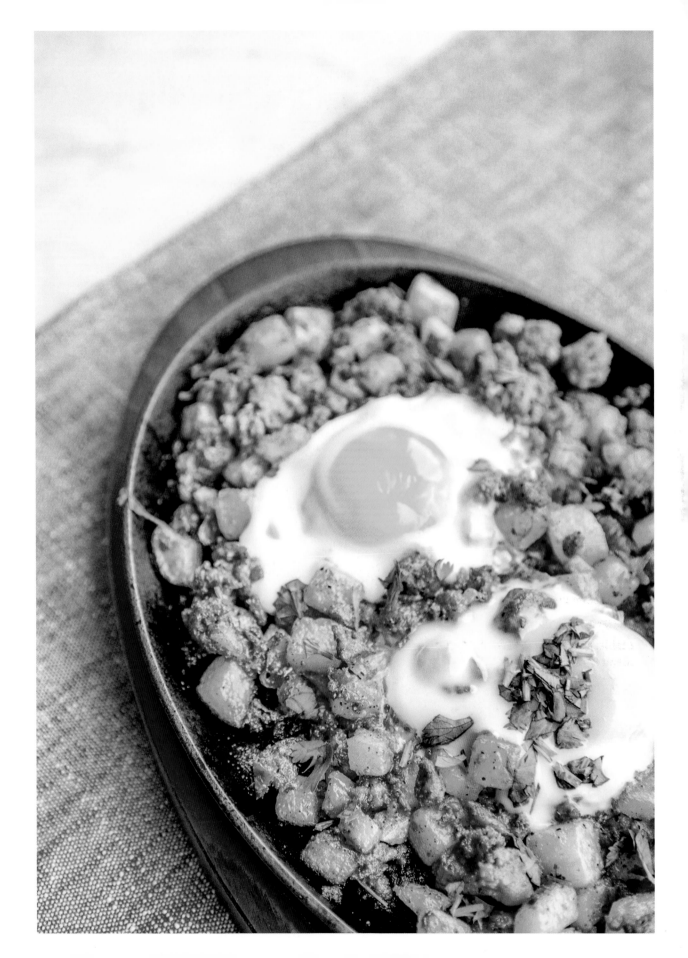

BACON & CARAMELIZED ONION BREAKFAST BAKE

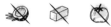

YIELD: nine 3-inch squares | **SERVING SIZE:** 1 square | **PREP TIME:** 5 minutes | **COOK TIME:** 35 minutes

This simple recipe uses just a few ingredients but is loaded with flavor. The bacon adds a salty lusciousness, of course, but the onions are where the magic is. Cooked down and caramelized in the bacon grease, they add a natural sweetness that perfectly complements the savory bacon and eggs.

½ cup chopped onions

6 slices bacon, chopped

½ teaspoon kosher salt

¼ teaspoon ground black pepper

10 large eggs

¼ cup filtered water

1 tablespoon chopped fresh parsley, for garnish (optional)

1. Preheat the oven to 375°F.

2. Put the onions, bacon, salt, and pepper in a large skillet. Cook, stirring occasionally, over medium heat for 10 minutes, or until the onions and bacon are golden brown.

3. Meanwhile, beat the eggs and water together in a large bowl until fully combined.

4. Transfer the bacon and onion mixture to a 9-inch square baking pan. Swirl the mixture around to grease the bottom and sides of the pan, then spread it evenly over the surface of the pan. Slowly pour the egg mixture into the pan, being careful not to displace the bacon mixture.

5. Bake for 25 minutes, or until firm to the touch in the center. Remove and let cool slightly before slicing into 9 squares. Garnish with the parsley if desired. Store leftovers in an airtight container in the refrigerator for up to 5 days or in the freezer for up to 3 months. Reheat in the microwave for 30 seconds to 1 minute before serving.

CALORIES: 146 **FAT:** 9g **PROTEIN:** 11g **CARBS:** 1g **FIBER:** 0g **NET CARBS:** 1g

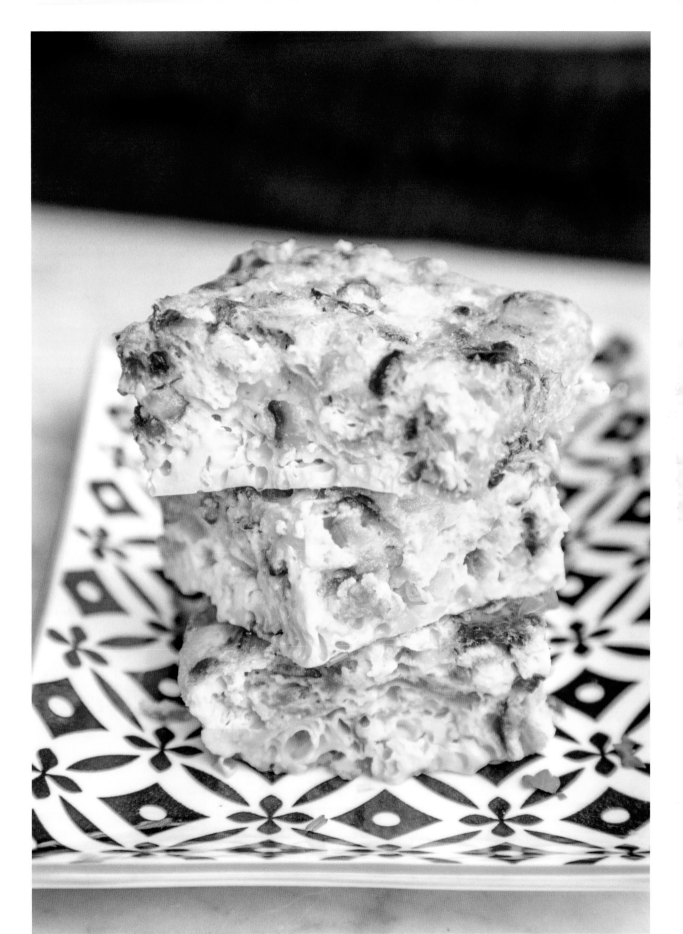

CINNAMON MAPLE GRANOLA

YIELD: 4 cups | **SERVING SIZE:** ½ cup | **PREP TIME:** 10 minutes | **COOK TIME:** 50 minutes

If you're missing cereal on your keto diet, then this granola will be a welcome addition. To keep it squeaky, there is no sweetener in this recipe, but the maple extract and naturally sweet coconut will trick your taste buds into thinking there is—especially if you add a handful of your favorite keto-friendly berries to the bowl. This tasty granola stays crispy in hemp milk for up to 15 minutes, so take your time and enjoy it!

1 cup unsalted sunflower seed butter (no sugar added), store-bought or homemade (page 78)

¼ cup coconut oil

2 large egg whites

2 tablespoons ground cinnamon

1 tablespoon maple extract

Pinch of kosher salt

1½ cups unsweetened shredded coconut

½ cup shelled hemp seeds (hemp hearts)

½ cup shelled raw pumpkin seeds (pepitas)

¼ cup sesame seeds

¼ cup psyllium husk powder

1. Preheat the oven to 325°F. Line a sheet pan with parchment paper.

2. Put the sunflower seed butter, coconut oil, egg whites, cinnamon, maple extract, and salt in a small blender and blend until smooth. Put the shredded coconut, shelled hemp seeds, pumpkin seeds, sesame seeds, and psyllium powder in a medium-sized bowl and stir to combine. Add the blended liquid and stir well until a clumpy "dough" forms.

3. Press the dough into the prepared sheet pan and bake for 30 minutes. Remove and break up the granola into bite-sized pieces. Return the pan to the oven and bake for an additional 20 minutes, or until crispy. Remove from the oven and let cool completely before eating. Store leftovers in an airtight container for up to 2 weeks.

Note: If not squeaky, you may sweeten the granola by adding granulated erythritol (about ⅓ cup should do it) when mixing the dry ingredients together in Step 2.

CALORIES: 491 | **FAT:** 44g | **PROTEIN:** 16g | **CARBS:** 15g | **FIBER:** 10g | **NET CARBS:** 5g

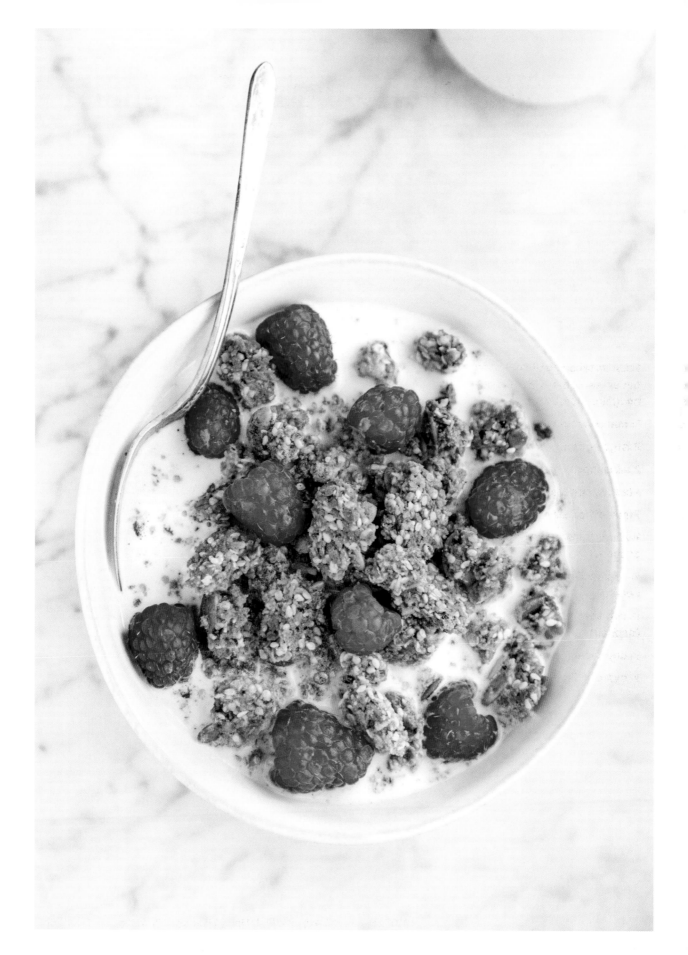

CRISPY RADISH CORNED BEEF HASH

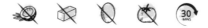

| **YIELD:** 4 servings | **SERVING SIZE:** ½ cup | **PREP TIME:** 5 minutes | **COOK TIME:** 18 minutes |

Perfect for when you have bacon fatigue (yep, it's a thing), this decadent corned beef hash uses radishes to stand in for the traditional potatoes! For you skeptics who aren't sure about radishes, I promise that cooking them mellows them out. The briny saltiness of the corned beef is what really stands out here. For extra protein, I like to enjoy this hash with a couple of fried eggs on the side.

1 tablespoon extra-virgin olive oil

1 cup diced radishes

¼ cup diced onions

½ teaspoon kosher salt

¼ teaspoon ground black pepper

1 (12-ounce) can corned beef, or 1 packed cup finely chopped corned beef

½ teaspoon dried oregano leaves

¼ teaspoon garlic powder

1. Heat the oil in a large skillet over medium heat. Add the radishes, onions, salt, and pepper and cook for 5 minutes, or until the radishes have started to soften.

2. To the pan, add the corned beef, oregano, and garlic powder and stir until well combined. Cook over medium-low heat, stirring occasionally, for 10 minutes, or until the radishes are soft and starting to brown.

3. Press the mixture into the bottom of the pan and cook over high heat for 3 minutes, or until crisp and brown on the bottom. Serve hot. Store leftovers in an airtight container in the refrigerator for up to 5 days.

CALORIES: 252   **FAT:** 16g   **PROTEIN:** 23g   **CARBS:** 3g   **FIBER:** 1g   **NET CARBS:** 2g

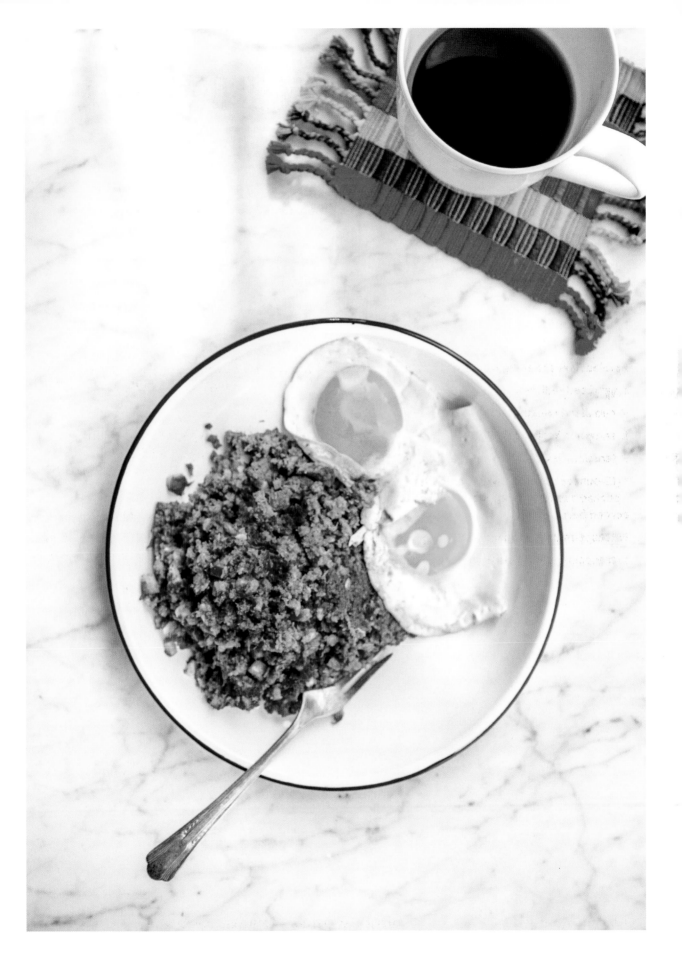

PROSCIUTTO & TOMATO OMELETTE

YIELD: 1 serving | PREP TIME: 5 minutes | COOK TIME: 5 minutes

Inspired by a ham-stuffed crepe we ate in Italy, this recipe makes a thin omelette that is folded twice to form a quarter circle, just like a crepe. No added salt is required; the prosciutto is salty enough to season the entire thing. This squeaky-friendly omelette tastes even more amazing with the Sun-Dried Tomato Sauce on page 102.

2 large eggs

1 tablespoon filtered water

1 teaspoon butter

4 slices prosciutto

4 slices tomato

5 fresh basil leaves

1. Whisk the eggs and water together in a small bowl.

2. Melt the butter in a 10-inch nonstick skillet over medium heat. When the butter is melted and sizzling, pour in the egg mixture and tilt the pan in a circular motion to cover the bottom with a thin layer of egg. Cook for 1 to 2 minutes, until mostly firm.

3. Place the slices of prosciutto on half of the egg circle. Carefully fold the empty side over the side with the prosciutto. Place the tomatoes and basil on half of the omelette. Carefully fold the empty half over the half with the tomatoes and basil, forming a quarter circle. Cook for an additional minute, or until no liquid is visible. Remove and serve immediately.

CALORIES: 242 FAT: 16g PROTEIN: 21g CARBS: 3g FIBER: 1g NET CARBS: 2g

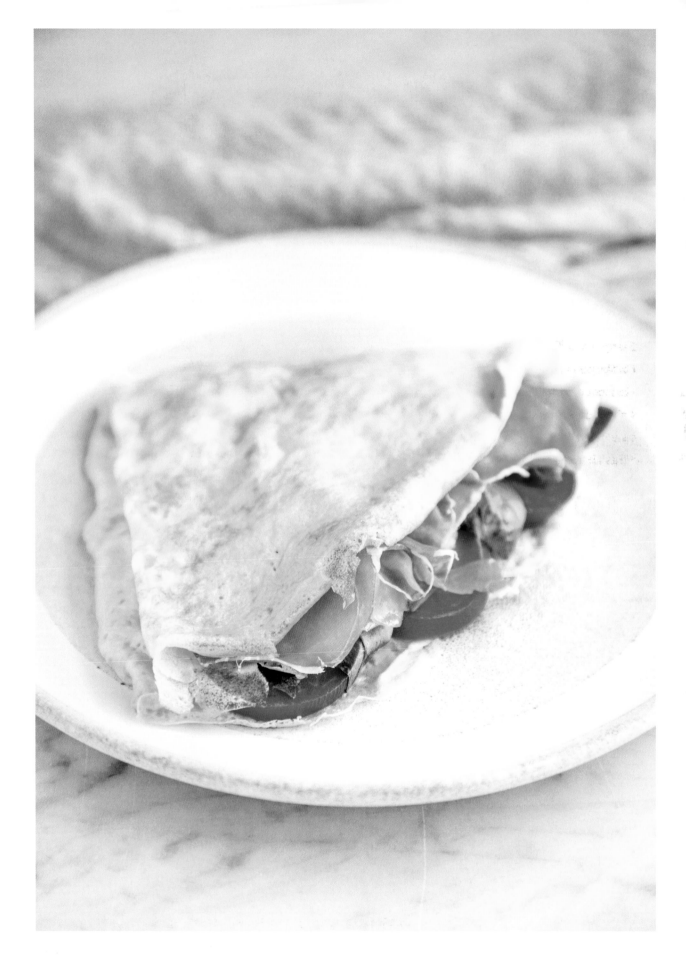

BAKED SCOTCH EGGS

YIELD: 6 pieces | SERVING SIZE: 1 piece | PREP TIME: 10 minutes | COOK TIME: 22 minutes

Mr. Hungry and I fell in love with Scotch eggs during a trip to London, and I started making them at home shortly after. I posted a recipe for a traditional version on my website, which starts with a soft-boiled egg that is then wrapped in sausage, breaded, and deep-fried. It's very tasty, but also time-consuming to make. This baked version is missing the bread-crumbs but is almost as satisfying and takes a lot less effort! Great for meal prep, these baked Scotch eggs are delicious hot or cold. I love them with a side of Quick-Pickled Red Onions (page 108).

1 pound breakfast sausage

6 medium eggs (see Note)

1. Preheat the oven to 375°F.

2. Divide the sausage into 12 equal portions. Press 6 pieces into the bottom and up the sides of 6 jumbo muffin cups (4-ounce capacity or greater). Break an egg into each cup. Press the remaining 6 sausage portions into disks with your hands and place one over each egg, pressing the edges lightly into the sausage to seal.

3. Bake for 22 minutes. Remove from the oven and let cool for 5 minutes before unmolding onto a serving plate. Store leftovers in an airtight container in the refrigerator for up to 5 days or in the freezer for up to 3 months. To reheat, place on a plate and microwave on high, covered, for 1 to 2 minutes.

Note: Most of the recipes in this book call for large eggs, but medium eggs give you a better ratio of yolk to white to sausage in this recipe.

CALORIES: 243   FAT: 15g   PROTEIN: 16g   CARBS: 1g   FIBER: 0g   NET CARBS: 1g

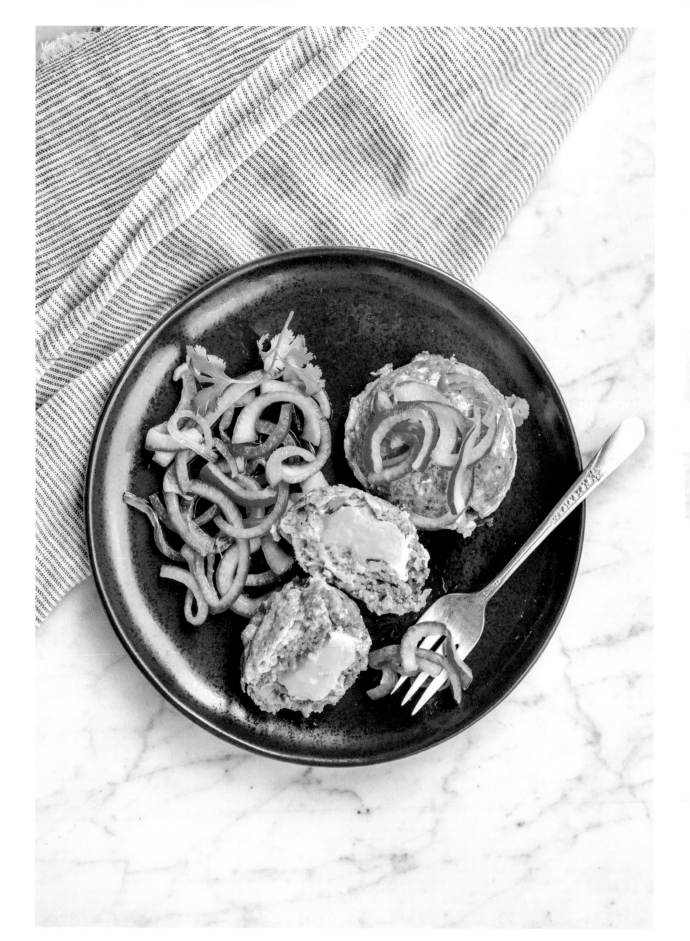

BREAKFAST BURRITO

YIELD: 1 serving | **PREP TIME:** 10 minutes

There's something about a fistful of breakfast burrito that's really satisfying to eat. This squeaky version is loaded with flavor and texture—you'll never miss the traditional flour tortilla!

1 Spinach Wrap (page 112)

2 eggs, scrambled

2 ounces breakfast sausage, crumbled and cooked (about ¼ cup)

¼ Hass avocado, cubed or sliced

2 tablespoons prepared salsa

1 tablespoon chopped fresh cilantro

1. Lay a 12-inch square sheet of parchment paper on the counter.

2. Place the spinach wrap in the center of the parchment. Spoon the scrambled eggs onto the wrap in a line about one-third of the way from the center on the side closest to you. Leave about 2 inches of the wrap empty on each side. Top the eggs with the sausage, avocado cubes, salsa, and cilantro.

3. Carefully fold in the left side of the wrap (not the parchment) and then the right side of the wrap to partially cover the toppings. While holding the sides in with your middle fingers, use your thumbs and index fingers to lift and roll the front edge of the wrap over the fillings and two sides. Continue rolling up and over until you have a roll with all the filling inside. Fold the left and right sides of the parchment into the middle and then roll the front of the parchment up and over to form a paper tube with the burrito inside. Cut through the middle and fold back the parchment to eat.

Note: You may use the meat of your choice in place of the sausage. If not squeaky, feel free to add cheese and/or sour cream.

CALORIES: 498 **FAT:** 36g **PROTEIN:** 31g **CARBS:** 11g **FIBER:** 5g **NET CARBS:** 6g

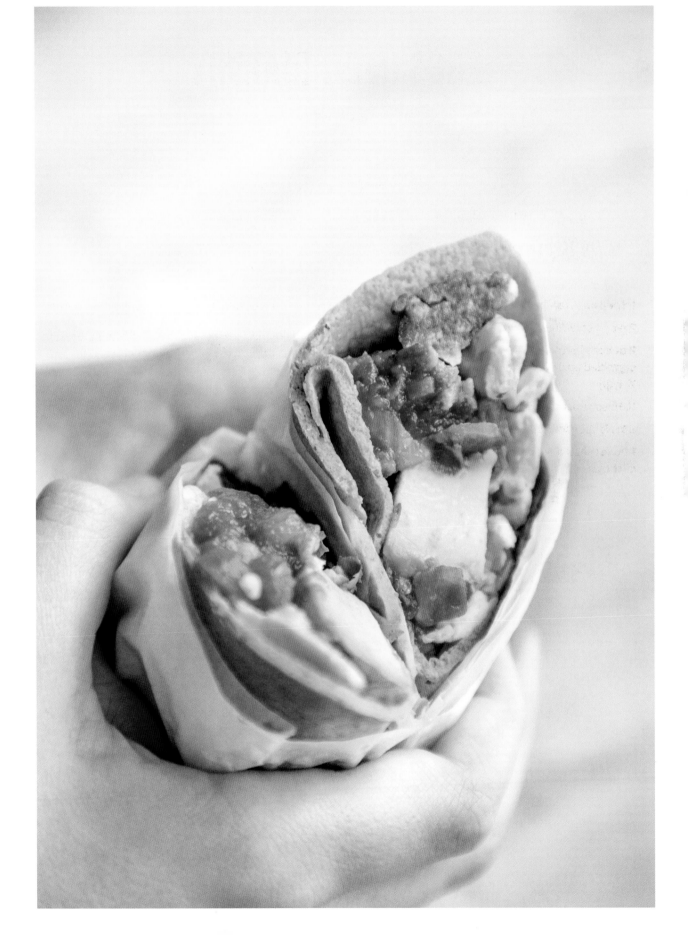

EGGS IN PURGATORY

YIELD: 5 servings | SERVING SIZE: ½ cup + 1 egg | PREP TIME: 10 minutes | COOK TIME: 35 minutes

A little spicy and a lot flavorful, this saucy baked egg dish is guaranteed to wake you up on even the most challenging of mornings!

1 pound Mexican-style fresh (raw) chorizo, casings removed

½ cup chopped poblano peppers

⅓ cup chopped onions

1 teaspoon minced garlic

1 teaspoon ground cumin

½ teaspoon kosher salt

¼ teaspoon ground black pepper

1 cup canned crushed tomatoes

5 large eggs

2 tablespoons chopped fresh cilantro, for garnish

1. Preheat the oven to 375°F.

2. Place the chorizo in a large ovenproof skillet and cook over medium heat, breaking into crumbles, for about 5 minutes. Add the poblanos, onions, garlic, cumin, salt, and black pepper and stir well. Cook for 5 minutes, or until the peppers and onions are soft. Stir in the tomatoes and simmer for 5 minutes, or until the mixture has thickened.

3. Make 5 depressions in the mixture using the back of a spoon and break an egg into each one. Transfer the skillet to the oven and bake for 18 minutes for a firm white with a runny yolk; if you prefer a solid yolk, bake for 20 minutes or longer. Garnish with the cilantro and serve hot. Store leftovers in an airtight container in the refrigerator for up to 5 days.

CALORIES: 343 FAT: 28g PROTEIN: 19g CARBS: 8g FIBER: 2g NET CARBS: 6g

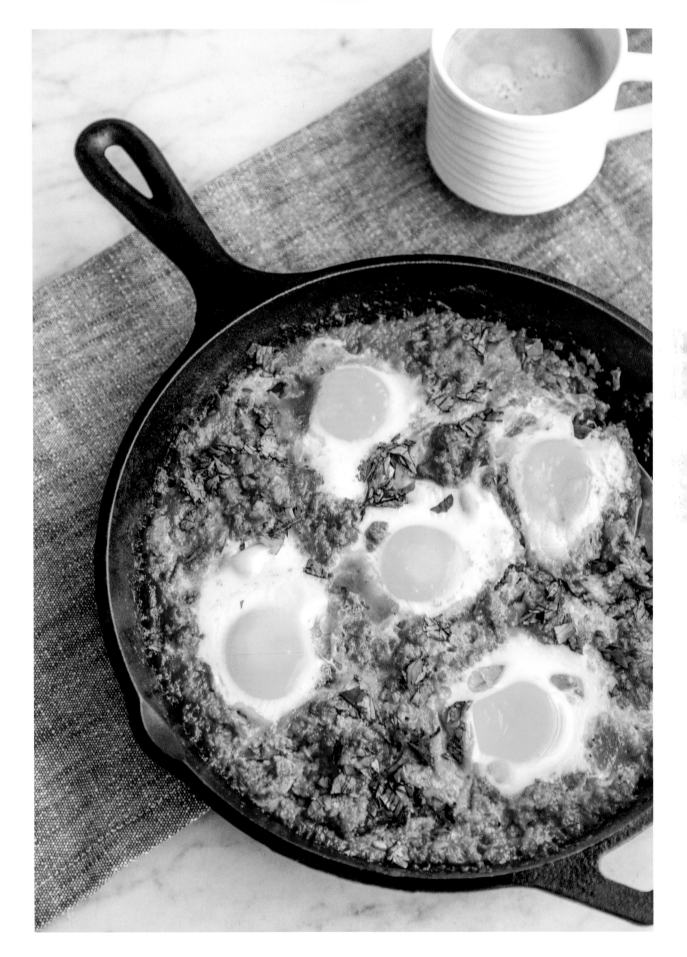

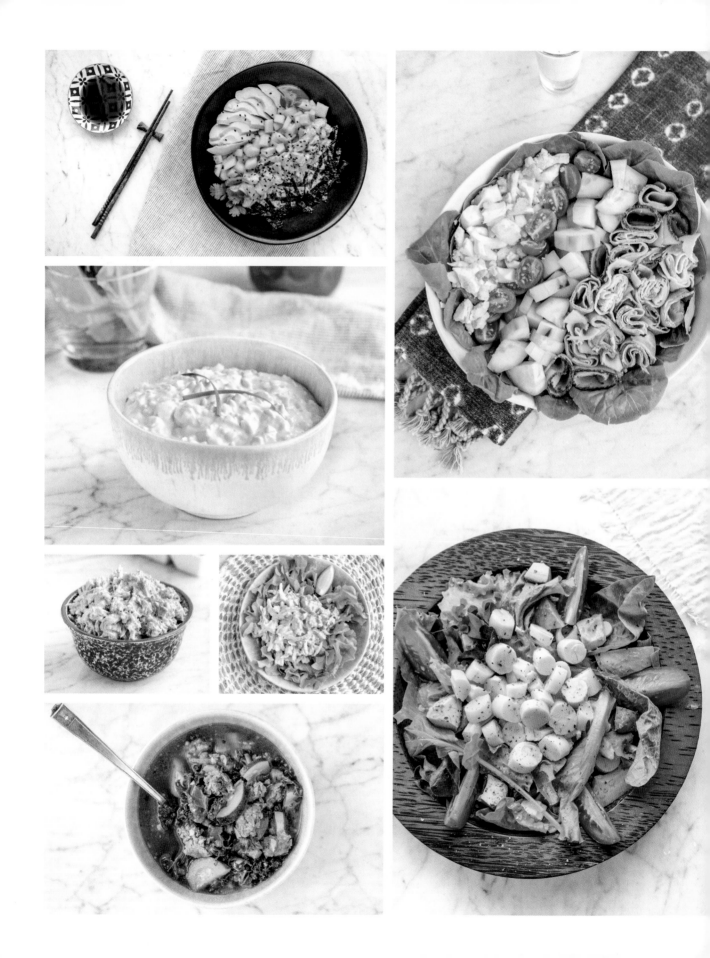

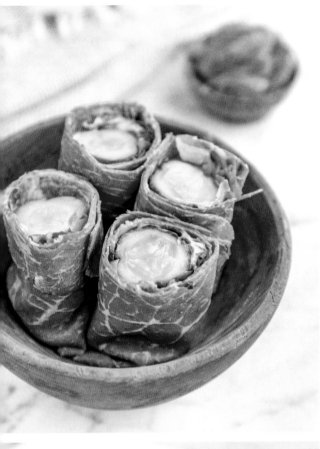

Soups, Salads & Wraps

Spicy Sausage & Kale Soup / 138

Roasted Cauliflower & Leek Soup / 140

Curried Turnip & Cauliflower Soup / 142

Chicken & Vegetable Soup / 144

Curried Chicken Salad / 146

Easy Tuna Salad / 148

Cobb Salad with Warm Bacon Vinaigrette / 150

Simple Egg Salad / 152

Spicy Shrimp Salad Sushi Bowl / 154

Buffalo Chicken Salad / 156

Chef's Salad / 158

Hearts of Palm Salad / 160

Muffuletta Wrap / 162

Chicken Club Wrap / 164

Pastrami Roll-Ups / 166

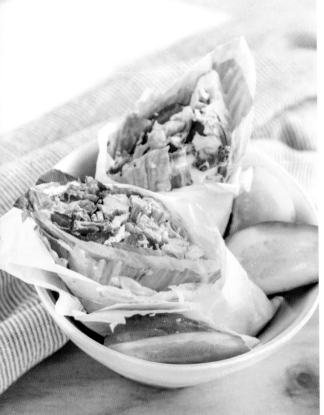

SPICY SAUSAGE & KALE SOUP

| YIELD: 3 quarts (12 cups) | SERVING SIZE: 1½ cups | PREP TIME: 10 minutes | COOK TIME: 28 minutes |

Salty, spicy, and so satisfying, this soup is loaded with hearty, healthy vegetables that also taste great! If you prefer to turn down the spice level, you can replace the hot Italian sausage with sweet.

1 tablespoon extra-virgin olive oil

1 pound hot Italian sausage, casings removed

½ cup chopped onions

2 cloves garlic, minced

3 cups chopped kale (about 1 bunch)

2 cups roughly chopped zucchini (about 2 medium zucchini)

4 cups chicken broth, store-bought or homemade (page 72)

4 cups filtered water

1 teaspoon kosher salt

¼ teaspoon ground black pepper

¼ teaspoon red pepper flakes (optional)

1. Put the olive oil and sausage in a large saucepan. Cook over medium heat for about 5 minutes, stirring and breaking up the sausage into crumbles with a wooden spoon. Add the onions and garlic and cook for 3 minutes, or until the onions are translucent.

2. Add the kale, zucchini, broth, water, salt, black pepper, and red pepper flakes, if using. Stir well and simmer for about 20 minutes, until the sausage is cooked through, the kale has softened, and the zucchini is fork-tender. Serve hot. Store leftovers in an airtight container in the refrigerator for up to 5 days or in the freezer for up to 3 months.

CALORIES: 186 **FAT:** 14g **PROTEIN:** 11g **CARBS:** 6g **FIBER:** 1g **NET CARBS:** 5g

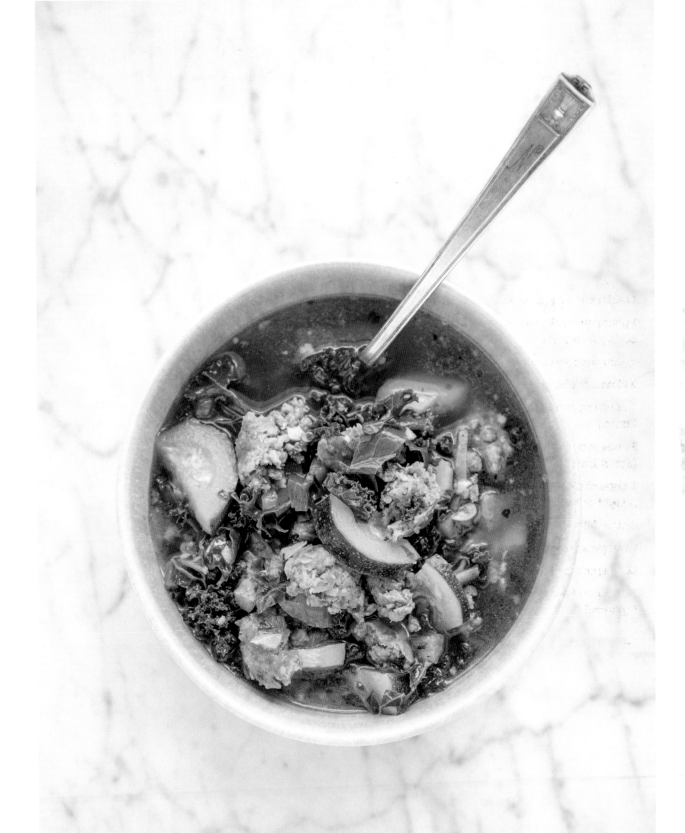

ROASTED CAULIFLOWER & LEEK SOUP

YIELD: 7½ cups | SERVING SIZE: 1¼ cups | PREP TIME: 15 minutes | COOK TIME: 40 minutes

More of a side dish or an appetizer as made, this luscious soup can be turned into a main dish with the addition of shredded cooked chicken or extra bacon. To make it vegetarian, replace the beef broth with vegetable broth and omit the bacon.

4 cups cauliflower florets (about 1 large head)

1 cup sliced leeks, washed (see Note)

1 clove garlic, peeled

2 tablespoons extra-virgin olive oil

2 teaspoons kosher salt, divided

¼ teaspoon ground black pepper

3 cups beef broth, store-bought or homemade (page 72)

3 cups filtered water

¼ teaspoon dried thyme leaves

⅛ teaspoon ground nutmeg

2 tablespoons butter

1 teaspoon white balsamic vinegar (no sugar added)

2 slices bacon, cooked and chopped

1. Preheat the oven to 400°F.

2. Place the cauliflower, cleaned leeks, garlic, olive oil, 1 teaspoon of the salt, and the pepper on a sheet pan. Stir to coat the vegetables with the oil and seasonings. Roast for 25 minutes, or until the cauliflower is slightly golden and fork-tender. Remove from the oven and transfer the roasted vegetables to a 5-quart pot.

3. To the pot, add the broth, water, thyme, and nutmeg. Cook, uncovered, over medium heat for 15 minutes, or until the cauliflower is soft enough to smash with a fork against the side of the pot.

4. Use an immersion blender to blend the soup until smooth. Add the butter, vinegar, and remaining teaspoon of salt. Stir and serve hot, garnished with the chopped cooked bacon. Store leftovers in an airtight container in the refrigerator for up to 5 days or in the freezer for up to 3 months.

Note: Because of the way leeks push through the soil when grown, dirt often gets trapped between the layers. It's important to clean them properly so that grit doesn't end up in your recipe. Simply cut off the dark green tops and then cut the white and light green stalks into ½-inch slices. Place the sliced leeks in a large bowl of water and use your fingers to break up the rings. The dirt will sink to the bottom, and the cleaned leeks will remain floating on the top to be scooped out and used. To get 1 cup of sliced leeks, you will need 2 large leeks (about 1 pound).

CALORIES: 142 FAT: 10g PROTEIN: 4g CARBS: 6g FIBER: 2g NET CARBS: 4g

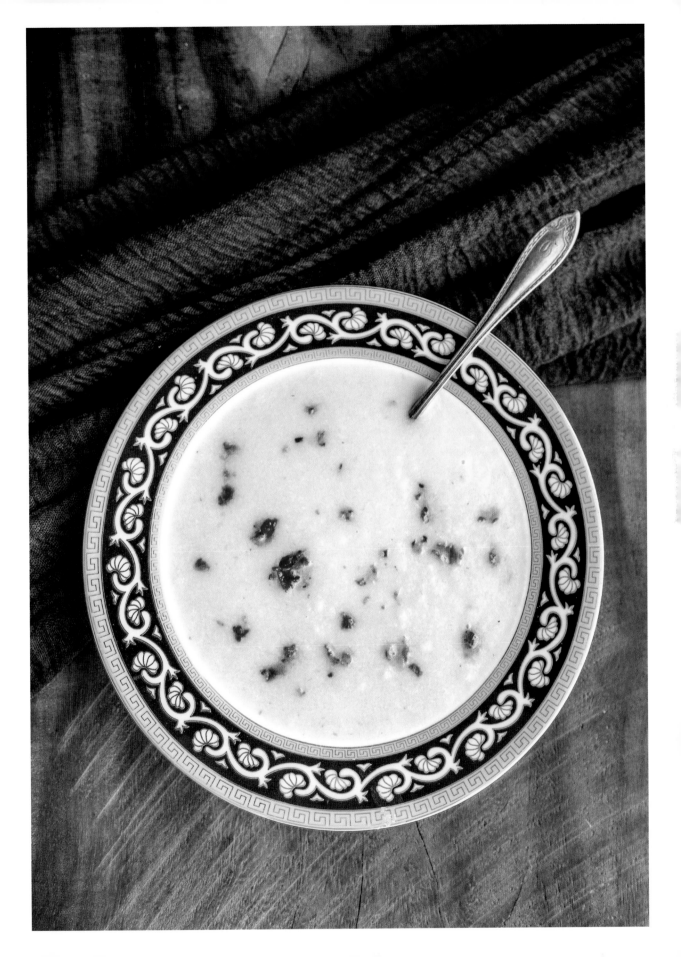

CURRIED TURNIP & CAULIFLOWER SOUP

YIELD: 7½ cups | **SERVING SIZE:** 1½ cups | **PREP TIME:** 8 minutes | **COOK TIME:** 25 minutes

Velvety and rich, this soup feels like cheating but isn't. The turnips mellow and sweeten when cooked, while the fragrant curry and other spices take over your kitchen in the best possible way. The soup is mildly spicy as is, but you can turn up the heat by adding a teaspoon of red pepper flakes while the soup simmers. If not squeaky, stir a tablespoon of sour cream or Greek yogurt into your bowl for a cool and creamy contrast.

1 tablespoon avocado oil or other light-tasting oil

3 cups peeled and chopped turnips (about 4 medium turnips)

3 cups cauliflower florets (about 1 medium head)

1 teaspoon chopped garlic

4 cups chicken broth, store-bought or homemade (page 72) (or vegetable broth for vegetarian)

1 tablespoon curry powder

1 teaspoon garam masala

1 teaspoon onion powder

1 teaspoon turmeric powder

1 teaspoon kosher salt

¼ teaspoon ground black pepper

1 cup canned coconut milk

1. Heat the oil in a large saucepan over medium heat. Add the turnips, cauliflower, and garlic and cook, stirring occasionally, for 5 minutes, or until the vegetables are slightly softened and turning golden.

2. Add the broth, curry powder, garam masala, onion powder, turmeric, salt, and pepper to the pan. Bring to a boil, then lower the heat and simmer for 20 minutes, or until the vegetables are soft enough to smash with a fork against the side of the pot.

3. Pour in the coconut milk and blend the soup with an immersion blender until smooth. Serve hot. Store leftovers in an airtight container in the refrigerator for up to 5 days or in the freezer for up to 3 months.

Note: If you don't have an immersion blender, carefully transfer the hot soup to a countertop blender and blend until smooth. Then pour it from the blender into soup bowls to serve.

CALORIES: 135 | **FAT:** 9g | **PROTEIN:** 3g | **CARBS:** 9g | **FIBER:** 3g | **NET CARBS:** 6g

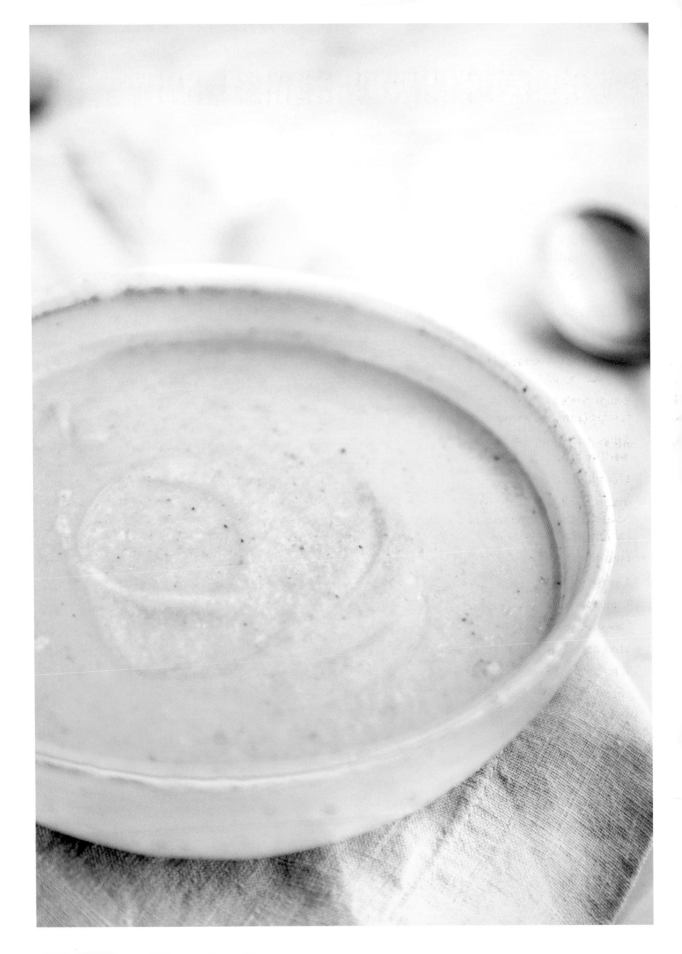

CHICKEN & VEGETABLE SOUP

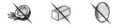

YIELD: 5 quarts (20 cups) | **SERVING SIZE:** 2 cups | **PREP TIME:** 20 minutes | **COOK TIME:** 35 minutes

While many people make this soup for the first time because it's the foundation of my popular 5-Day Keto Soup Diet (find the plan on pages 64 to 67), it quickly becomes a family favorite and goes into the regular rotation. Perfectly balanced in macros and flavor, this nutrient-packed soup will keep you satisfied for hours.

4 slices bacon, chopped

1 tablespoon extra-virgin olive oil

1 cup sliced white mushrooms

¼ cup sun-dried tomatoes, chopped

¼ cup chopped onions

1 tablespoon minced garlic

2 quarts chicken broth, store-bought or homemade (page 72)

3 cups filtered water

1 small celery root (about 14 ounces), peeled and cut into ½-inch cubes (about 2 cups)

4 cups chopped cooked chicken breast (about 4 breasts)

6 ounces green beans, cut into 1-inch pieces (about 1 cup)

4 cups chopped Swiss chard leaves and stems (about 1 large bunch)

2 cups roughly chopped yellow squash

2 tablespoons red wine vinegar

2 teaspoons kosher salt

½ teaspoon ground black pepper

¼ cup chopped fresh basil leaves

1. In a stockpot (at least 6 quarts), cook the bacon in the olive oil over medium heat for 2 minutes. Add the mushrooms, sun-dried tomatoes, onions, and garlic and cook for 5 minutes, or until the onions are translucent.

2. Pour in the broth and water, then add the celery root and cooked chicken. Bring to a boil, then lower the heat and simmer for 15 minutes, or until the celery root is fork-tender. Add the green beans, Swiss chard, and yellow squash and simmer for 10 minutes, or until the beans and squash are softened but not mushy.

3. Add the vinegar and season with the salt and pepper. Stir in the fresh basil just before serving. Store leftovers in an airtight container in the refrigerator for up to 5 days or in the freezer for up to 3 months.

CALORIES: 170 **FAT:** 5g **PROTEIN:** 23g **CARBS:** 9g **FIBER:** 4g **NET CARBS:** 5g

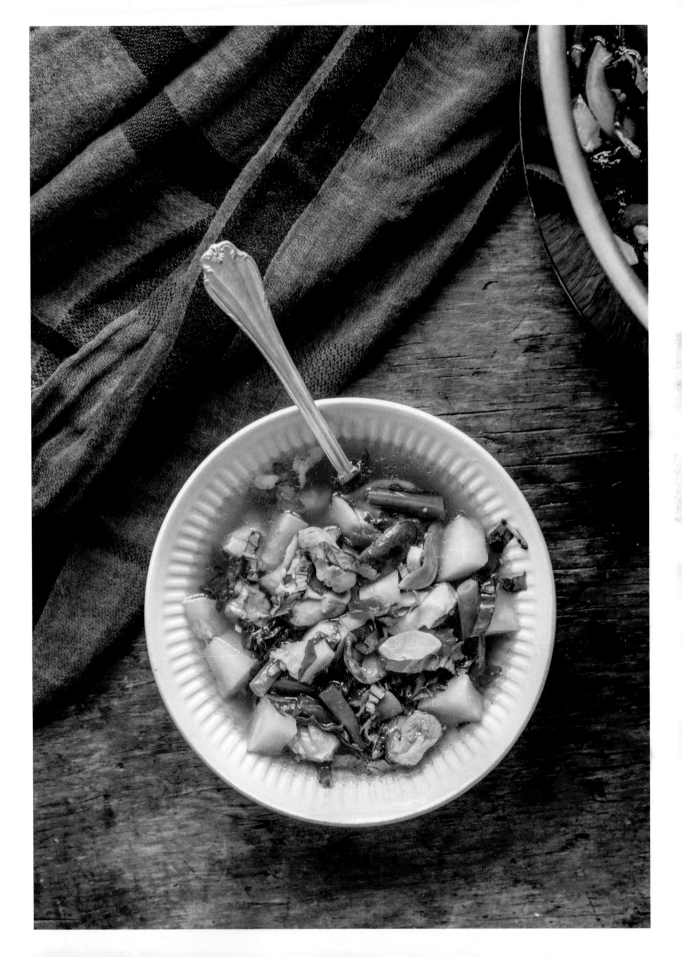

CURRIED CHICKEN SALAD

YIELD: 2½ cups	**SERVING SIZE:** ½ cup	**PREP TIME:** 10 minutes

This super easy chicken salad is redolent with curry, has a pleasing crunch from the pumpkin seeds and small amount of chopped apples, and finishes with a punch of fresh herbs. Salty, sweet, chewy, rich—this tasty chicken salad will quickly become your new go-to.

2 cups cubed cooked chicken

½ cup chopped Granny Smith apples

⅓ cup mayonnaise

3 tablespoons shelled raw pumpkin seeds (pepitas)

1 tablespoon chopped fresh cilantro

1 tablespoon chopped fresh mint

1 tablespoon curry powder

½ teaspoon kosher salt

¼ teaspoon ground black pepper

Put all the ingredients in a large bowl and stir well. Store leftovers in an airtight container in the refrigerator for up to 5 days.

Note: To make this recipe even more convenient and prevent the need for any cooking on your end, pick up a rotisserie chicken at the grocery store. One bird will provide more than enough chicken for this recipe.

CALORIES: 246 **FAT:** 19g **PROTEIN:** 19g **CARBS:** 2g **FIBER:** 0g **NET CARBS:** 2g

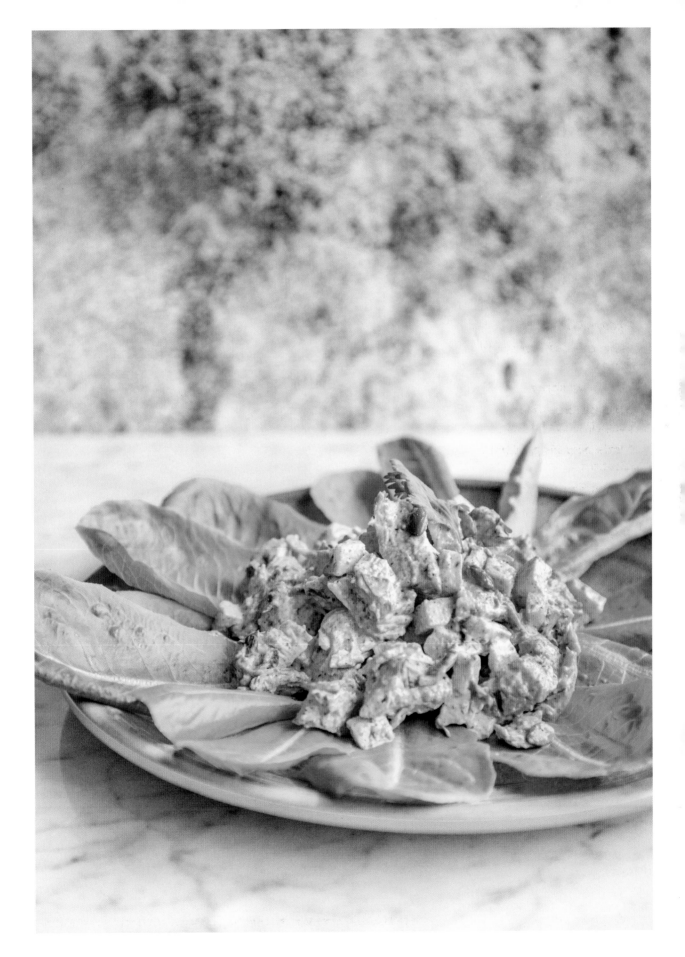

EASY TUNA SALAD

YIELD: 1 cup | **SERVING SIZE:** ½ cup | **PREP TIME:** 5 minutes

---

Not that you can't figure out how to make tuna salad on your own—but I will say that this simple version is pretty delicious. It's my son's favorite, and the secret is the dried onion flakes. They add a punch of flavor without the harsh sulfur burn of fresh onions that can turn some people off. When you eat the salad immediately, the onion flakes also provide a crunchy texture that we really enjoy. I like to dress up this tuna salad with pepperoncini, chopped pickles, and/or some of my Quick-Pickled Red Onions (page 108).

2 (5-ounce) cans tuna, drained

3 tablespoons mayonnaise

1 teaspoon dried onion flakes

¼ teaspoon kosher salt

¼ teaspoon ground black pepper

Put all the ingredients in a small bowl and stir well to combine. Taste and add more salt if desired. Store leftovers in an airtight container in the refrigerator for up to 5 days.

CALORIES: 248 **FAT:** 19g **PROTEIN:** 20g **CARBS:** 2g **FIBER:** 0g **NET CARBS:** 2g

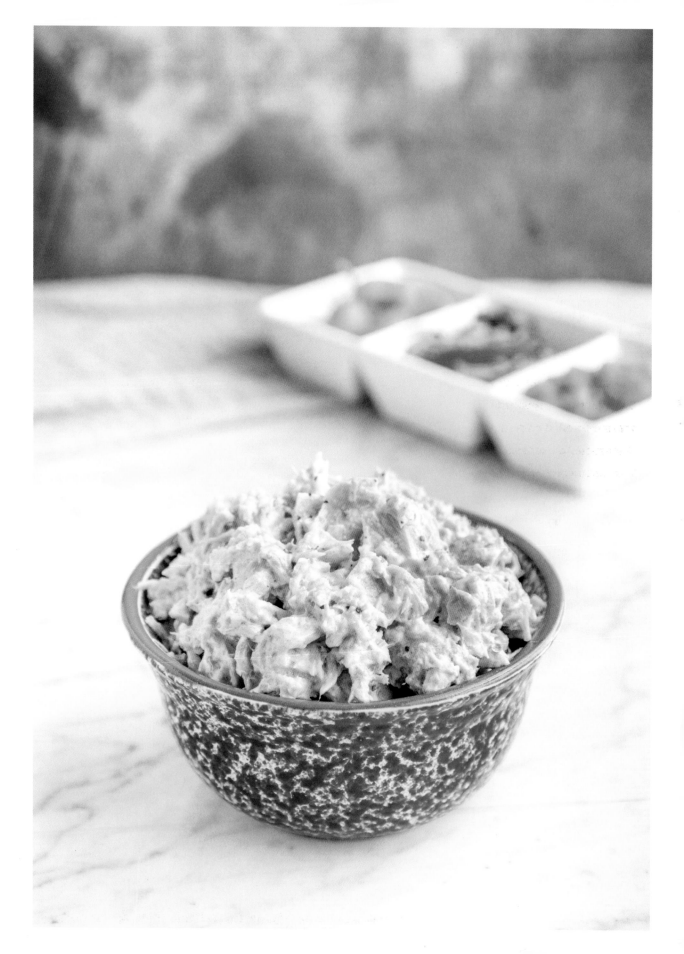

COBB SALAD WITH WARM BACON VINAIGRETTE

YIELD: 1 serving | **SERVING SIZE:** 1 salad + 2 tablespoons vinaigrette | **PREP TIME:** 10 minutes

---

This classic cobb salad is hearty and packed with protein and healthy fats. The warm bacon dressing is homey and delicious, making this already tasty salad a winner on all counts. This recipe makes enough vinaigrette for three salads and will keep in the fridge for up to a month.

For the salad:

2 cups mixed spring greens

2 hard-boiled eggs, quartered

¼ cup chopped tomatoes

½ cup chopped Hass avocado (about 1 large avocado)

¼ cup chopped cooked bacon

2 tablespoons Quick-Pickled Red Onions (page 108; optional)

For the vinaigrette:

(Makes 6 tablespoons)

¼ cup warm bacon grease

1 tablespoon white balsamic vinegar (no sugar added)

1 teaspoon Dijon mustard

¼ teaspoon kosher salt

Spread the greens on a plate and top with the egg quarters, tomatoes, avocado, bacon, and pickled onions, if using. Put the vinaigrette ingredients in a small bowl and whisk to combine. Spoon 2 tablespoons of the dressing over the salad and serve immediately. Store the remaining dressing in an airtight container in the refrigerator for up to 1 month. Reheat in the microwave for 15 seconds before serving.

SALAD: **CALORIES:** 363 **FAT:** 27g **PROTEIN:** 22g **CARBS:** 10g **FIBER:** 6g **NET CARBS:** 4g

VINAIGRETTE: **CALORIES:** 190 **FAT:** 19g **PROTEIN:** 0g **CARBS:** 2g **FIBER:** 0g **NET CARBS:** 2g

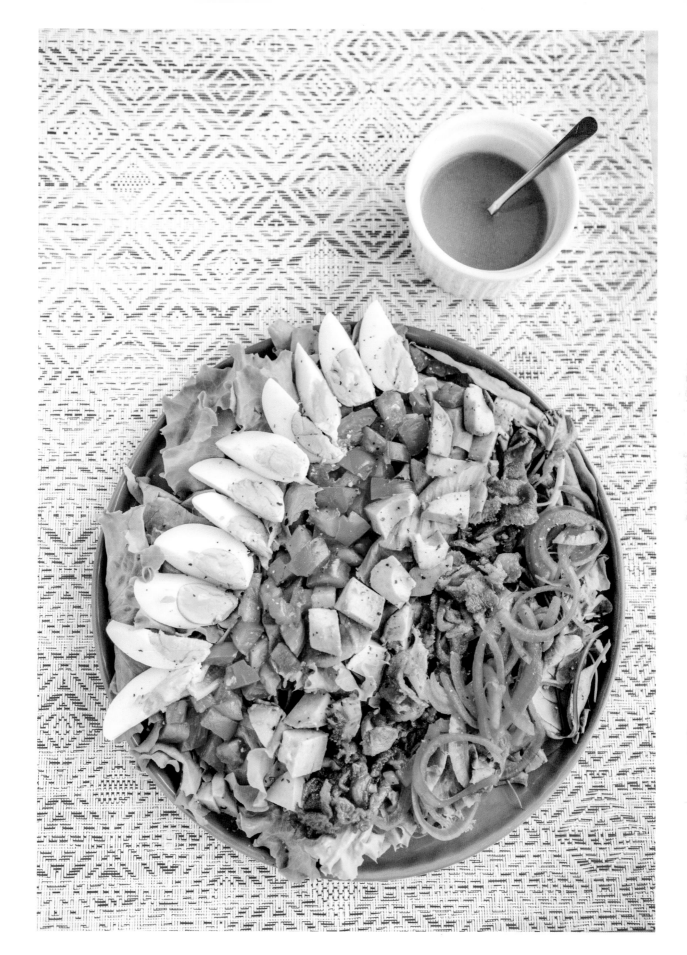

SIMPLE EGG SALAD

| YIELD: 1½ cups | SERVING SIZE: ½ cup | PREP TIME: 10 minutes | COOK TIME: 10 minutes |

This simple yet delicious egg salad is an easily packable and budget-friendly lunch option. Prep it on the weekend for no-fuss lunches all week. One of my favorite ways to enjoy this salad is wrapped in a romaine lettuce leaf with a slice of cooked bacon and some Quick-Pickled Red Onions (page 108).

6 large eggs

2 tablespoons mayonnaise

1 teaspoon Dijon mustard

1 teaspoon fresh lemon juice

½ teaspoon kosher salt

¼ teaspoon ground black pepper

1. Place the eggs in a medium-sized saucepan. Add cold water until the eggs are covered by about an inch. Bring to a boil, then lower the heat and simmer uncovered for 10 minutes. Turn off the heat and let the eggs and water cool for 30 minutes. Remove the eggs from the pan and peel them under cold running water.

2. Put the eggs in a food processor and pulse until chopped. Stir in the mayonnaise, mustard, lemon juice, salt, and pepper. Taste and adjust the seasoning as desired. Store leftovers in an airtight container in the refrigerator for up to 5 days.

CALORIES: 222 **FAT:** 19g **PROTEIN:** 13g **CARBS:** 1g **FIBER:** 0g **NET CARBS:** 1g

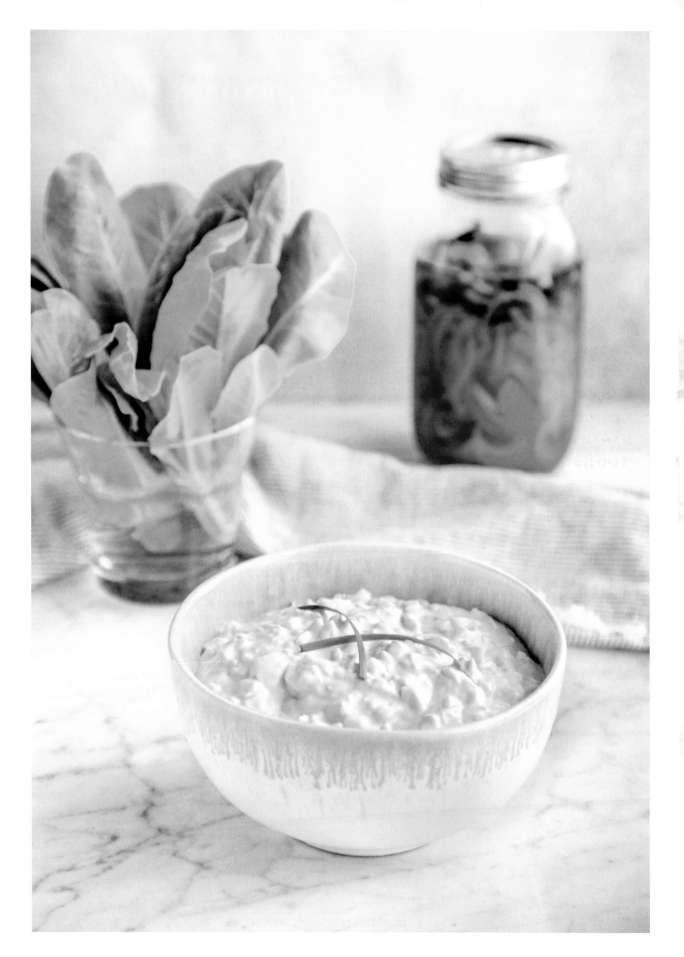

SPICY SHRIMP SALAD SUSHI BOWL

| YIELD: 4 servings | SERVING SIZE: 1 bowl + 2 tablespoons dressing | PREP TIME: 10 minutes |

This tasty bowl has all the flavors and textures of your favorite spicy sushi roll, but without the carbs, raw fish, or tedious wrapping. If you prep and refrigerate all the components in advance, then you'll be able to throw them into a bowl at a moment's notice for lunches during the week.

For the spicy shrimp salad:

1 pound large shrimp, cooked, peels and tails removed (see Note)

⅓ cup mayonnaise

2 tablespoons Sriracha sauce, plus more for serving if desired

1 teaspoon chopped fresh cilantro, plus more for garnish if desired

1 teaspoon coconut aminos

1 teaspoon fresh lime juice

For the dressing:

¼ cup plus 1 tablespoon filtered water

1 tablespoon coconut aminos

1 tablespoon rice wine vinegar (no sugar added)

1 tablespoon toasted sesame oil

For assembly:

2 cups cooked cauliflower rice

2 cups chopped cucumbers

2 ripe Hass avocados, sliced

¼ cup thinly sliced nori (dried seaweed sheets)

4 teaspoons sesame seeds (black or white)

1. *Make the spicy shrimp salad:* Chop the shrimp into bite-sized pieces, then put it in a medium-sized bowl along with the mayonnaise, Sriracha, cilantro, coconut aminos, and lime juice. Mix well until combined. Place in the refrigerator to chill for 10 minutes, or until ready to use. Store leftover shrimp salad in an airtight container in the refrigerator for up to 5 days.

2. *Make the dressing:* Put the dressing ingredients in a small bowl and whisk with a fork until well mixed. Set aside until ready to serve. Store leftover dressing in an airtight container in the refrigerator for up to 2 weeks.

3. *Assemble the bowl:* Place ½ cup of the cauliflower rice in a serving bowl. Top with ½ cup of the shrimp salad, ½ cup of the chopped cucumbers, and about one-quarter of the avocado slices (½ avocado). Sprinkle 1 tablespoon of the sliced nori over the entire bowl or, for a fancier presentation, arrange the slices in a crisscross pattern at one end. Sprinkle the bowl with 1 teaspoon of the sesame seeds and garnish with cilantro if desired. Serve with 2 tablespoons of the dressing and extra Sriracha sauce if desired.

Note: Buying shrimp raw and cooking it yourself will result in better flavor and texture than purchasing precooked frozen shrimp and thawing it. While the frozen option can work in a pinch, I recommend starting with raw if time allows. To cook raw shrimp for this recipe, peel and devein the shrimp and remove their tails. Bring a large saucepan of water to a boil and drop the shrimp into the boiling water. Cook for 2 to 3 minutes, until the shrimp are bright white and curled into C-shapes. Drain and let cool before chopping.

| CALORIES: 407 | FAT: 34g | PROTEIN: 17g | CARBS: 13g | FIBER: 7g | NET CARBS: 6g |

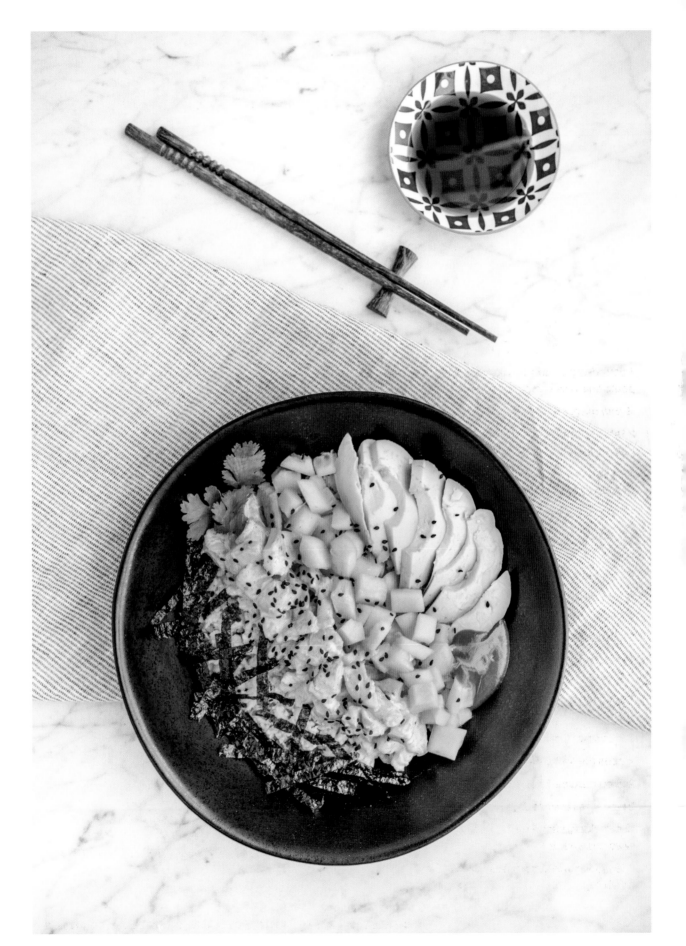

BUFFALO CHICKEN SALAD

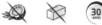

| YIELD: 2½ cups | SERVING SIZE: ½ cup | PREP TIME: 5 minutes |

This easy chicken salad delivers the flavors of everybody's favorite classic Buffalo wings—without the mess. Just a few ingredients and a couple of minutes spent in the kitchen, and you've got lunch prepared for the whole week. Look at you go!

2 cups chopped cooked chicken

½ cup thinly sliced celery (about 1 stalk)

⅓ cup mayonnaise

2 tablespoons Louisiana-style hot sauce

Combine all the ingredients in a large bowl. Serve warm or cold. Store leftovers in an airtight container in the refrigerator for up to 5 days.

Note: If not squeaky, you can add ¼ cup of crumbled blue cheese.

CALORIES: 173 **FAT:** 14g **PROTEIN:** 13g **CARBS:** 0g **FIBER:** 0g **NET CARBS:** 0g

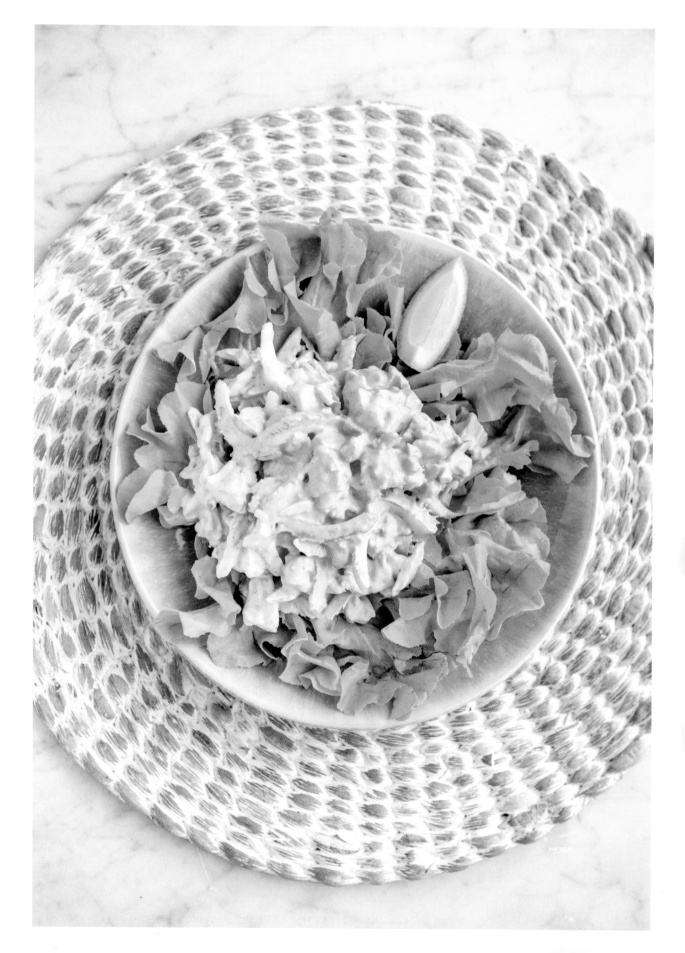

CHEF'S SALAD

YIELD: 1 serving | PREP TIME: 8 minutes

A salad on its own isn't always enough food to keep you going from lunch until dinner. This hearty chef's salad is loaded with satiating protein that will definitely get you through the afternoon—especially if you throw in a 3 p.m. bulletproof coffee (page 324), and I never say no to coffee.

2 cups torn romaine lettuce leaves (about 4 ounces)

3 ounces deli ham

3 ounces deli turkey

2 hard-boiled eggs, chopped

1 cup chopped cucumbers (about 1 small cucumber)

5 cherry tomatoes, cut in half

Spread the lettuce over a large plate or put it in a serving bowl. Top with the ham, turkey, eggs, cucumbers, and tomatoes.

Note: My Garlicky Lemon & Tarragon Dressing on page 91 is a great choice for this salad, but you can use any squeaky dressing you like; just remember to factor in the per-serving nutrition information for the dressing.

CALORIES: 348 FAT: 14g PROTEIN: 42g CARBS: 10g FIBER: 4g NET CARBS: 6g

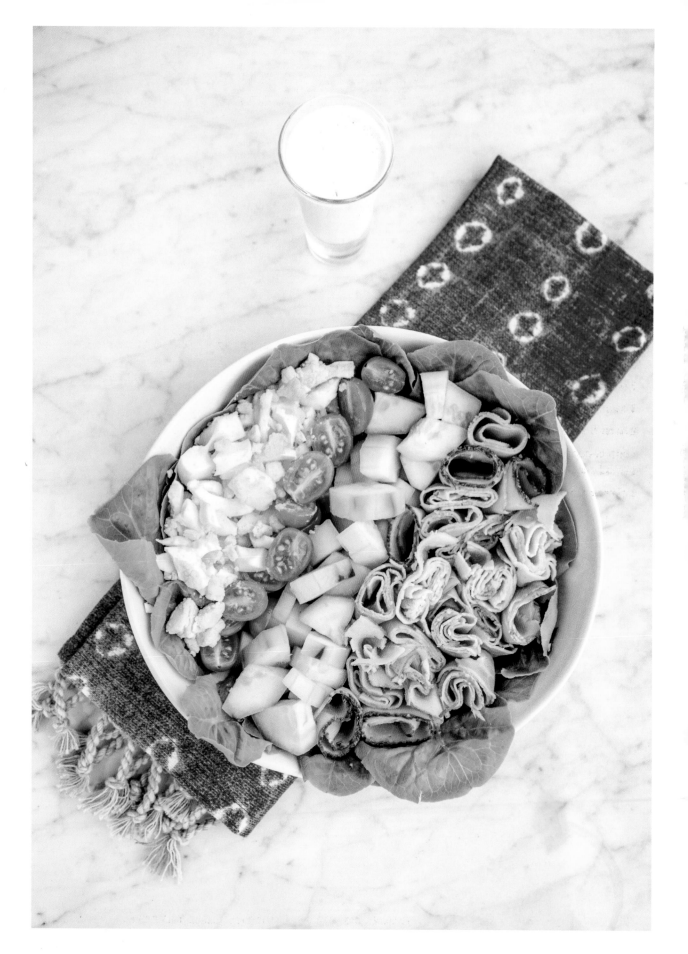

HEARTS OF PALM SALAD

YIELD: 1 serving | **PREP TIME:** 8 minutes

Common here in Central America, hearts of palm salad (always accompanied by avocado and tomato) is a fantastic option when you're looking for an easy and healthy plant-based lunch. Hearts of palm are high in vitamin C and have a semisoft starchy texture that makes them hearty and satisfying in a salad or as a snack—all with only 3 grams of net carbs per half cup.

2 cups spring greens

½ Hass avocado, chopped

½ cup sliced canned hearts of palm (about ½ [14-ounce] can)

½ plum tomato, quartered

1 tablespoon extra-virgin olive oil

1 teaspoon fresh lemon juice

¼ teaspoon kosher salt

¼ teaspoon ground black pepper

Spread the greens on a large plate. Top with the avocado, hearts of palm, and tomato. Drizzle with the olive oil and lemon juice, then sprinkle with the salt and pepper. Serve immediately.

CALORIES: 282 **FAT:** 25g **PROTEIN:** 6g **CARBS:** 14g **FIBER:** 8g **NET CARBS:** 6g

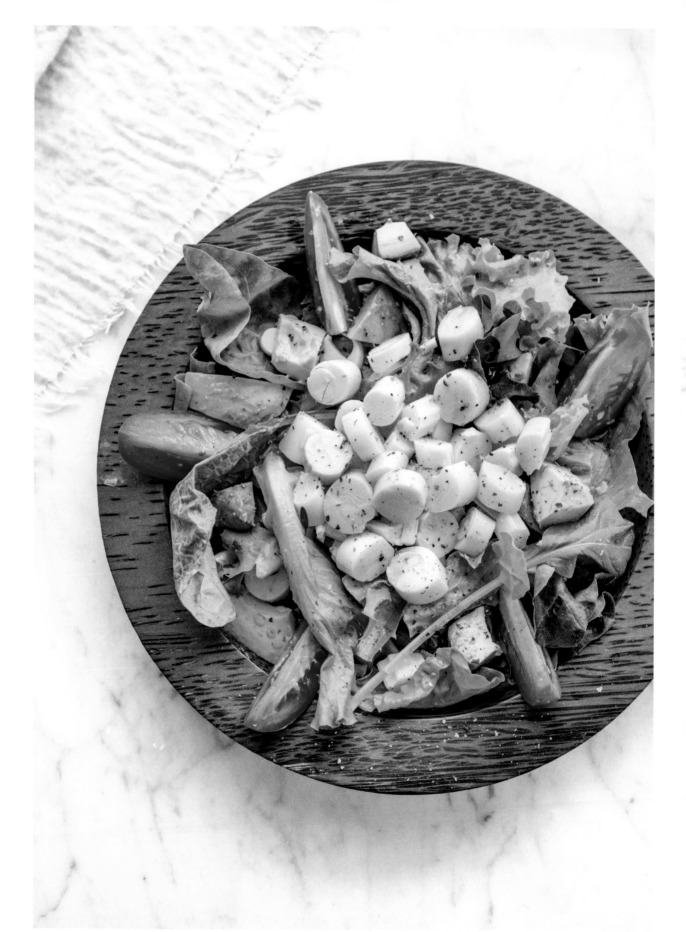

MUFFULETTA WRAP

YIELD: 1 serving | **PREP TIME:** 5 minutes

The muffuletta is a famous sandwich from New Orleans that traditionally contains cold cuts, cheese, and the ubiquitous briny olive salad that gives the muffuletta its distinctive flavor. This squeaky version doesn't contain cheese, and it's made on a homemade spinach wrap instead of bread, but it's a solid contender and one of my favorite recipes in this book.

1 Spinach Wrap (page 112)

1 ounce sliced Genoa salami

1 ounce sliced prosciutto or other ham

1 ounce sliced mortadella or bologna

1 tablespoon mayonnaise

¼ cup Olive Salad (page 110)

1. Lay a 12-inch square sheet of parchment paper or aluminum foil on the counter. Place the spinach wrap in the center of the parchment. Spread the salami in a line of overlapping slices across the bottom one-third of the wrap on the side closest to you. Top with a row of prosciutto and then a row of mortadella. Smear the mayonnaise in a line across the top of the meat slices. Spoon the olive salad in a line across the top of the mayonnaise.

2. Carefully fold the left and right sides over the toppings by about 2 inches (they won't meet in the center) and then, using your thumbs and index fingers, roll up the end closest to you over the middle to enclose the two side folds. Continue rolling until a tube is formed. Fold the parchment paper over the sides of the roll and then roll up from the side closest to you until the wrap is totally enclosed in parchment. Cut in half and fold the parchment down to eat the wrap.

CALORIES: 544 **FAT:** 45g **PROTEIN:** 26g **CARBS:** 4g **FIBER:** 2g **NET CARBS:** 2g

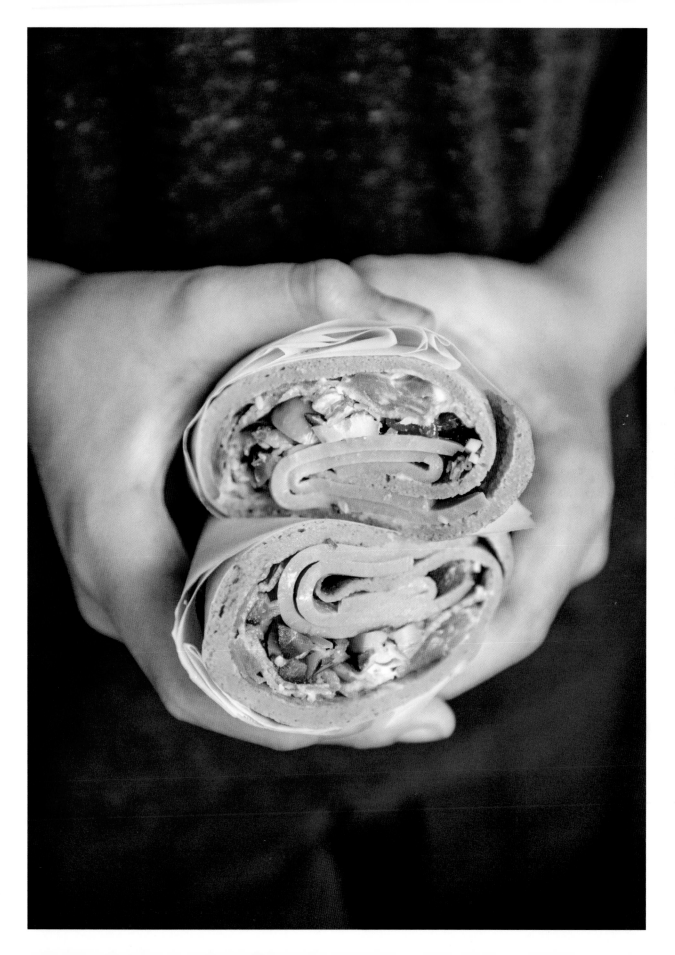

CHICKEN CLUB WRAP

YIELD: 1 serving | **PREP TIME:** 8 minutes

I love a good club sandwich, but unfortunately, the bread and cheese are a no-no on Squeaky Clean Keto. The good news is that the best parts of the sandwich (chicken, bacon, tomatoes, and mayonnaise, oh my) can be wrapped in crunchy lettuce leaves and enjoyed (almost) as much as the real thing.

2 large iceberg or green leaf lettuce leaves

2 ounces cooked chicken breast, sliced

4 thin wedges plum tomato

2 slices bacon, cooked

2 tablespoons mayonnaise

Kosher salt and ground black pepper

1. Lay a 12-inch square sheet of parchment paper on the counter. Place the lettuce leaves, overlapping by about one-third, on the parchment. Spread the chicken in a line about 8 inches long near the end closest to you. Place the tomato wedges along the line of chicken. Top with the bacon slices. Spread the mayonnaise on the lettuce along the edge of the bacon. Sprinkle the entire surface with salt and pepper.

2. Starting from the edge closest to you, carefully roll the lettuce and filling into a tight roll and slide toward you on the parchment paper. Roll the parchment tightly around the lettuce wrap, folding in the two sides to contain the edges. Cut the roll through the middle and fold down the edges of the parchment as you eat the roll.

Note: This wrap is reminiscent of a classic club, and it's super tasty as is. But if you like to get creative and change things up once in a while, try some add-ins. Here are my favorites: chopped fresh basil or dill, avocado wedges, Quick-Pickled Red Onions (page 108), Dijon mustard, dill pickles, or dill pickle relish.

CALORIES: 354 **FAT:** 29g **PROTEIN:** 19g **CARBS:** 5g **FIBER:** 2g **NET CARBS:** 3g

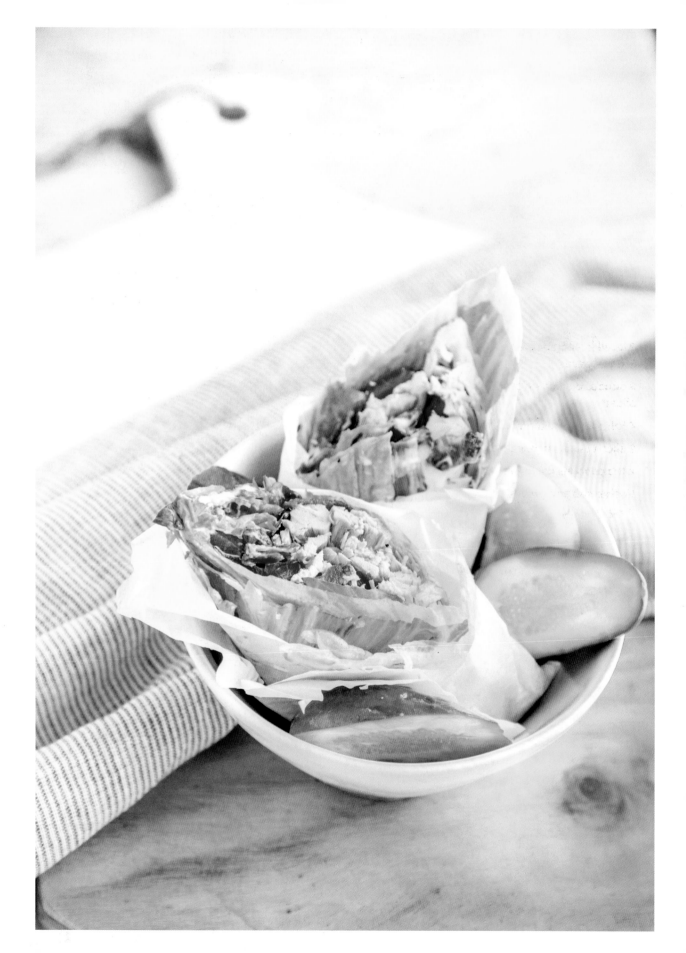

PASTRAMI ROLL-UPS

YIELD: 4 rolls (8 pieces) | **SERVING SIZE:** 1 roll (2 pieces) | **PREP TIME:** 8 minutes

These easy and convenient roll-ups contain all the enticing flavors of a pastrami-on-rye sandwich, without the carbs! The pickles in the middle give them a fun crunch, and if you use the caraway seeds, you'll get a hint of rye bread flavor that makes it even more authentic.

¼ cup mayonnaise

1 tablespoon spicy brown mustard

½ teaspoon caraway seeds (optional)

8 slices pastrami

4 large lettuce leaves

4 kosher dill pickles

Put the mayonnaise, mustard, and caraway seeds, if using, in a small bowl and mix well. Place 2 pastrami slices, slightly overlapping, on a cutting board. Top with a lettuce leaf and a pickle. Spread 1 tablespoon of the mayonnaise mixture over the pickle. Roll up and slice in half. Repeat 3 times for a total of 4 rolls (8 pieces). Store leftovers in an airtight container in the refrigerator for up to 3 days.

CALORIES: 179 **FAT:** 13g **PROTEIN:** 12g **CARBS:** 1g **FIBER:** 0g **NET CARBS:** 1g

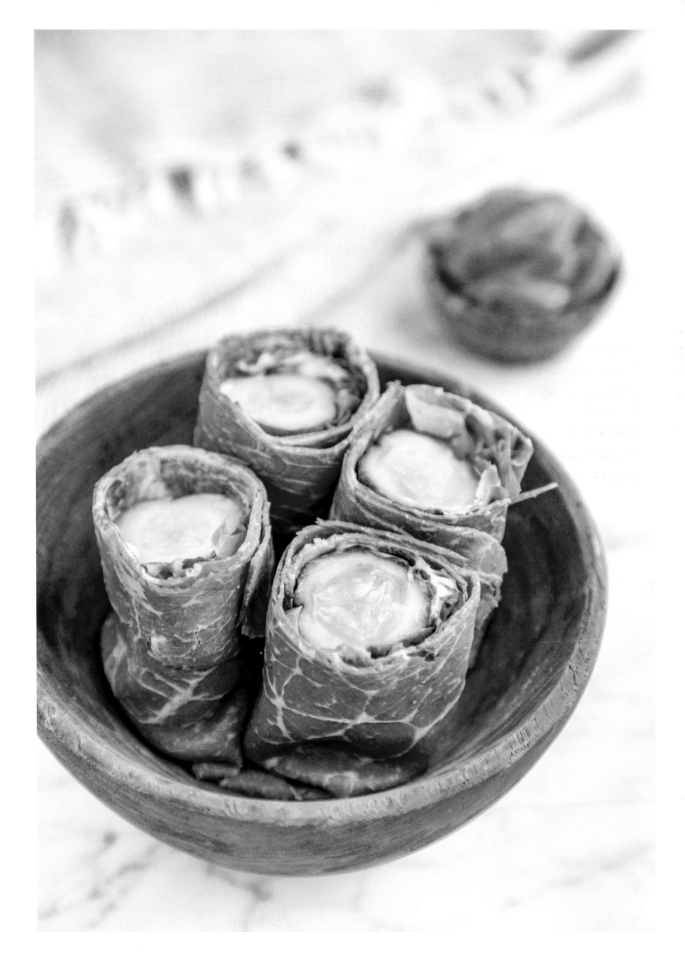

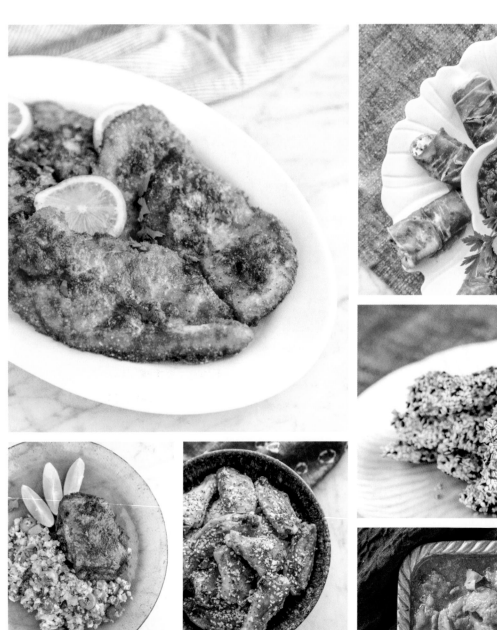

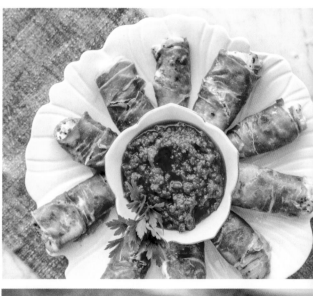

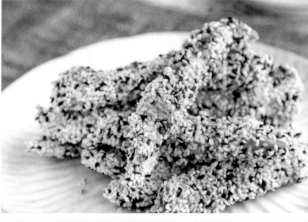

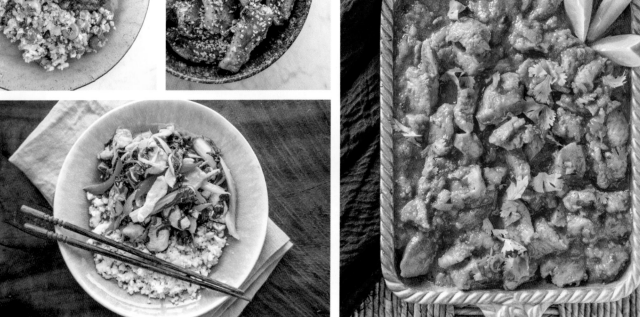

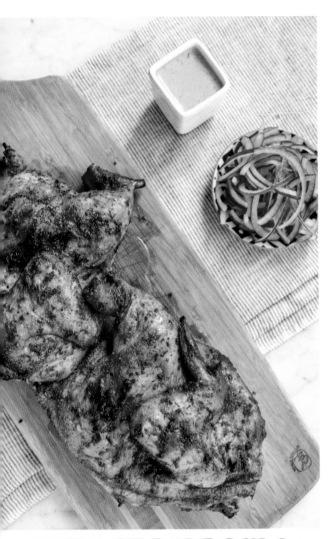

Chicken

Tuscan Chicken with Zoodles / 170

Prosciutto-Wrapped Chicken Tenders / 172

Chicken Chop Suey / 174

Chicken Korma / 176

Everything Chicken Wings / 178

Sesame Chicken Fingers / 180

Simply Roasted Chicken Breasts / 182

Arroz con Pollo / 184

Butter Chicken / 186

Peruvian Chicken / 188

Chicken Jalfrezi / 190

Crispy Lemon Chicken / 192

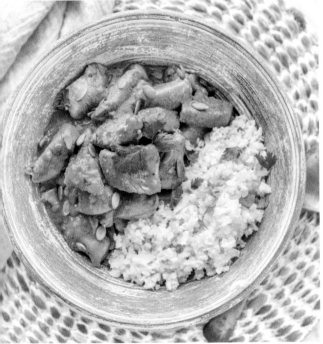

TUSCAN CHICKEN WITH ZOODLES

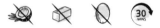

| YIELD: 4 servings | SERVING SIZE: 2 cups | PREP TIME: 10 minutes | COOK TIME: 8 minutes |

You can have this super easy one-pan meal on the table in 20 minutes or less—perfect for busy weeknights! It's a little spicy, a lot garlicky, and ultra-satisfying after a long day. If your family isn't keto, you can serve this chicken with regular pasta for them; if you aren't squeaky or dairy-free, then I recommend adding a liberal sprinkling of freshly grated Parmesan cheese over the top just before serving.

3 tablespoons extra-virgin olive oil

1 pound boneless, skinless chicken breasts, cut into bite-sized pieces

2 tablespoons chopped sun-dried tomatoes

2 teaspoons minced garlic

1 teaspoon kosher salt

½ teaspoon red pepper flakes

¼ teaspoon dried oregano leaves

¼ teaspoon ground black pepper

6 cups zucchini noodles (about 4 medium zucchini)

¼ cup fresh basil leaves, roughly chopped

1. Heat the oil in a large skillet over medium heat. Add the chicken, sun-dried tomatoes, garlic, salt, red pepper flakes, oregano, and black pepper and stir well. Cook for about 5 minutes, until the chicken pieces are cooked through and turning golden brown.

2. Add the zucchini noodles and stir well. Cook for 2 minutes, or until the zucchini is slightly softened but not mushy. Remove from the heat and stir in the basil. Serve hot. Store leftovers in an airtight container in the refrigerator for up to 5 days.

CALORIES: 260 | FAT: 12g | PROTEIN: 29g | CARBS: 8g | FIBER: 3g | NET CARBS: 5g

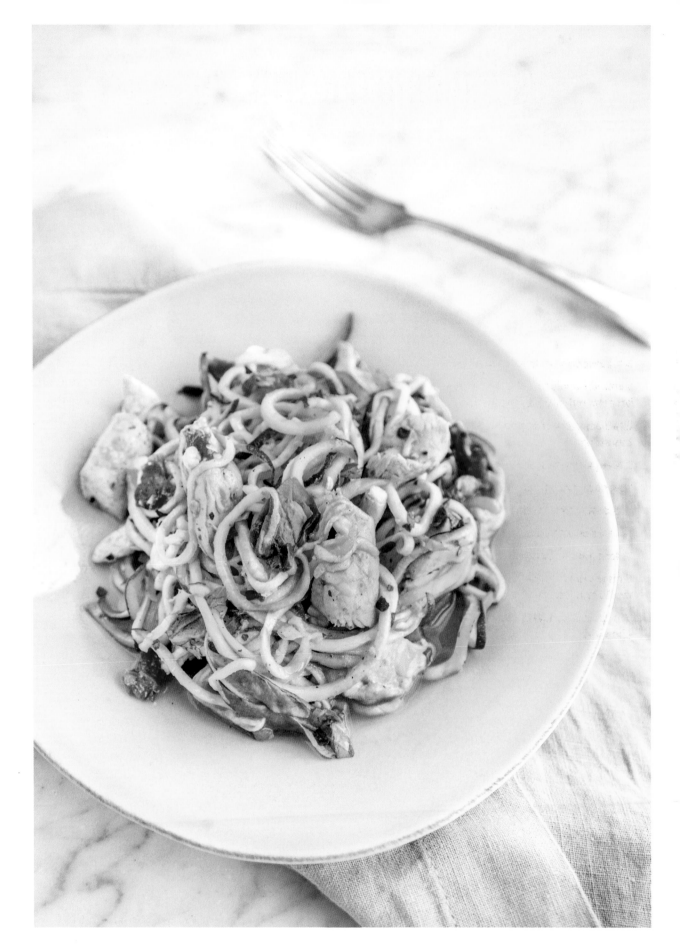

PROSCIUTTO-WRAPPED CHICKEN TENDERS

YIELD: 6 servings | **SERVING SIZE:** 2 tenders | **PREP TIME:** 8 minutes | **COOK TIME:** 20 minutes

Salty prosciutto wrapped around tender chunks of herbed chicken makes for a fun and tasty finger food that even picky kids will enjoy! Whether you're serving these as an appetizer or a main course, you'll want to make extra for your weekly meal prep since they can easily be eaten cold on the go or used to bulk up salads with some healthy protein. Shown here with Sun-Dried Tomato Sauce (page 102), they also pair well with Roasted Red Pepper Sauce (page 94) or Creamy Garlic Sauce (page 106).

1 tablespoon extra-virgin olive oil

1 teaspoon dried oregano leaves

1 teaspoon kosher salt

½ teaspoon garlic powder

½ teaspoon red pepper flakes

¼ teaspoon ground black pepper

12 chicken tenders (about 1½ pounds) (see Note)

12 slices prosciutto

1. Preheat the oven to 375°F. Line a sheet pan with parchment paper.

2. Put the olive oil, oregano, salt, garlic powder, red pepper flakes, and black pepper in a large bowl and stir well. Add the chicken, stirring until all the pieces are coated.

3. Wrap each tender in a slice of prosciutto and place on the prepared sheet pan. Bake for 20 minutes, or until a meat thermometer inserted in the center of a tender reads 165°F. Remove and serve warm. Store leftovers in an airtight container in the refrigerator for up to 5 days.

Note: If your grocer doesn't carry chicken tenders, you can cut boneless, skinless chicken breasts into pieces 4 inches long by 1 inch thick.

CALORIES: 270 **FAT:** 10g **PROTEIN:** 31g **CARBS:** 0g **FIBER:** 0g **NET CARBS:** 0g

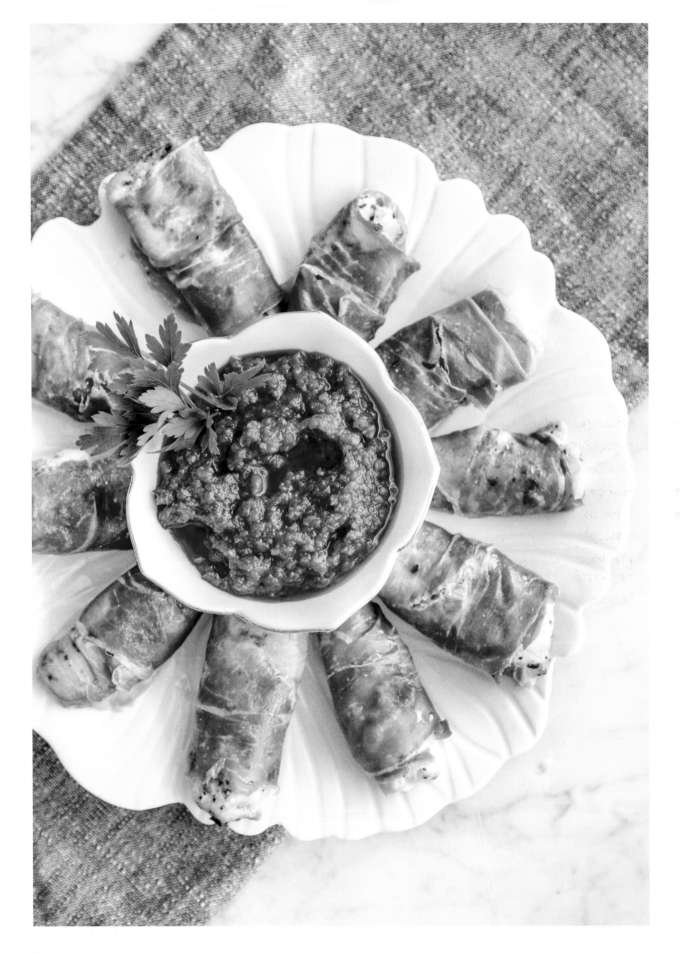

CHICKEN CHOP SUEY

| YIELD: 4 servings | SERVING SIZE: 1½ cups | PREP TIME: 10 minutes | COOK TIME: 15 minutes |

The perfect balance of salty and slightly sweet, this Chinese restaurant classic boasts tender slices of chicken and lots of healthy veggies, all swimming in a delicious velvety sauce. It is shown served with cauliflower rice and of course chopsticks for a more authentic experience!

2 tablespoons avocado oil or other light-tasting oil

1 teaspoon toasted sesame oil

2 teaspoons minced garlic

1 pound boneless, skinless chicken breasts, thinly sliced

3 cups roughly chopped bok choy, leaves and stems separated (about 2 heads)

1 cup thinly sliced celery (about 2 stalks)

1 red bell pepper, cut into strips

½ cup canned bean sprouts, drained (about ½ [14-ounce] can)

½ cup sliced scallions

½ cup filtered water

1 tablespoon coconut aminos

1 tablespoon fish sauce (no sugar added)

½ teaspoon xanthan gum

1. Heat the avocado oil and sesame oil in a large skillet over medium-high heat until shimmering. Add the garlic and fry for about 1 minute, until fragrant. Add the chicken and sauté for 2 to 3 minutes, until golden. Next, add the bok choy stems, celery, and bell pepper. Sauté for 5 minutes, or until the bok choy stems are turning translucent. Finally, add the bean sprouts, scallions, and bok choy leaves and stir.

2. In a small bowl, whisk together the water, coconut aminos, fish sauce, and xanthan gum. Pour the mixture into the pan with the chicken and vegetables. Simmer for about 5 minutes, until the sauce is reduced and slightly thickened. Store leftovers in an airtight container in the refrigerator for up to 5 days or in the freezer for up to 3 months.

CALORIES: 228 FAT: 11g PROTEIN: 24g CARBS: 6g FIBER: 2g NET CARBS: 4g

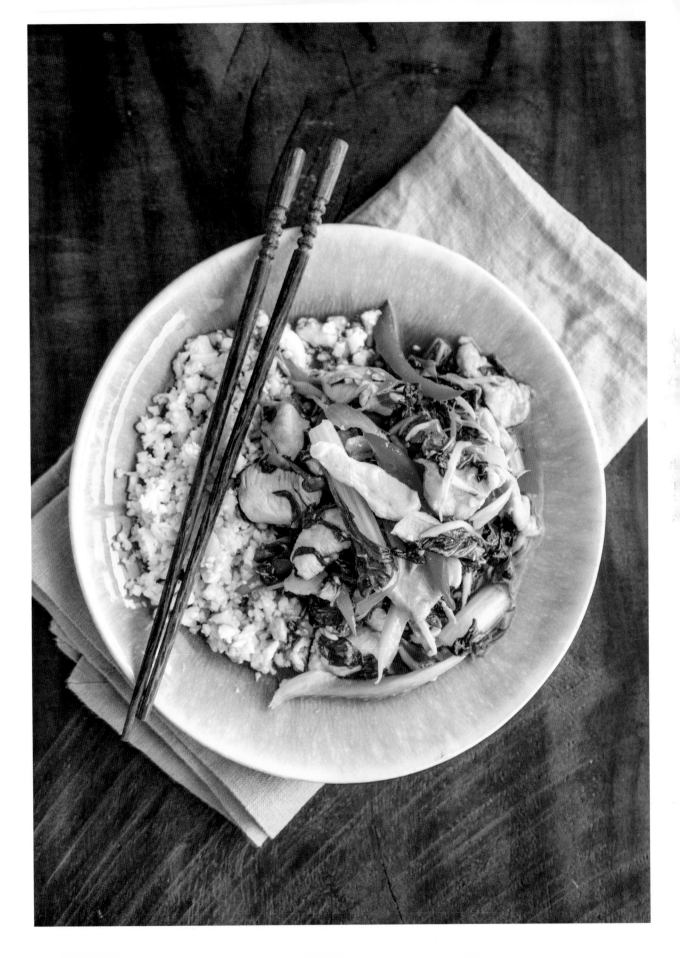

CHICKEN KORMA

| **YIELD:** 6 servings | **SERVING SIZE:** ¾ cup | **PREP TIME:** 15 minutes | **COOK TIME:** 17 minutes |

An Indian takeout classic, korma is one of my favorite curries. Mildly spicy and very decadent, korma is typically thickened with yogurt or cream. Since dairy is a no-no while eating Squeaky Clean Keto, I've thickened this version with coconut milk, and it is just as creamy as the real thing. You can substitute lamb or goat for the chicken for an even richer, meatier flavor. I often serve it with cauliflower rice to soak up all that delicious sauce.

2 tablespoons coconut oil

1 cup chopped onions

4 cloves garlic, peeled

2 tablespoons chopped fresh ginger

1 tablespoon ground coriander

1 tablespoon ground cumin

2 teaspoons garam masala

1½ teaspoons kosher salt

1 teaspoon turmeric powder

½ teaspoon cayenne pepper

½ teaspoon ground cardamom

¼ teaspoon ground black pepper

1½ pounds boneless, skinless chicken breasts, cut into bite-sized pieces

½ cup chopped tomatoes

¼ cup (½ stick) butter

1 cup canned coconut milk

1 cup chicken broth, store-bought or homemade (page 72)

¼ cup roughly chopped fresh cilantro leaves, for garnish

¼ cup shelled raw pumpkin seeds (pepitas), for garnish

1. Put the coconut oil, onions, garlic, ginger, coriander, cumin, garam masala, salt, turmeric, cayenne, cardamom, and black pepper in a small blender or food processor and blend until mostly smooth.

2. Heat a large skillet over medium heat. Put the spice paste in the pan and cook, stirring often, for about 2 minutes, until fragrant. Add the chicken, tomatoes, and butter and cook, stirring occasionally, for about 5 minutes, until the chicken is golden brown. Pour in the coconut milk and broth and stir well, scraping any bits from the bottom of the pan into the sauce.

3. Simmer over low heat for 10 minutes, or until the sauce has reduced by half. Garnish with the cilantro and pumpkin seeds. Store leftovers in an airtight container in the refrigerator for up to 5 days or in the freezer for up to 3 months.

CALORIES: 319 **FAT:** 24g **PROTEIN:** 17g **CARBS:** 6g **FIBER:** 1g **NET CARBS:** 5g

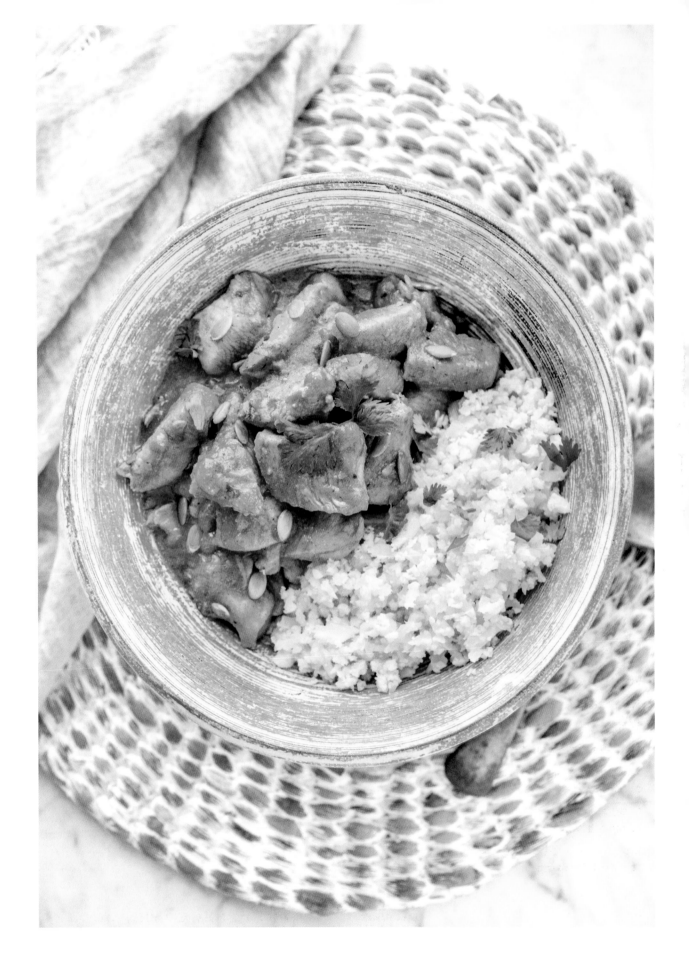

EVERYTHING CHICKEN WINGS

YIELD: 6 servings | **SERVING SIZE:** about 6 wings | **PREP TIME:** 5 minutes | **COOK TIME:** 45 minutes

These are the easiest chicken wings I've ever made—and thanks to the everything bagel seasoning, also the tastiest! As a side note, if you're not basting your baked chicken wings with melted butter after cooking them, what are you even doing with your life? Adding another layer of rich flavor, the butter also acts as a glue to hold the seasoning on. Once you try them, you'll never want to eat wings any other way. If you're a dipper like me, these wings go nicely with my All-Purpose Green Sauce (page 98).

3 pounds chicken wings, trimmed and separated into wingettes and drumettes (see page 38)

3 tablespoons butter, melted

3 tablespoons Everything Bagel Seasoning (page 80)

1. Preheat the oven to 400°F.

2. Spread out the chicken wing pieces on a sheet pan. Bake for 45 minutes, or until the wings are golden and crispy. Remove from the oven and transfer the wings to a serving bowl.

3. Pour the melted butter over the wings, then stir or toss to coat the wings in the butter. Sprinkle the seasoning over the wings and shake to coat them evenly in the seasoning. Serve immediately. Store leftovers in an airtight container in the refrigerator for up to 5 days. To reheat, heat 2 tablespoons of avocado oil in a large skillet over medium heat. Add the wings and cook for about 2 minutes per side, until crisp and heated through.

CALORIES: 481 | **FAT:** 37g | **PROTEIN:** 32g | **CARBS:** 1g | **FIBER:** 0g | **NET CARBS:** 1g

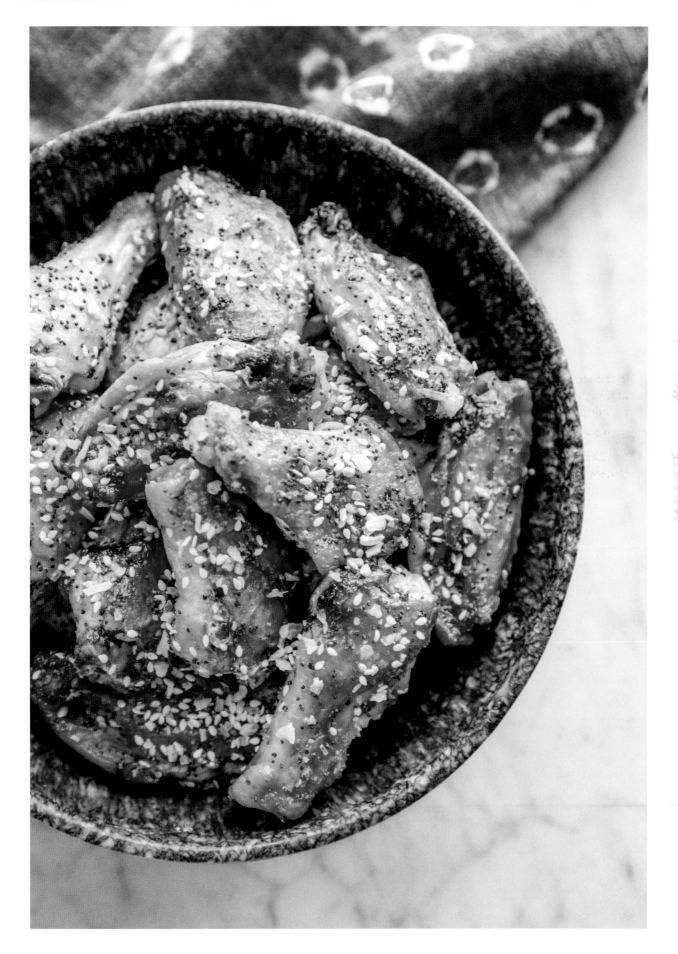

SESAME CHICKEN FINGERS

YIELD: 4 servings | **SERVING SIZE:** 4 ounces | **PREP TIME:** 10 minutes | **COOK TIME:** 20 minutes

I don't know about you, but I've never outgrown my childhood love of chicken fingers! Now that I'm adulting, I make them a little fancier—but I still love the act of dipping and eating them with my hands. Baked, not fried, these Asian-inspired gems go perfectly with the Sesame Ginger Dressing on page 90.

1 large egg

1 teaspoon fish sauce (no sugar added)

1 teaspoon toasted sesame oil

1 teaspoon kosher salt

½ teaspoon Chinese five-spice powder

1 pound boneless, skinless chicken breasts, cut lengthwise into long strips

⅓ cup white sesame seeds

2 tablespoons black sesame seeds (optional)

1. Preheat the oven to 375°F. Line a sheet pan with parchment paper.

2. Put the egg, fish sauce, sesame oil, salt, and five-spice powder in a medium-sized bowl. Stir well. Add the chicken strips to the egg mixture and stir to coat.

3. Put the sesame seeds in a flat dish; if using both white and black sesame seeds, stir them together until evenly mixed. One by one, dip the egg-washed chicken strips into the sesame seeds and roll to coat. Place the coated chicken on the prepared sheet pan.

4. Bake for 20 minutes, or until the sesame seeds are turning golden and the chicken is cooked through. Remove from the oven and serve. Store leftovers in an airtight container in the refrigerator for up to 5 days or in the freezer for up to 3 months. Leftovers can be eaten cold or reheated in the microwave for 1 minute.

CALORIES: 199 | **FAT:** 10g | **PROTEIN:** 24g | **CARBS:** 3g | **FIBER:** 2g | **NET CARBS:** 1g

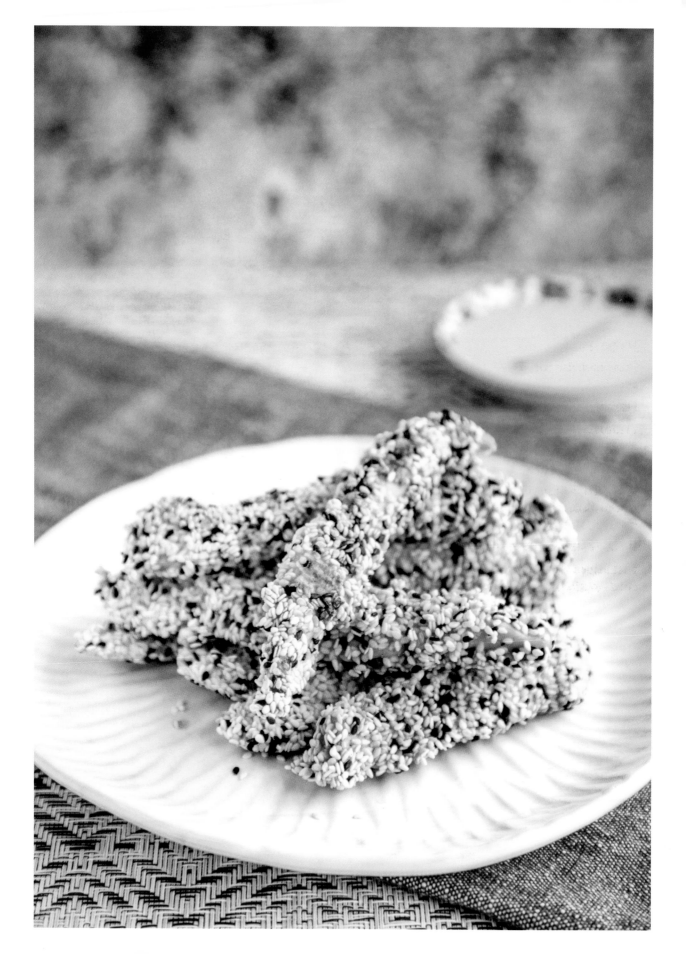

SIMPLY ROASTED CHICKEN BREASTS

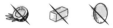

| YIELD: 2 servings | SERVING SIZE: 1 chicken breast | PREP TIME: 5 minutes | COOK TIME: 40 minutes |

While chicken is a blank canvas for so many flavors and cooking methods, you can't go wrong with the timeless classic of simply roasting it with the skin on. Roasting chicken on the bone results in juicier and more flavorful meat, which is perfectly complemented by the bright and herby Charmoula Sauce (page 87) shown here. The basic but tasty spice mix on this chicken produces a crispy and delicious skin that will be the highlight of the meal—but if you really want to, you can use boneless, skinless breasts and reduce the cooking time to 20 minutes.

1 teaspoon kosher salt

½ teaspoon garlic powder

½ teaspoon smoked paprika

½ teaspoon turmeric powder

¼ teaspoon ground black pepper

1 tablespoon extra-virgin olive oil

2 (8-ounce) bone-in, skin-on chicken breasts

1. Preheat the oven to 400°F.

2. Put the salt and spices in a small bowl and stir to combine. Rub the chicken breasts with the olive oil, then rub the spice mixture all over the chicken. Place the chicken in a baking dish.

3. Roast for 40 minutes, or until a thermometer inserted in the thickest part of a breast reads 165°F. Remove from the oven and let rest for 10 minutes before serving. Store leftovers in an airtight container in the refrigerator for up to 5 days.

CALORIES: 320 FAT: 21g PROTEIN: 31g CARBS: 0g FIBER: 0g NET CARBS: 0g

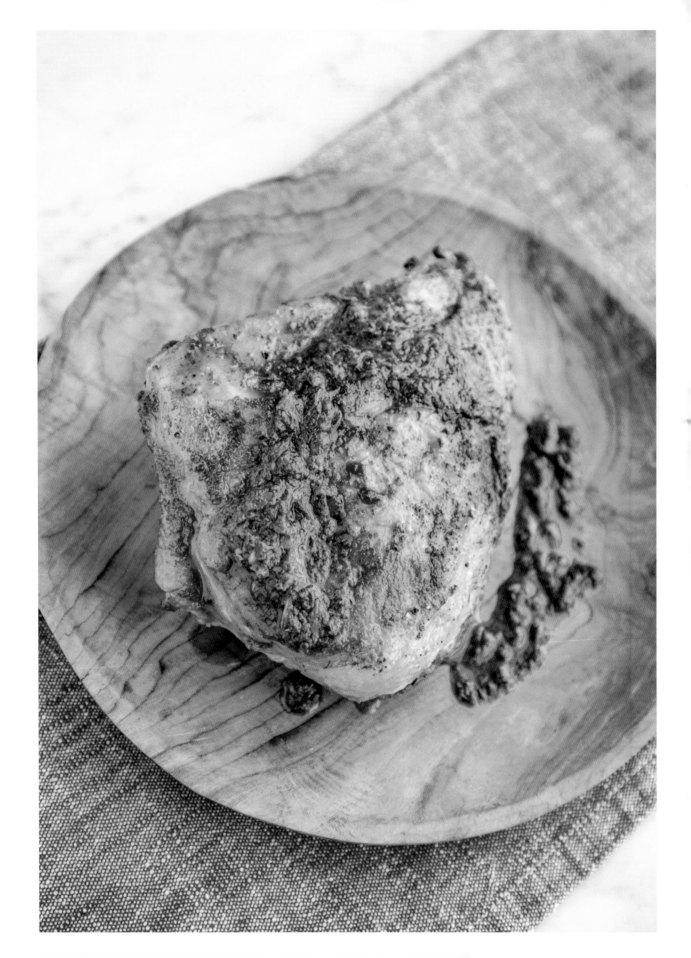

ARROZ CON POLLO

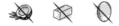

| YIELD: 6 servings | SERVING SIZE: 1 chicken thigh + ¾ cup cauliflower rice | PREP TIME: 10 minutes | COOK TIME: 30 minutes |

Arroz con pollo, meaning simply "rice with chicken," is a staple where we live in Central America. While the flavor profile can vary by region, it almost always includes liberally spiced baked chicken with a side of rice that is flavored with lots of garlic, onion, bell pepper, and tomatoes—often referred to as "sofrito." I took the liberty of adding capers and pimento-stuffed olives to my version, giving it a Spanish flair and a slightly briny flavor that masks any lingering cauliflower skunkiness. You'll want to put this homey and comforting dish in your regular rotation!

For the seasoning blend:

1 tablespoon ground cumin

2 teaspoons kosher salt

2 teaspoons smoked paprika

1 teaspoon dried oregano leaves

1 teaspoon garlic powder

1 teaspoon ground coriander

1 teaspoon onion powder

½ teaspoon dried thyme leaves

½ teaspoon ground black pepper

½ teaspoon turmeric powder

6 bone-in, skin-on chicken thighs

3 tablespoons extra-virgin olive oil

⅓ cup chopped onions

¼ cup chopped red or orange bell peppers

1 teaspoon minced garlic

4 cups riced cauliflower

1 teaspoon kosher salt

¼ teaspoon ground black pepper

½ cup canned diced tomatoes

10 pimento-stuffed olives, sliced in half

1 teaspoon capers, drained

¼ cup chopped fresh cilantro, for garnish

Lime wedges, for serving

1. Combine the ingredients for the seasoning blend in a small bowl. Rub the mixture all over the chicken thighs.

2. Heat the oil in a large skillet over medium heat. Fry the chicken for 5 minutes per side, or until golden and crisp. Remove the chicken from the pan and set aside.

3. Add the onions, bell peppers, and garlic to the skillet and cook for 5 minutes, or until fragrant and translucent. Add the riced cauliflower, salt, and pepper and cook for 5 minutes, stirring occasionally. Add the tomatoes, olives, and capers and stir well. Top with the cooked chicken and simmer uncovered for 10 minutes, or until the liquid has evaporated and the chicken is cooked to 165°F in its thickest part. Garnish with the cilantro and serve with lime wedges. Store leftovers in an airtight container in the refrigerator for up to 5 days or in the freezer for up to 3 months.

CALORIES: 451 FAT: 30g PROTEIN: 36g CARBS: 6g FIBER: 2g NET CARBS: 4g

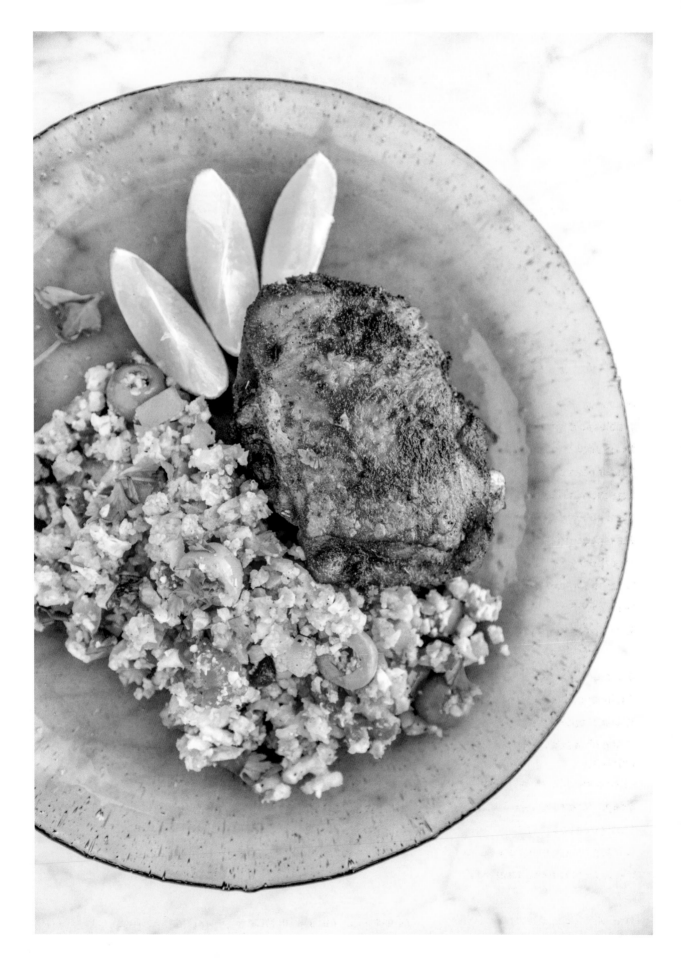

BUTTER CHICKEN

YIELD: 6 servings | **SERVING SIZE:** 1 cup | **PREP TIME:** 10 minutes | **COOK TIME:** 25 minutes

Easily one of the most popular Indian curries, especially with kids, butter chicken is mildly sweet thanks to the inclusion of tomato paste and cinnamon. This dairy-free version gets its creamy consistency from coconut milk and a rich umami flavor from coconut aminos. Unlike many curries that benefit from long cooking times, this butter chicken comes together relatively quickly. Serve it with cauliflower rice to soak up every drop of the delicious sauce.

½ cup (1 stick) butter

2 pounds boneless, skinless chicken breasts, cut into bite-sized pieces

1 teaspoon kosher salt

¼ teaspoon ground black pepper

⅓ cup chopped onions

1 teaspoon minced garlic

2 tablespoons tomato paste

1 tablespoon minced fresh ginger

1 tablespoon garam masala

2 teaspoons paprika

1 teaspoon ground coriander

½ teaspoon ground cardamom

¼ teaspoon ground cinnamon

1 cup canned coconut milk

1 tablespoon coconut aminos or fish sauce (no sugar added)

1 tablespoon fresh lime juice

¼ cup chopped fresh cilantro, for garnish

6 lime wedges, for serving

1. Melt the butter in a large skillet over medium-high heat. Add the chicken, salt, and pepper and cook for 5 minutes, or until the chicken is turning golden brown. Remove the chicken from the pan and set aside.

2. Reduce the heat to medium and add the onions, garlic, tomato paste, ginger, garam masala, paprika, coriander, cardamom, and cinnamon to the pan and cook for 2 minutes, or until fragrant. Return the chicken to the pan and stir to coat. Cook for 3 minutes, or until the chicken is hot and fragrant.

3. Pour the coconut milk, coconut aminos, and lime juice into the pot. Simmer over low heat, stirring occasionally, for about 15 minutes, until the sauce has thickened slightly. Taste and season with additional salt if desired. Garnish with the cilantro and serve with lime wedges. Store leftovers in an airtight container in the refrigerator for up to 5 days or in the freezer for up to 3 months.

CALORIES: 375 **FAT:** 25g **PROTEIN:** 30g **CARBS:** 5g **FIBER:** 1g **NET CARBS:** 4g

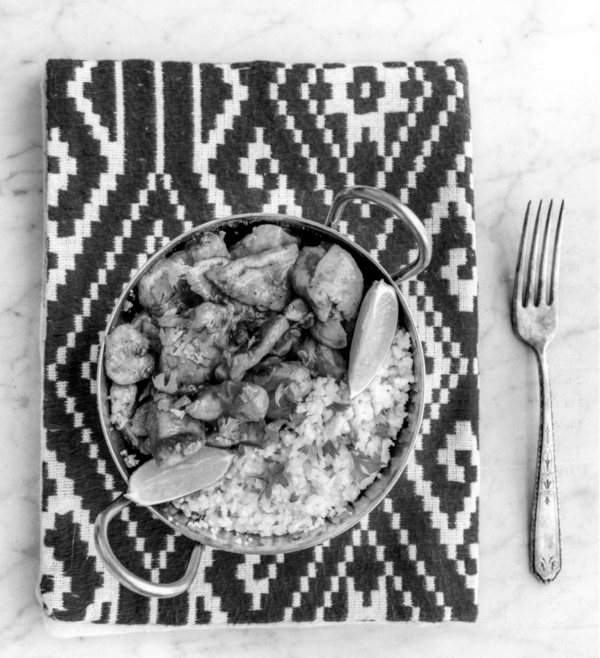

PERUVIAN CHICKEN

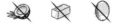

YIELD: 6 servings | SERVING SIZE: 4 to 6 ounces | PREP TIME: 10 minutes | COOK TIME: 70 minutes

Peruvian "fast" food restaurants are among my absolute favorites, and I always order the same thing—wood fire–roasted chicken, pickled red onions with cilantro, and extra green sauce. While this version isn't wood-fired, the rich spice mix is on point, and the end result is always a crowd-pleaser. You simply must serve this chicken with Quick-Pickled Red Onions (page 108) and All-Purpose Green Sauce (page 98) to get the full experience!

For the marinade:

3 tablespoons extra-virgin olive oil

1 teaspoon grated lime zest

2 teaspoons fresh lime juice

2 teaspoons minced garlic

1 tablespoon ground cumin

1 tablespoon kosher salt

1 tablespoon paprika

1 teaspoon dried oregano leaves

½ teaspoon ground black pepper

½ teaspoon onion powder

1 (5- to 6-pound) whole chicken

1. Preheat the oven to 400°F.

2. Put all the marinade ingredients in a small blender or food processor and process until you have a mostly smooth paste. Rub the paste all over the inside and outside of the chicken, including under the skin of the breast and legs as far as you can reach.

3. Place the chicken in a roasting pan. Roast the chicken uncovered for 70 minutes, or until a thermometer inserted in the center of a thigh reads 165°F. Remove from the oven and let rest uncovered for 15 minutes before cutting and serving. Store leftovers in an airtight container in the refrigerator for up to 5 days.

Note: Do not cover the chicken while it's resting or the skin will lose its crispness.

1 THIGH: **CALORIES:** 358 **FAT:** 22g **PROTEIN:** 36g **CARBS:** 0g **FIBER:** 0g **NET CARBS:** 0g

1 DRUMSTICK: **CALORIES:** 233 **FAT:** 12g **PROTEIN:** 29g **CARBS:** 0g **FIBER:** 0g **NET CARBS:** 0g

1 BREAST: **CALORIES:** 193 **FAT:** 8g **PROTEIN:** 29g **CARBS:** 0g **FIBER:** 0g **NET CARBS:** 0g

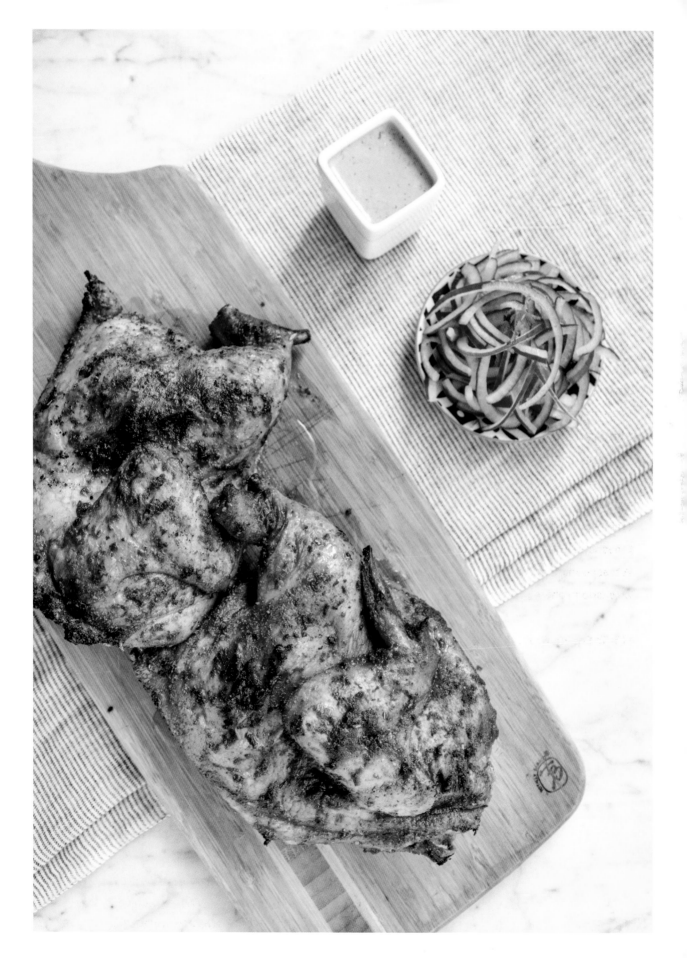

CHICKEN JALFREZI

YIELD: 4 servings | **SERVING SIZE:** 1¼ cups | **PREP TIME:** 10 minutes | **COOK TIME:** 15 minutes

Easily the fastest of the curries in this book, jalfrezi relies on a quick sauté and plenty of spices to achieve its bold flavor. More stewlike than creamy, this curry will make your nose run. If you want to dial back the spice, reduce the amount of red pepper flakes to 1 teaspoon, but I'll be sad for you. Like all the curries in this book, you can serve this one over cauliflower rice to bulk it up and make it a complete meal.

1 teaspoon kosher salt

1 tablespoon ground coriander

1 tablespoon ground cumin

1 tablespoon garam masala

2 teaspoons red pepper flakes

1 teaspoon turmeric powder

½ teaspoon ground black pepper

1½ pounds boneless, skinless chicken breasts, cut into bite-sized pieces

2 tablespoons avocado oil or other light-tasting oil, for frying

½ cup chopped onions

2 tablespoons minced fresh ginger

1 teaspoon minced garlic

1 cup canned crushed tomatoes

2 tablespoons butter

¼ cup chopped fresh cilantro, for garnish

4 lime wedges, for serving

1. Combine the salt and spices in a small bowl, then toss the chicken pieces in the spice blend and set aside.

2. Heat the oil in a large skillet over medium-high heat until shimmering. Add the onions, ginger, and garlic and cook for 2 minutes, or until fragrant. Add the chicken and cook, stirring occasionally, for 5 minutes, or until cooked through.

3. Add the tomatoes and butter and simmer for 5 minutes, or until the sauce has thickened enough to coat the back of a spoon. Garnish with the cilantro and serve with lime wedges. Store leftovers in an airtight container in the refrigerator for up to 5 days or in the freezer for up to 3 months.

CALORIES: 315 **FAT:** 17g **PROTEIN:** 33g **CARBS:** 5g **FIBER:** 1g **NET CARBS:** 4g

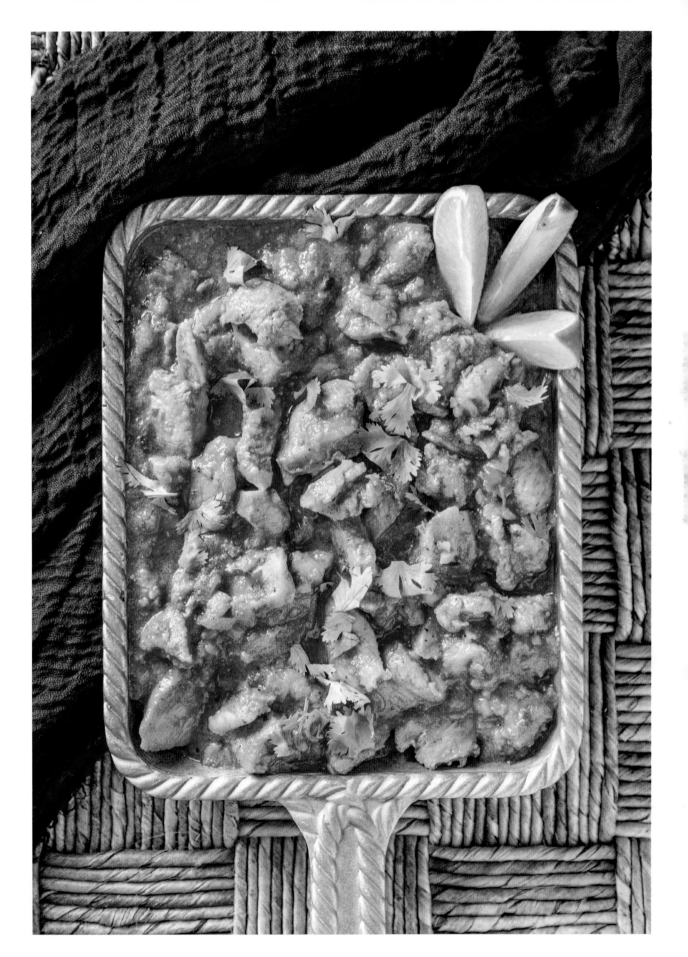

CRISPY LEMON CHICKEN

YIELD: 6 servings | SERVING SIZE: 1 cutlet + 1 tablespoon lemon butter | PREP TIME: 10 minutes | COOK TIME: 15 minutes

Lemon and chicken are a classic pairing that never gets old. Throw in a crunchy coating and a liberal amount of butter, and let's just say there is nothing you and your family won't love about this easy chicken dinner that you can have on the table in under 30 minutes.

6 (6-ounce) chicken cutlets

⅓ cup mayonnaise

⅓ cup Sun-Flour (page 74)

2 tablespoons coconut flour

1 teaspoon grated lemon zest

1 teaspoon kosher salt

¼ teaspoon garlic powder

¼ teaspoon ground black pepper

2 tablespoons extra-virgin olive oil

¼ cup (½ stick) butter

2 tablespoons fresh lemon juice

6 lemon slices, for garnish (optional)

2 tablespoons chopped fresh parsley, for garnish

1. Put the chicken and mayonnaise in a medium-sized bowl. Stir well to coat the entire surface of the chicken with mayonnaise.

2. Put the flours, lemon zest, salt, garlic powder, and black pepper in a small bowl and stir well. Dredge each chicken piece in the flour mixture so that all the surfaces are completely coated.

3. Heat the oil in a large skillet over medium heat until shimmering. Cook the chicken cutlets, 3 at a time, for about 3 minutes per side, until golden brown and cooked through. Remove the cooked chicken to a serving platter. Wipe any burned bits of coating from the skillet with a paper towel.

4. Add the butter and lemon juice to the skillet and cook for 2 minutes, or until the butter is melted and the mixture has thickened slightly. Pour the hot lemon butter over the chicken, garnish with the lemon slices (if using) and parsley, and serve immediately. Store leftovers in an airtight container in the refrigerator for up to 5 days.

Note: I use mayonnaise rather than beaten eggs as the "glue" for the coating, which helps keep it from falling off during frying.

CALORIES: 400　FAT: 17g　PROTEIN: 41g　CARBS: 3g　FIBER: 2g　NET CARBS: 1g

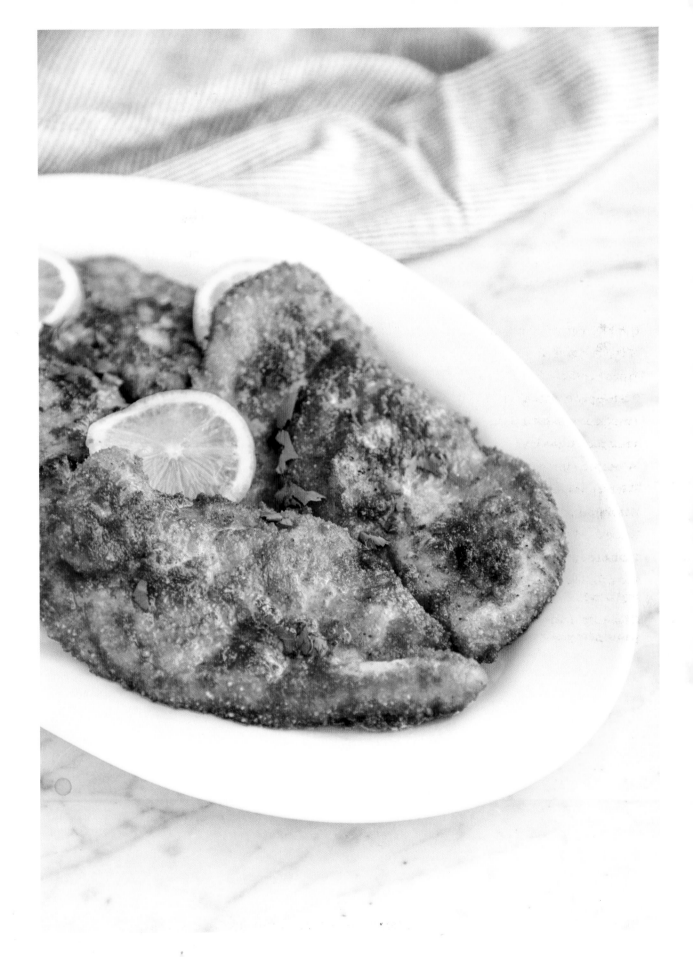

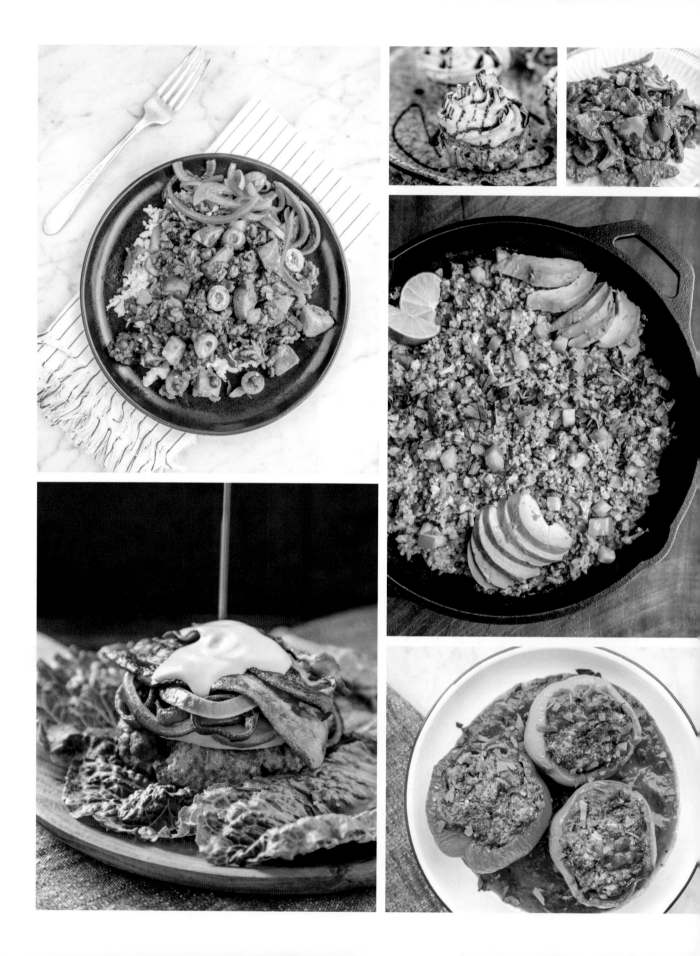

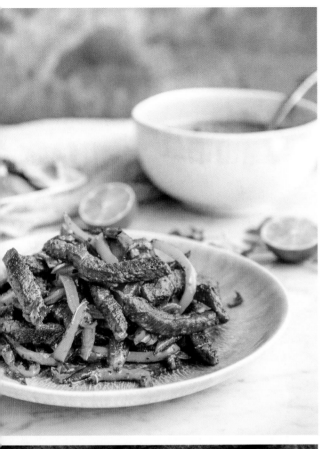

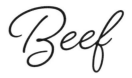

Beef

Instant Pot Beef Curry / 196

Spanish Rice Hamburger Skillet / 198

Beef Picadillo / 200

Chili Dog Skillet / 202

Sheet Pan Steak Fajitas / 204

Beef Kofta Meatballs / 206

Sheet Pan Meatballs with Zoodles / 208

Meatloaf Cupcakes / 210

Italian-Style Stuffed Peppers / 212

Ginger Beef Stir-Fry / 214

Sheet Pan Bacon Burgers / 216

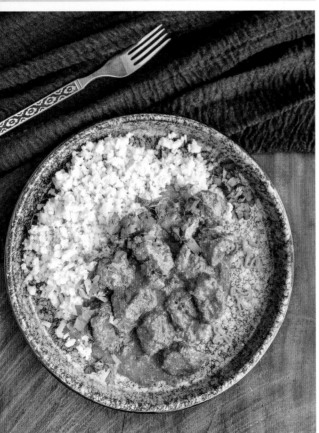

INSTANT POT BEEF CURRY

YIELD: 6 servings | **SERVING SIZE:** 1 cup | **PREP TIME:** 15 minutes | **COOK TIME:** 55 minutes

This rich and mildly spicy beef curry becomes meltingly tender in under an hour when cooked in an Instant Pot or other pressure cooker. The end result is a crowd-pleasing dinner that reheats well all week long. If you like your curry really spicy, like I do, you can double the habanero. I recommend serving this curry over cauliflower rice, as shown.

For the curry paste:

2 tablespoons ground coriander

1 tablespoon ground cumin

2 teaspoons kosher salt

2 teaspoons turmeric powder

1 teaspoon garam masala

½ teaspoon ground black pepper

2 cloves garlic, minced

2 teaspoons minced fresh ginger

2 teaspoons grated lime zest

2 tablespoons extra-virgin olive oil

3 pounds stew beef, cut into 1-inch pieces

½ cup diced tomatoes

1 teaspoon minced habanero peppers

¾ cup beef broth, store-bought or homemade (page 72)

1 tablespoon apple cider vinegar

⅓ cup Sun-Flour (page 74)

2 teaspoons coconut milk powder

1 teaspoon garam masala

¼ cup fresh cilantro leaves, for garnish

1. In a large bowl, stir together the ingredients for the curry paste until fully combined. Add the beef and stir well until all the pieces are coated in the paste.

2. Turn on the Instant Pot to the Sauté function to preheat the insert. Put half of the beef in the pot and cook for 2 to 3 minutes, until browned. Remove and repeat with the remaining beef.

3. Return all the browned beef to the Instant Pot, then add the tomatoes, habanero peppers, broth, and vinegar. Cover the pot with the lid and lock it in place. Make sure the steam vent is closed. Set the pot to Manual/High Pressure for 40 minutes. When the cooking is done, wait for the pressure to release naturally (if you aren't sure what that means, read your Instant Pot manual carefully to avoid accidents), then carefully remove the lid. Remove the meat from the pot with a slotted spoon and set aside.

4. Turn the Instant Pot back on and set it to Sauté. Add the flour, coconut milk powder, and garam masala. Simmer, stirring occasionally, for 5 to 7 minutes, until thickened and reduced by about half. Return the meat to the pot and stir well. Taste and season with additional salt if desired. Serve garnished with the cilantro. Store leftovers in an airtight container in the refrigerator for up to 5 days or in the freezer for up to 3 months.

CALORIES: 481 **FAT:** 35g **PROTEIN:** 43g **CARBS:** 3g **FIBER:** 1g **NET CARBS:** 2g

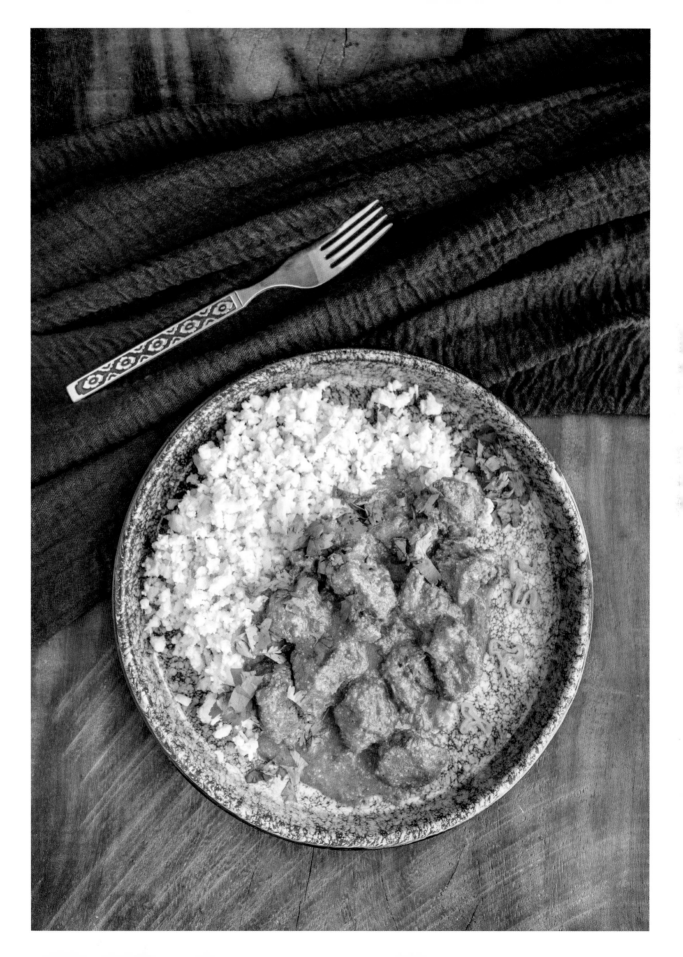

SPANISH RICE HAMBURGER SKILLET

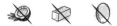

| **YIELD:** 4 servings | **SERVING SIZE:** 1½ cups | **PREP TIME:** 15 minutes | **COOK TIME:** 16 minutes |

This is one of those quick and easy family-friendly dinners that you'll want to make regularly once you try it. It is mild as is, but you can add chopped fresh jalapeños or habaneros to up the heat. While it doesn't necessarily need it, you can also spruce up this skillet meal with chopped fresh cilantro, diced fresh tomatoes, avocado slices, and lime wedges according to your preference. And of course, if you're not squeaky or avoiding dairy, you can top it with shredded cheese and sour cream to make it even tastier.

2 tablespoons extra-virgin olive oil

1 tablespoon dried onion flakes

1 teaspoon minced garlic

2 teaspoons ground cumin

1 teaspoon kosher salt

½ teaspoon dried oregano leaves

¼ teaspoon ground black pepper

1 pound ground beef (80/20)

3 cups riced cauliflower

½ cup canned diced tomatoes

1 (4-ounce) can chopped green chilis

⅓ cup chicken broth, store-bought or homemade (page 72)

Heat the oil in a large skillet over medium heat. Add the onion flakes and garlic and cook for 1 minute, or until fragrant. Add the cumin, salt, oregano, pepper, and ground beef. Cook, stirring occasionally, for about 5 minutes, until the meat is browned. Add the riced cauliflower, tomatoes, green chilis, and broth. Stir well and simmer, uncovered, for 10 minutes, or until the rice is soft, the liquid has evaporated, and the mixture is mostly dry. Store leftovers in an airtight container in the refrigerator for up to 5 days or in the freezer for up to 3 months.

CALORIES: 368 **FAT:** 29g **PROTEIN:** 21g **CARBS:** 6g **FIBER:** 2g **NET CARBS:** 4g

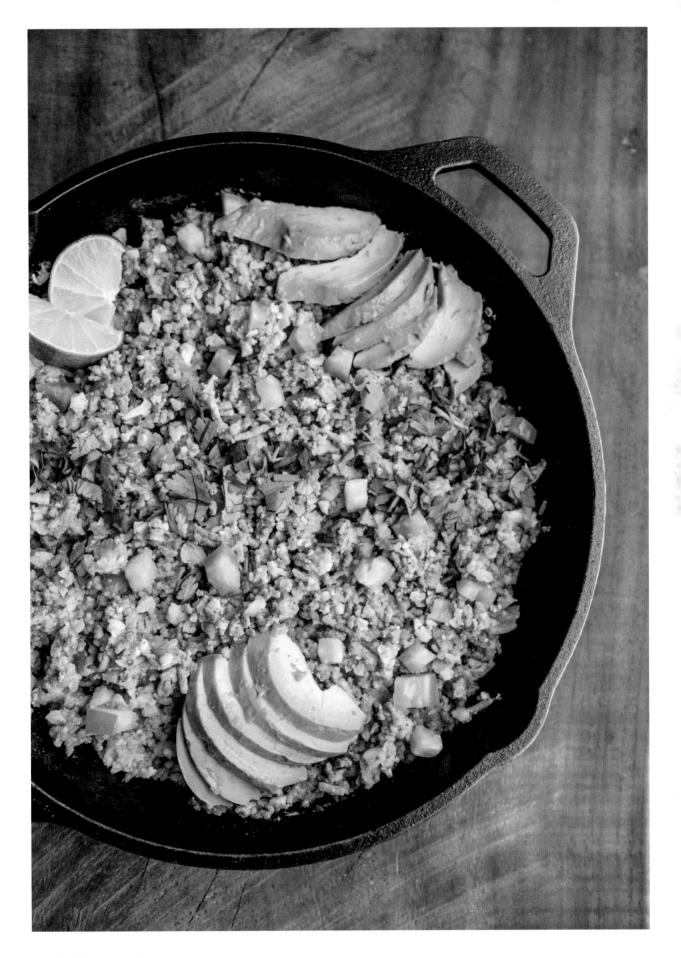

BEEF PICADILLO

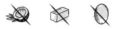

YIELD: 6 servings | SERVING SIZE: 1 cup | PREP TIME: 15 minutes | COOK TIME: 25 minutes

This Spanish-inspired dish is tangy, sweet, briny, savory perfection. If you're sick of the same old ground beef dishes, then you're going to love this unique and delicious flavor profile. While picadillo traditionally gets its sweetness from raisins, I use chopped prunes instead, which have a little less carbs—plus, you'll be super regular! You can omit them to save a few grams, but in my opinion, doing so would adversely affect the balance of the recipe. I recommend going for it as written, at least the first time. I like to serve this dish with Quick-Pickled Red Onions (page 108) and cauliflower rice, as shown.

2 tablespoons extra-virgin olive oil

⅓ cup chopped onions

1 teaspoon minced garlic

2 cups chopped radishes

2 teaspoons ground cumin

½ teaspoon kosher salt

½ teaspoon ground black pepper

1 pound ground beef (80/20)

1 (4-ounce) can chopped green chilis

½ cup pimento-stuffed green olives

½ cup canned crushed tomatoes

¼ cup chopped prunes

½ cup chicken broth, store-bought or homemade (page 72)

2 tablespoons capers, drained

¼ cup chopped fresh cilantro, for garnish

1. Heat the oil in a large skillet over medium heat. Add the onions and garlic and cook for 2 to 3 minutes, until fragrant and beginning to soften. Add the radishes and cook for 3 to 5 minutes, stirring occasionally, until they begin to turn translucent. Add the cumin, salt, pepper, and ground beef. Cook, stirring frequently, until the beef is browned, about 5 minutes.

2. To the skillet, add the green chilis, olives, tomatoes, prunes, and broth and stir well. Simmer for 5 minutes, or until the radishes have softened. Stir in the capers and cook for an additional 3 to 5 minutes, until most of the liquid has evaporated and has turned a glossy reddish brown color. Remove from the heat and serve garnished with the cilantro. Store leftovers in an airtight container in the refrigerator for up to 5 days or in the freezer for up to 3 months.

CALORIES: 290 FAT: 22g PROTEIN: 14g CARBS: 9g FIBER: 2g NET CARBS: 7g

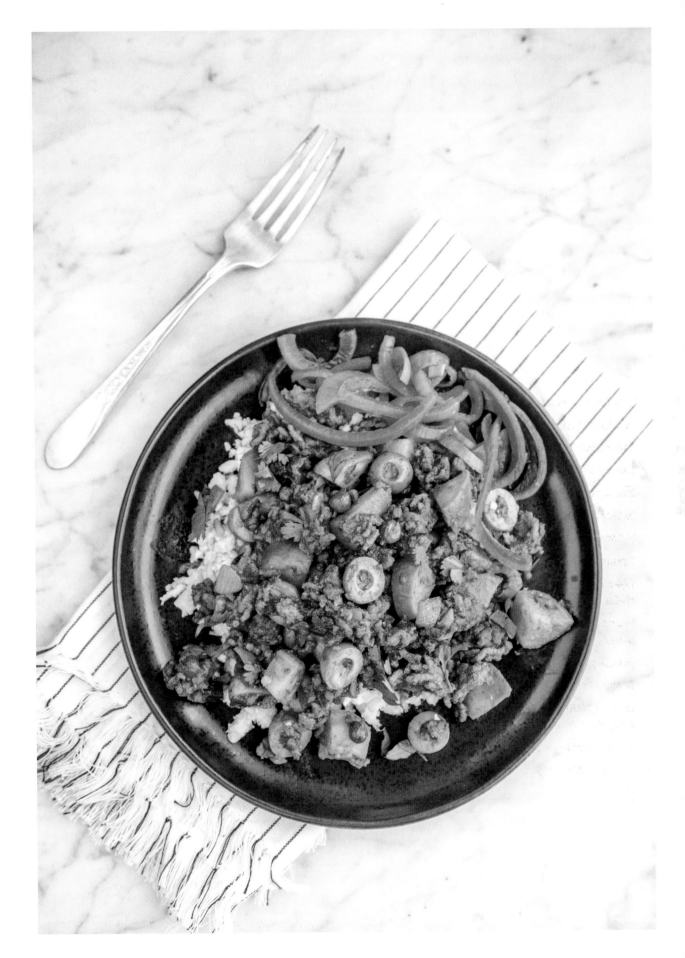

CHILI DOG SKILLET

YIELD: 6 servings | **SERVING SIZE:** 1¾ cups | **PREP TIME:** 10 minutes | **COOK TIME:** 30 minutes

If you love a great chili dog, then you'll love this easy skillet meal. It combines all the best elements of a chili dog (except the bun, sorry) in a tasty dinner that reheats like a dream all week long. There are lots of ways to garnish this dish, but my favorites are a liberal sprinkling of Quick-Pickled Red Onions (page 108), sauerkraut, and some chopped avocado.

1 pound ground beef (80/20)

½ cup prepared salsa

1 teaspoon coconut aminos

1 teaspoon Dijon mustard

1 teaspoon kosher salt

1 teaspoon ground cumin

½ teaspoon garlic powder

¼ teaspoon ground black pepper

4 hot dogs, sliced diagonally, ½ inch thick

4 cups cauliflower florets (about 1 large head)

¼ cup filtered water

2 tablespoons mayonnaise

Put everything except the mayonnaise in a large skillet and stir well to break up the ground beef. Cook, covered, over medium heat, stirring occasionally, for 30 minutes, or until the cauliflower is fork-tender. Remove the pan from the heat and stir in the mayonnaise. Serve hot garnished with your favorite squeaky-friendly chili dog toppings. Store leftovers in an airtight container in the refrigerator for up to 5 days or in the freezer for up to 3 months.

Note: If not squeaky, you can add ½ cup of shredded cheddar cheese in the last 5 minutes of cooking.

CALORIES: 329 **FAT:** 25g **PROTEIN:** 19g **CARBS:** 7g **FIBER:** 2g **NET CARBS:** 5g

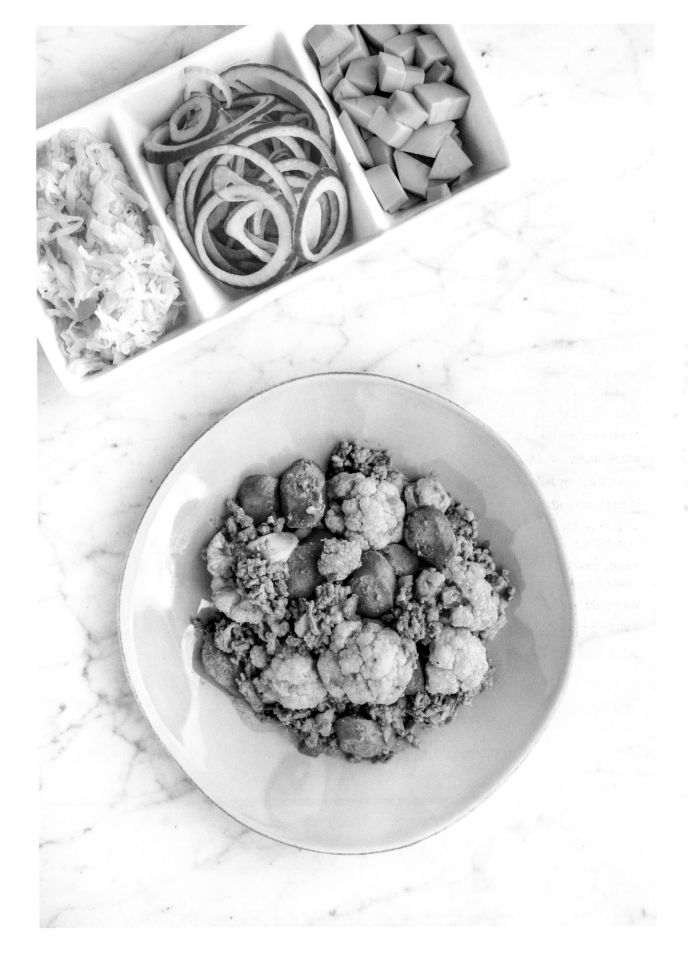

SHEET PAN STEAK FAJITAS

YIELD: 4 servings | SERVING SIZE: ¾ cup | PREP TIME: 15 minutes | COOK TIME: 20 minutes

Oh sheet pan meal, how I love thee. Easy to make and a cinch to clean up—sheet pan dinners are a staple in my house. This fajitas recipe is one of my favorites because I can keep it squeaky for me but serve tortillas, cheese, and sour cream to my family and friends without a lot of extra work. It's also a great one to prep in advance and freeze when you need dinner on the table fast (see Notes below).

3 tablespoons avocado oil or other light-tasting oil

1 cup sliced bell peppers (any color)

1 cup sliced poblano peppers

½ cup sliced red onions

1 teaspoon sliced garlic

1 teaspoon kosher salt

1 tablespoon ground cumin

1 teaspoon chili powder

½ teaspoon garlic powder

½ teaspoon ground black pepper

1 pound lean boneless beef steak, such as sirloin or flank, sliced into thin strips

1. Preheat the oven to 400°F.

2. Pour the oil onto a sheet pan. Place the bell peppers, poblanos, onions, and garlic on the pan and stir to coat them in the oil.

3. Put the salt and spices in a large bowl and stir to combine. Add the steak to the bowl and stir well to coat. Transfer the steak to the sheet pan and stir to combine with the veggies. Spread out in a thin layer.

4. Bake for 20 minutes, or until the vegetables are crisp-tender and the meat is cooked through. Store leftovers in an airtight container in the refrigerator for up to 5 days.

Notes: You can substitute chicken, pork, or shrimp for the steak. Chicken or pork would have the same cook time as the beef; if using shrimp, add it to the pan during the last 10 minutes of cooking.

For a freezer meal, combine all the ingredients except the oil in a gallon-sized freezer bag and seal tightly. Freeze for up to 3 months. To cook, thaw and then drain any liquid before spreading the meat and vegetables on a sheet pan. Coat with 3 tablespoons of oil and bake as directed above.

CALORIES: 266 | FAT: 9g | PROTEIN: 32g | CARBS: 5g | FIBER: 1g | NET CARBS: 4g

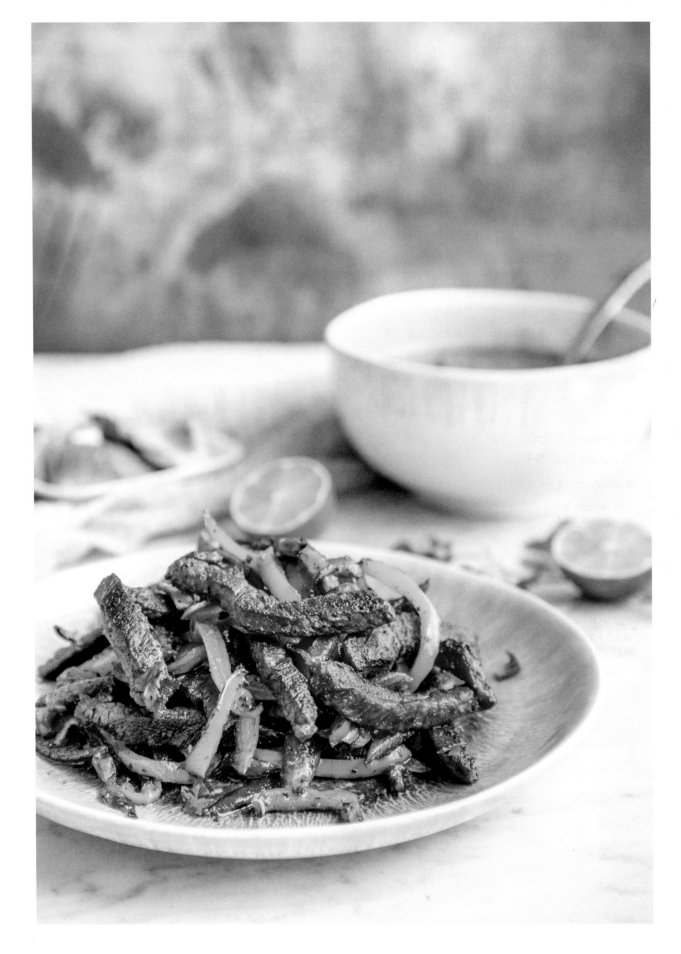

BEEF KOFTA MEATBALLS

YIELD: 4 servings | **SERVING SIZE:** 3 meatballs | **PREP TIME:** 15 minutes | **COOK TIME:** 15 minutes

Kofta is a Middle Eastern dish consisting of minced meat flavored with onion and spices that is commonly served as meatballs or kebabs. I went with beef for these meatballs, but you can also make them with ground lamb if you can get it. To keep these meatballs SCK friendly, I used hemp seeds to bulk them up and mayonnaise to bind them. The hemp seeds lighten up the meat mixture beautifully, and, as an added bonus, they are loaded with healthy fats and important nutrients like magnesium. The mayonnaise makes these meatballs super silky and adds a subtle tang. They're especially tasty paired with cauliflower rice and Dairy-Free Tzatziki (page 96); you won't want to stop at just three!

1 pound ground beef (80/20)

¼ cup mayonnaise

¼ cup shelled hemp seeds (hemp hearts)

¼ cup chopped fresh cilantro

¼ cup chopped fresh parsley, plus more for garnish if desired

1 teaspoon grated lemon zest

1 teaspoon dried oregano leaves

1 teaspoon ground coriander

1 teaspoon ground cumin

1 teaspoon kosher salt

1 teaspoon onion powder

1 teaspoon smoked paprika

½ teaspoon ground allspice

½ teaspoon ground black pepper

½ teaspoon garlic powder

1. Preheat the oven to 400°F. Oil a sheet pan.

2. Put all the ingredients in a medium-sized bowl and mix well with your hands. Form into 12 meatballs about 1½ inches in diameter. Place the meatballs on the prepared sheet pan.

3. Bake for 15 minutes, or until browned and firm to the touch. Remove from the oven and garnish with parsley if desired. Store leftovers in an airtight container in the refrigerator for up to 5 days or in the freezer for up to 3 months.

CALORIES: 360 **FAT:** 19g **PROTEIN:** 24g **CARBS:** 2g **FIBER:** 1g **NET CARBS:** 1g

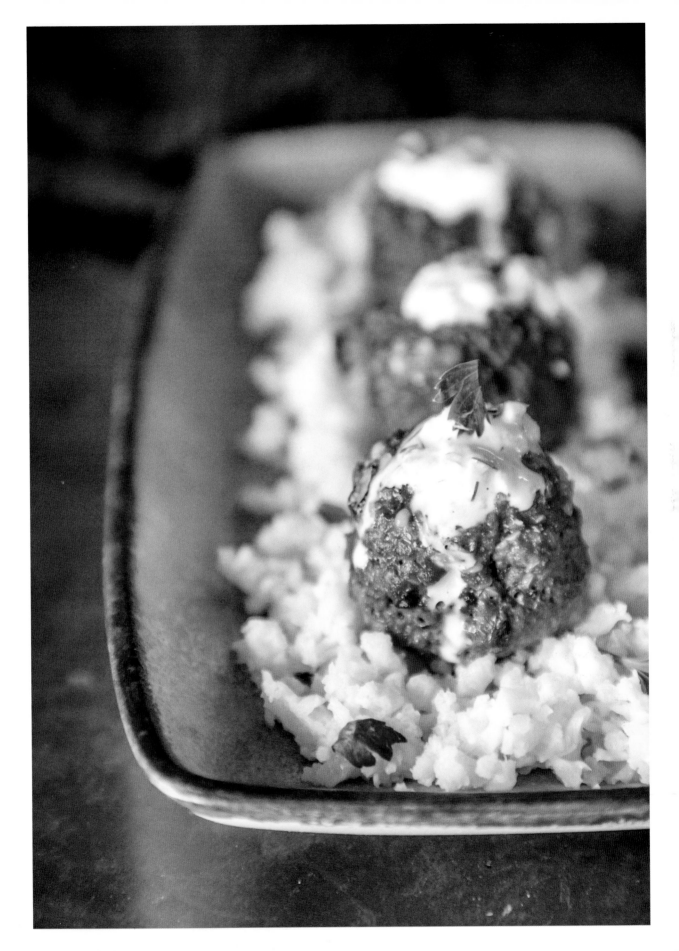

SHEET PAN MEATBALLS WITH ZOODLES

YIELD: 4 servings | **SERVING SIZE:** 3 meatballs + 1 cup zoodles with sauce | **PREP TIME:** 15 minutes | **COOK TIME:** 15 minutes

Hearty and soul-satisfying, these tasty meatballs are super easy to make because they are baked on a sheet pan instead of fried. While they don't contain the Parmesan cheese I'd typically use in an Italian meatball, the hemp seeds give them a similar texture, and plenty of herbs and spices provide all the flavor you're looking for. Even non-keto family and friends will enjoy this dish, and you can easily substitute regular pasta for them and add a sprinkle of Parmesan while keeping it squeaky for you.

2 tablespoons extra-virgin olive oil, for the pan

For the meatballs:

1 pound ground beef (80/20)

¼ cup shelled hemp seeds (hemp hearts)

¼ cup mayonnaise

¼ cup finely chopped fresh parsley

1 teaspoon kosher salt

½ teaspoon dried oregano leaves

½ teaspoon garlic powder

½ teaspoon onion powder

¼ teaspoon ground black pepper

6 cups zucchini noodles (about 4 medium zucchini)

1½ cups marinara sauce, store-bought or homemade (page 84)

Fresh basil sprigs, for garnish (optional)

1. Preheat the oven to 400°F. Pour the olive oil onto a sheet pan.

2. Put all the meatball ingredients in a medium-sized bowl and mix well with your hands. Form into 12 meatballs about 1½ inches in diameter. Place the meatballs on the sheet pan and gently roll each one in the oil to coat. Arrange the meatballs on half of the sheet pan and bake for 10 minutes.

3. Remove the meatballs from the oven and spread the zucchini noodles over the empty half of the sheet pan. Stir the zucchini to coat the noodles with any oil or juices on the pan. Spoon the marinara sauce over the zucchini.

4. Return the pan to the oven for 5 to 7 minutes, until the zucchini is done to your liking. Remove from the oven, transfer the meatballs to a serving dish, and gently tilt one corner of the pan over a bowl to drain any excess liquid from the zucchini. Serve the meatballs and zoodles hot, garnished with fresh basil if desired. Store leftovers in an airtight container in the refrigerator for up to 5 days.

CALORIES: 501 | **FAT:** 40g | **PROTEIN:** 25g | **CARBS:** 9g | **FIBER:** 4g | **NET CARBS:** 5g

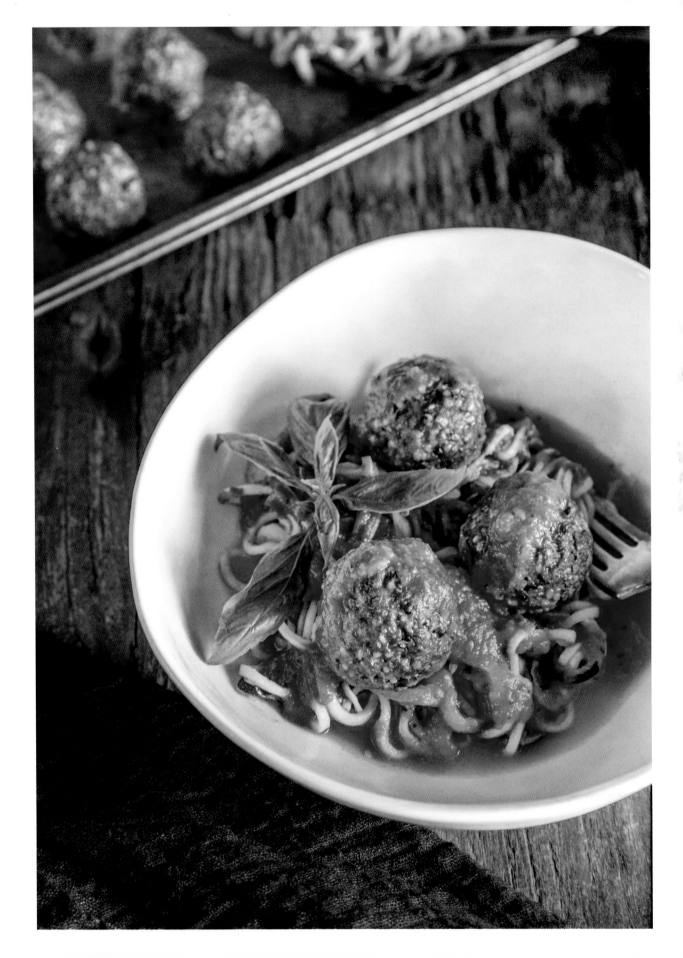

MEATLOAF CUPCAKES

YIELD: 8 mini meatloaves | **SERVING SIZE:** 2 mini meatloaves | **PREP TIME:** 8 minutes | **COOK TIME:** 20 minutes

These tasty gems are fun to make and easy to eat, with the added bonus of built-in portion control! Even the kids will love this dish, and it's a great recipe for your lil' chef-in-training to get hands-on experience with mixing the meat and pressing it into the cups. While you can eat these with other side dishes, I highly recommend topping them with Duchess Cauliflower and a drizzle of Easy Balsamic Glaze for a complete meal that will bring the house down every time.

1 tablespoon extra-virgin olive oil, for the pan

1 pound ground beef (80/20)

½ cup grated zucchini

¼ cup mayonnaise

¼ cup shelled hemp seeds (hemp hearts)

1 tablespoon dried parsley

1 teaspoon kosher salt

1 teaspoon onion powder

½ teaspoon garlic powder

½ teaspoon ground black pepper

For serving (optional):

8 pieces Duchess Cauliflower (page 302)

1 tablespoon Easy Balsamic Glaze (page 86)

1. Preheat the oven to 375°F. Brush 8 standard-size muffin cups with the olive oil.

2. Put the remaining ingredients in a medium-sized bowl and stir well. Divide the meat mixture evenly among the prepared muffin cups. Press down and flatten with the back of a spoon. Bake for 20 minutes, or until cooked through. Serve topped with the Duchess Cauliflower pieces and a drizzle of balsamic glaze if desired. Store leftovers in an airtight container in the refrigerator for up to 5 days.

Note: For this recipe, grated or very finely grated zucchini works best because it blends easily into the ground beef. I grate the zucchini using the smallest holes on my box grater, the side normally used for grating hard cheese.

CALORIES: 394 **FAT:** 20g **PROTEIN:** 23g **CARBS:** 2g **FIBER:** 1g **NET CARBS:** 1g

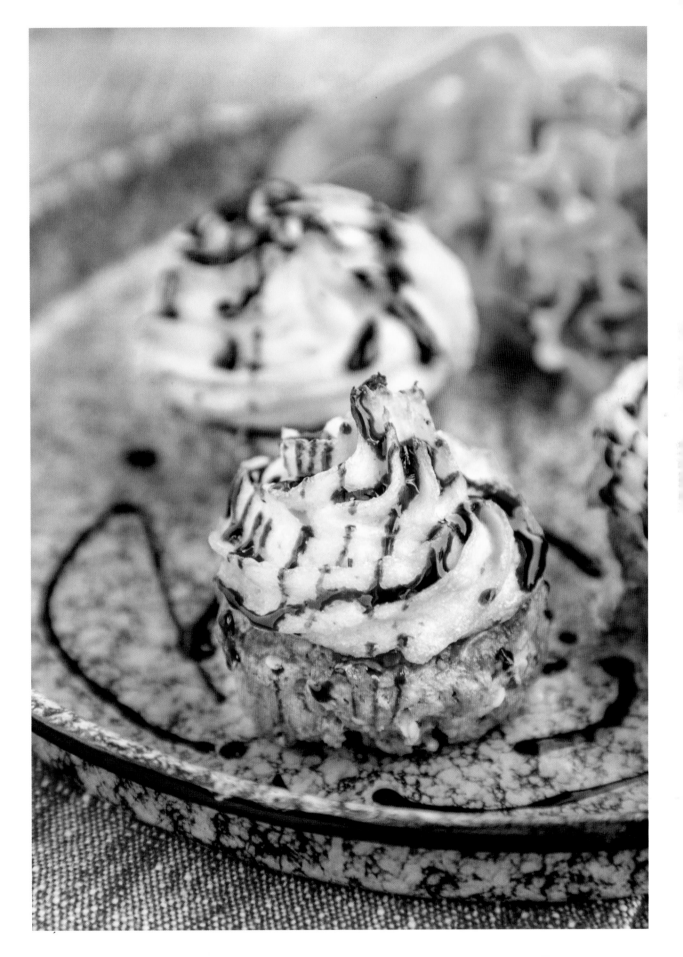

ITALIAN-STYLE STUFFED PEPPERS

YIELD: 4 stuffed peppers | **SERVING SIZE:** 1 stuffed pepper + 2 tablespoons sauce | **PREP TIME:** 15 minutes | **COOK TIME:** 34 minutes

---

There's something inherently fun about eating one food stuffed into another food, and this stuffed peppers recipe is no exception. This squeaky version boasts savory ground beef mixed with riced cauliflower and spices, which is pressed into sweet bell peppers and baked in a tangy tomato sauce. Baking makes the peppers even sweeter, and all that tasty beef juice soaks into the sauce, so nothing is wasted. This is next-level comfort food!

4 large bell peppers (any color)

1 pound ground beef (80/20)

¾ cup riced cauliflower

2 tablespoons chopped fresh parsley, plus more for garnish if desired

¼ cup mayonnaise

1 teaspoon kosher salt

1 teaspoon garlic powder

½ teaspoon onion powder

½ teaspoon dried oregano leaves

¼ teaspoon ground black pepper

½ cup canned crushed tomatoes

1 tablespoon extra-virgin olive oil

1 teaspoon balsamic vinegar (no sugar added)

1. Preheat the oven to 400°F.

2. Slice the tops off the bell peppers and scoop out any seeds from the insides. Place on a microwave-safe plate and microwave for 4 minutes, or until softened.

3. Put the ground beef, riced cauliflower, parsley, mayonnaise, salt, garlic powder, onion powder, oregano, and black pepper in a large bowl and mix well. Divide the mixture evenly into 4 balls and stuff a ball into each pepper, pressing until the meat has filled the cavity.

4. Put the crushed tomatoes, olive oil, and vinegar in a 9-inch square baking dish and stir. Spread out the mixture and set the stuffed peppers in the pan on top of the sauce.

5. Bake for 30 minutes, or until the meat in the centers of the peppers reaches 160°F. Remove from the oven and serve hot, with the tomato sauce spooned over the top. Garnish with fresh parsley if desired. Store leftovers in an airtight container in the refrigerator for up to 5 days or in the freezer for up to 3 months.

CALORIES: 397 **FAT:** 33g **PROTEIN:** 23g **CARBS:** 9g **FIBER:** 3g **NET CARBS:** 6g

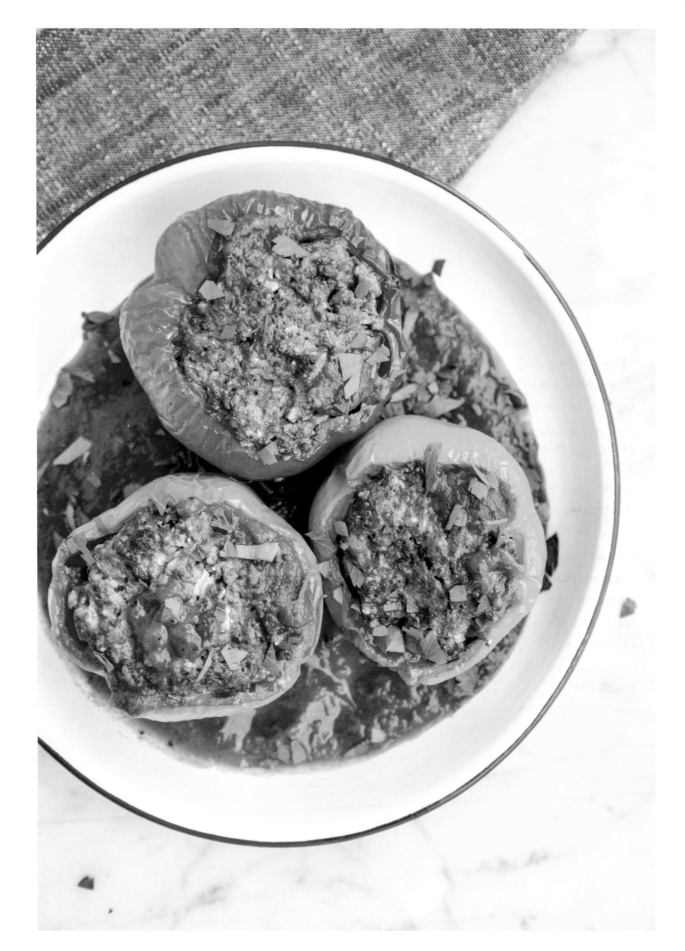

GINGER BEEF STIR-FRY

YIELD: 4 servings | SERVING SIZE: 1 cup | PREP TIME: 8 minutes | COOK TIME: 10 minutes

Skip the takeout (and the carbs) and make a delicious stir-fry at home instead. Easy to whip up at a moment's notice, this ginger beef dish is tangy and slightly sweet, with plenty of protein and healthy veggies included. To bulk it up even more, you can serve it on a bed of cauliflower rice or spaghetti squash.

2 tablespoons avocado oil or other light-tasting oil

1 teaspoon toasted sesame oil

1 tablespoon minced fresh ginger

2 teaspoons minced garlic

1 cup broccoli florets

1 cup sliced red bell peppers

1 pound lean boneless beef steak, such as sirloin or flank, thinly sliced

1 tablespoon coconut aminos

1 tablespoon white vinegar

1 teaspoon fish sauce (no sugar added)

½ teaspoon kosher salt

¼ teaspoon ground black pepper

¼ cup filtered water

¼ teaspoon xanthan gum

1 cup sliced scallions, green parts only

1. Heat the avocado oil and sesame oil in a large skillet over medium-high heat. Add the ginger and garlic and stir-fry for 1 minute. Add the broccoli and bell peppers and stir-fry for 3 minutes, or until the broccoli is bright green and starting to soften. Add the beef, coconut aminos, vinegar, fish sauce, salt, and black pepper to the pan and stir well. Cook for 2 minutes, or until the beef is beginning to brown.

2. To the skillet, add the water and xanthan gum and stir well. Stir-fry for another 3 minutes, or until the beef is fully cooked and the broccoli is fork-tender. Remove the pan from the heat and stir in the scallions. Serve hot. Store leftovers in an airtight container in the refrigerator for up to 5 days.

CALORIES: 289 FAT: 14g PROTEIN: 33g CARBS: 6g FIBER: 2g NET CARBS: 4g

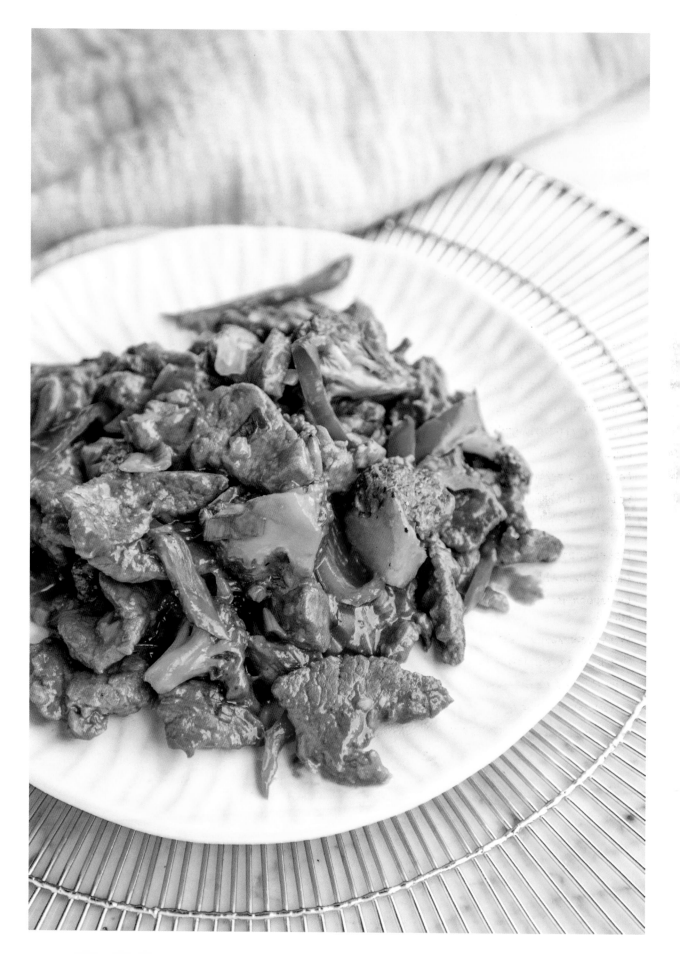

SHEET PAN BACON BURGERS

YIELD: 4 burgers | **SERVING SIZE:** 1 burger + 2 tablespoons sauce | **PREP TIME:** 15 minutes | **COOK TIME:** 20 minutes

Can we all just take a minute and appreciate that a) sheet pan meals are life right now, and b) this sheet pan burger recipe proves that you don't need a grill or a lot of hands-on cooking time to indulge that burger craving? This recipe is tried and tested, not just by my family and friends, but by the many people who have made the recipe from my website and reported back with rave reviews.

1½ pounds ground beef (80/20)

1 teaspoon kosher salt

½ teaspoon garlic powder

¼ teaspoon ground black pepper

6 slices bacon, cut in half crosswise

4 slices red onion (about ¼ inch thick)

2 jalapeño peppers, sliced into rings, seeded if desired

½ cup Creamy Sriracha Dipping Sauce (page 93)

1. Preheat the oven to 425°F.

2. Put the ground beef, salt, garlic powder, and black pepper in a medium-sized bowl and mix well with your hands. Form into 4 equal-size patties about 5 inches in diameter and 1 inch thick and place the patties on a sheet pan. Put the bacon, onion slices, and jalapeño rings on the same sheet pan.

3. For medium-done burgers, bake for 20 minutes or until the burgers reach 160°F; bake longer if you prefer your burgers more well-done. Remove from the oven.

4. Build each plate with 1 patty, 3 pieces of bacon, 1 slice of onion, the desired amount of jalapeños, and a 2-tablespoon drizzle of the sauce. Serve warm. Store leftovers in an airtight container in the refrigerator for up to 5 days.

Notes: If, after 20 minutes, the bacon and veggies aren't crisp enough for your liking, remove the patties from the sheet pan so they don't overcook, then broil the bacon and veggies for 2 minutes or until the desired crispness is reached.

If you're an avocado fan like I am, you may wish to add a couple of slices to this burger like I did here. If you do, be sure to account for the difference in the nutrition; the avocado is not included in my calculations below.

CALORIES: 510 **FAT:** 39g **PROTEIN:** 36g **CARBS:** 4g **FIBER:** 1g **NET CARBS:** 4g

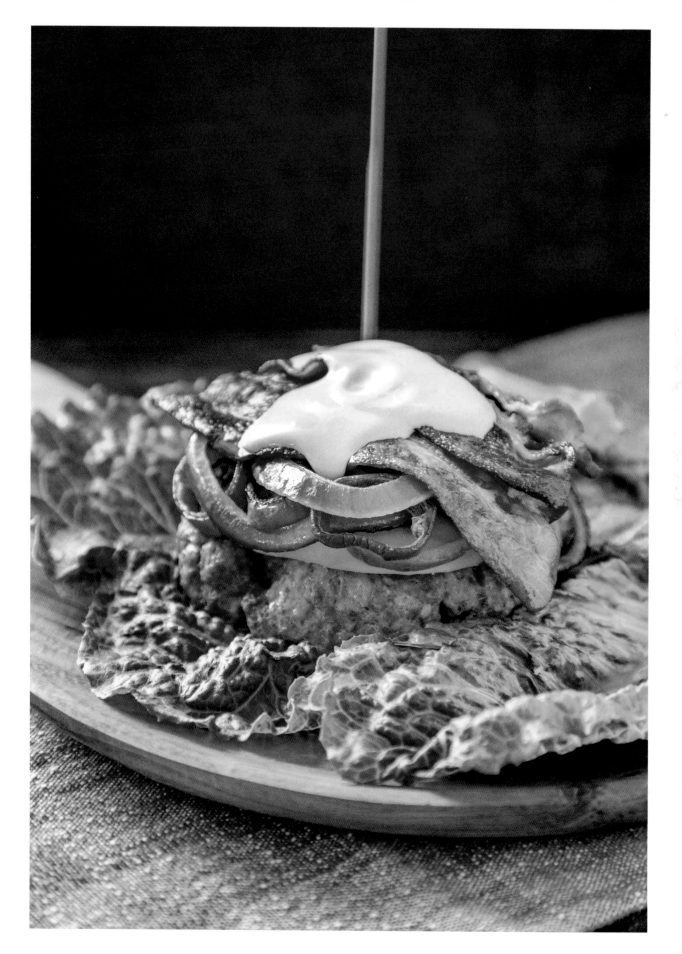

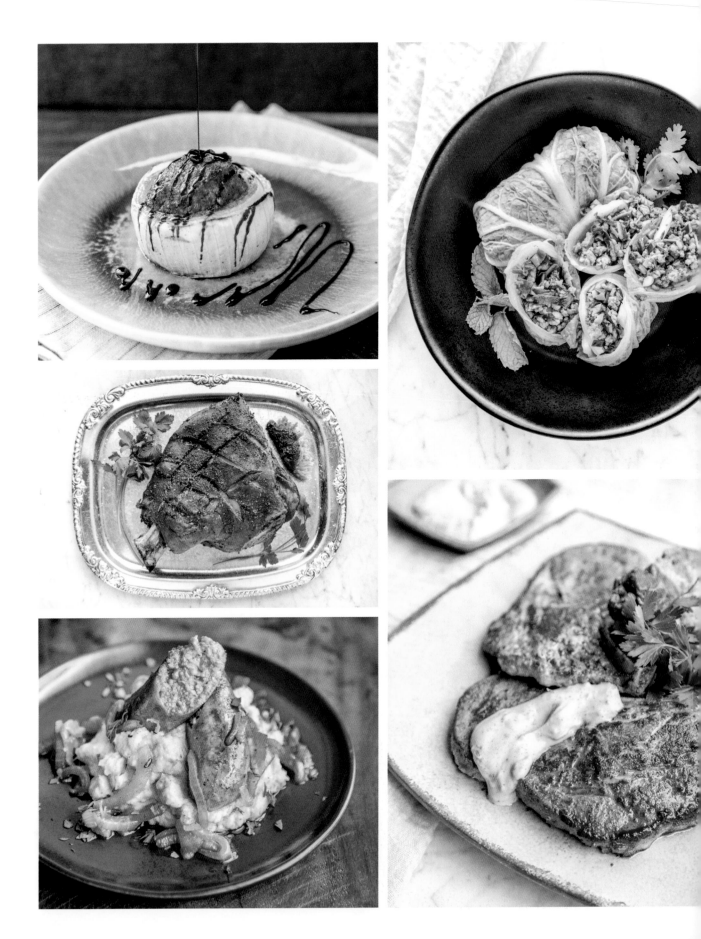

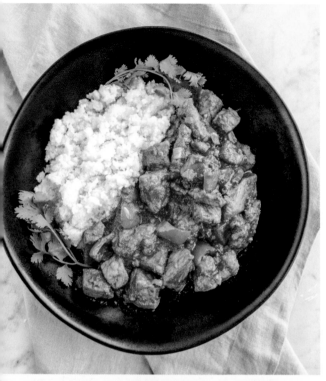

Pork

Pork & Pine Nut Eggplant Rollatini / 220

Ham Steaks with Redeye Gravy / 222

Bangers & Mash / 224

Inside-Out Egg Rolls / 226

Slow-Roasted Pork Shoulder / 228

Five-Spice Pork Chops / 230

Vindaloo / 232

Cajun Pork Tenderloin / 234

Sausage-Stuffed Onions with Balsamic Glaze / 236

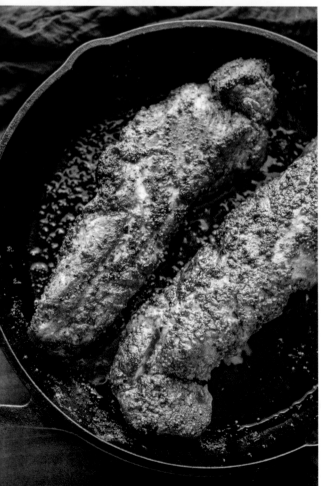

PORK & PINE NUT EGGPLANT ROLLATINI

YIELD: 5 servings | **SERVING SIZE:** 6 or 7 rolls + 3 tablespoons sauce | **PREP TIME:** 20 minutes | **COOK TIME:** 35 minutes

Go outside your comfort zone with this one—you'll be glad you did! This recipe is a little more labor-intensive than most of the others in this book, but the bold and unique flavors of these eggplant roll-ups make them worth the extra time. The spices give the pork filling a distinctive Middle Eastern flair, which is well complemented by the tangy tomato sauce and cooling effect of the fresh mint. If the eggplant is too stiff to roll, microwave it, uncovered, for 30 seconds or until just pliable. You can replace the eggplant with zucchini if you prefer.

For the sauce:

1 cup canned crushed tomatoes

2 tablespoons extra-virgin olive oil

1 tablespoon chopped fresh mint

1 teaspoon balsamic vinegar (no sugar added)

1 teaspoon dried onion flakes

½ teaspoon kosher salt

¼ teaspoon garlic powder

¼ teaspoon ground black pepper

For the filling:

1 pound ground pork

3 tablespoons pine nuts, roughly chopped

1 teaspoon kosher salt

1 teaspoon garam masala

½ teaspoon garlic powder

½ teaspoon ground coriander

½ teaspoon ground cumin

¼ teaspoon ground allspice

¼ teaspoon ground black pepper

4 long narrow eggplants, sliced lengthwise into 6-inch-long strips about ¼ inch thick

Roughly chopped fresh mint, for garnish

Pine nuts, for garnish

1. Preheat the oven to 375°F.

2. Put all the ingredients for the sauce in a medium-sized bowl. Stir well to combine, then spoon half of the sauce into a 10-inch ovenproof skillet or casserole dish. Set the remaining sauce aside.

3. Put all the ingredients for the filling in a separate medium-sized bowl. Mix with your hands or a spoon until fully combined.

4. Lay a slice of eggplant on a cutting board with a short end facing you. Spoon about 1 tablespoon of the pork filling onto the end closest to you, then roll up the eggplant and place the roll upright in the skillet. Repeat with the remaining eggplant slices and filling. If you have any extra eggplant, reserve it for another use. Spoon the remaining sauce over the eggplant rolls.

5. Bake for 35 minutes, or until the tops have turned golden brown and a thermometer inserted into the center of a roll reads 165°F. Serve hot. Garnish with fresh mint and extra pine nuts if desired. Store leftovers in an airtight container in the refrigerator for up to 5 days.

CALORIES: 300 **FAT:** 19g **PROTEIN:** 19g **CARBS:** 9g **FIBER:** 5g **NET CARBS:** 4g

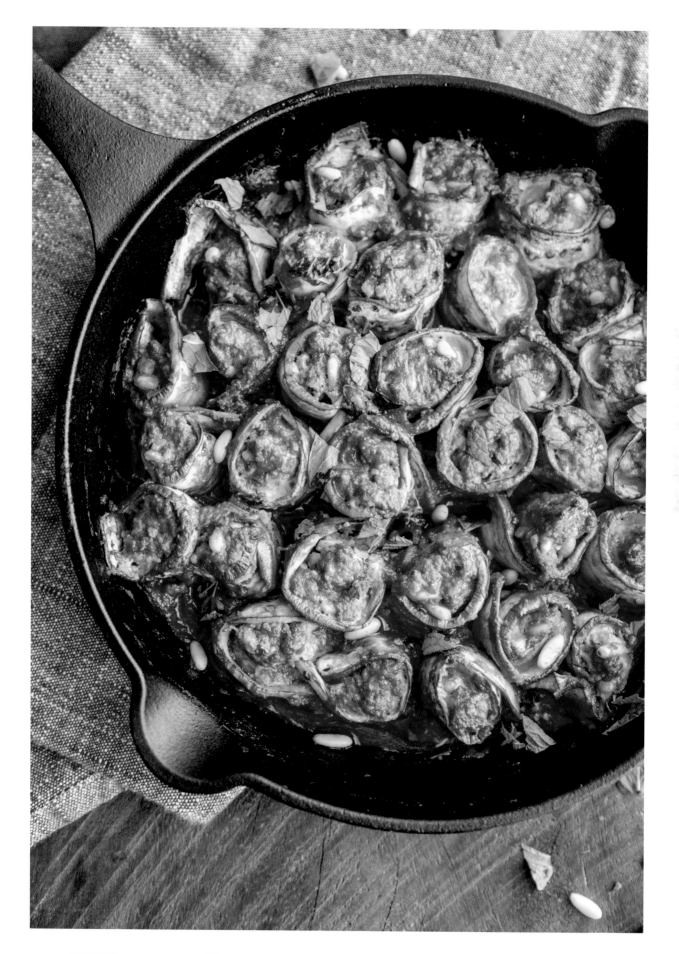

HAM STEAKS WITH REDEYE GRAVY

YIELD: 4 servings | **SERVING SIZE:** 1 steak + 2 tablespoons gravy | **PREP TIME:** 2 minutes | **COOK TIME:** 10 minutes

This recipe was inspired by a classic Southern dish of ham steaks served with a gravy made with coffee (hear me out) and bacon grease. Typically, it also contains molasses to make it sweet, but since molasses is a no-no on keto, I've used balsamic vinegar to give the gravy depth and a hint of sweetness while still being squeaky clean. This quick and easy recipe falls into the "don't knock it 'til you try it" category—salty ham and bitter coffee are a perfect match, made even better when you add a fluffy pile of my Garlic & Chive Cauliflower Mash (page 290) to the plate!

1 tablespoon bacon grease

4 (6-ounce) ham steaks, about ½ inch thick

¼ cup brewed coffee

¼ cup filtered water

1 tablespoon balsamic vinegar (no sugar added)

3 tablespoons cold butter, cut into 6 slices

1. Melt the bacon grease in a large skillet over medium-high heat. Add the ham steaks and cook for 3 minutes per side, or until golden brown. Remove the ham steaks to a serving platter.

2. Pour the coffee, water, and vinegar into the pan and bring to a boil. Scrape any bits of ham stuck to the bottom of the pan into the gravy. Cook for 2 minutes more, or until the liquid has reduced by about one-third. Remove the pan from the heat and whisk the cold butter into the gravy until melted. Pour the gravy over the ham steaks and serve immediately. Store leftovers in an airtight container in the refrigerator for up to 5 days.

CALORIES: 228 **FAT:** 15g **PROTEIN:** 20g **CARBS:** 3g **FIBER:** 0g **NET CARBS:** 3g

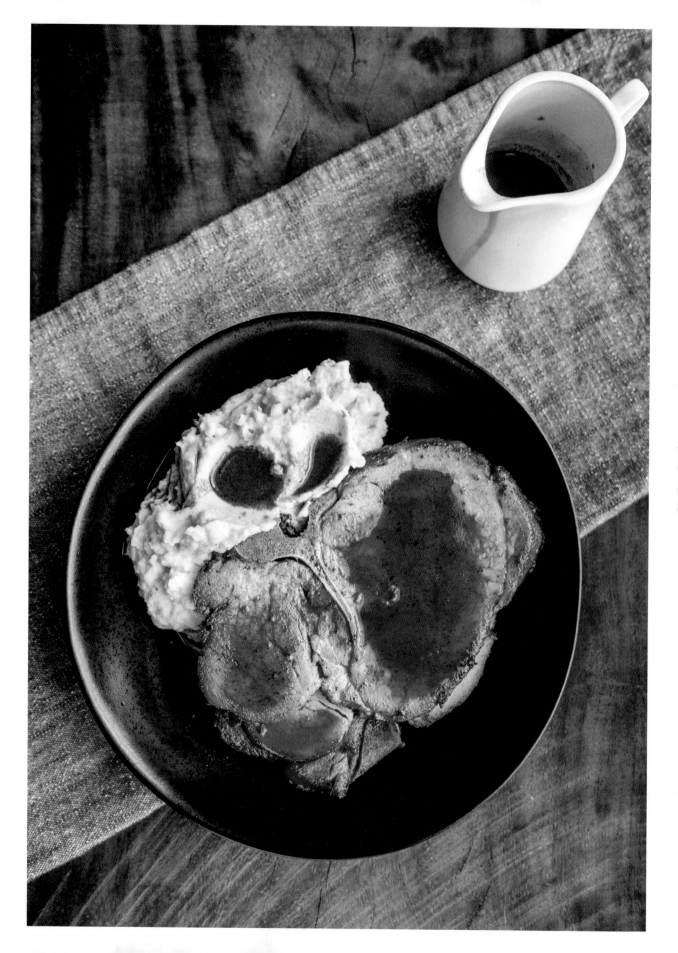

BANGERS & MASH

YIELD: 4 servings | SERVING SIZE: ½ cup mash + 1 sausage + 2 tablespoons gravy | PREP TIME: 5 minutes | COOK TIME: 20 minutes

Bangers and mash is a dish of British origin that traditionally consists of a bed of mashed potatoes topped with cooked sausage and a creamy onion gravy. My keto version is just as hearty and crave-worthy, but it uses my Garlic & Chive Cauliflower Mash as a base and omits the cream in the gravy to keep it squeaky. Fun fact: they call the sausages "bangers" because most sausages were made with a higher proportion of water during World War I when meat was rationed and hard to come by. Due to the water content, they had a tendency to explode during cooking. That's what we call dinner AND a show.

4 fresh pork sausages (about 6 ounces each)

1 cup sliced onions

2 tablespoons butter

1 tablespoon extra-virgin olive oil

⅓ cup chicken broth, store-bought or homemade (page 72)

1 teaspoon red wine vinegar

½ teaspoon kosher salt

¼ teaspoon ground black pepper

1 batch Garlic & Chive Cauliflower Mash (page 290), hot

2 tablespoons chopped fresh parsley, for garnish

1. Place the sausages in a large skillet and cook over medium heat for about 3 minutes per side, until golden brown and cooked through. Remove from the pan and set aside.

2. Add the onions, butter, and olive oil to the skillet and cook, still over medium heat, for about 7 minutes, until the onions have browned and softened. Add the broth, vinegar, salt, and pepper to the pan and simmer over low heat for 5 minutes, or until the gravy has thickened enough to coat a spoon.

3. Cut the sausages in half crosswise and return them to the pan. Cook for 2 minutes, or until heated through. To serve, place ½ cup of the hot cauliflower mash on a plate. Top with 2 sausage halves and 2 tablespoons of the onion gravy. Garnish with fresh parsley. Store leftovers in an airtight container in the refrigerator for up to 5 days.

CALORIES: 510   FAT: 44g   PROTEIN: 17g   CARBS: 12g   FIBER: 4g   NET CARBS: 8g

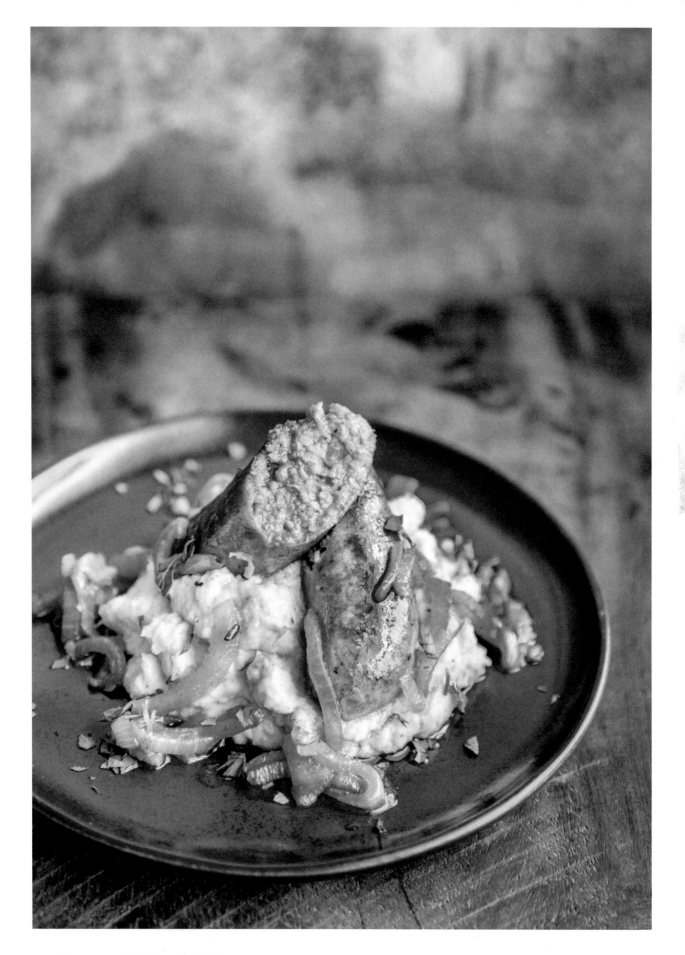

INSIDE-OUT EGG ROLLS

YIELD: 8 rolls | **SERVING SIZE:** 2 rolls | **PREP TIME:** 20 minutes | **COOK TIME:** 10 minutes

This recipe for inside-out egg rolls is one of my favorites in this book. These beauties are loaded with luscious ground pork, all your favorite Asian flavors, lots of texture from the chopped chestnuts, and a medley of fresh herbs to finish. They are bright, fresh, and fun to eat—you'll want to make them over and over again!

For the filling:

1 tablespoon toasted sesame oil

¼ cup chopped water chestnuts

1 tablespoon minced fresh ginger

1 teaspoon minced garlic

1 pound ground pork

1 cup shredded napa cabbage

½ cup shredded red cabbage

1 tablespoon coconut aminos

1 tablespoon fish sauce (no sugar added)

1 tablespoon rice wine vinegar (no sugar added)

1 tablespoon Sriracha sauce

½ teaspoon kosher salt

¼ cup sliced scallions

¼ cup roughly chopped fresh cilantro

¼ cup roughly chopped fresh mint

8 large napa cabbage leaves, for wrapping

1. Heat the sesame oil in a large skillet over medium heat. Add the water chestnuts, ginger, and garlic and cook, stirring occasionally, for 2 minutes, or until fragrant. Add the ground pork and cook, stirring frequently to break it up, until the meat is browned and cooked through, about 5 minutes. Add the shredded napa and red cabbage, coconut aminos, fish sauce, vinegar, Sriracha, and salt. Stir and cook for 3 minutes, or until the cabbage is wilted. Stir in the scallions, cilantro, and mint and remove the pan from the heat.

2. Rinse the napa cabbage leaves well and microwave on a large microwave-safe plate, uncovered, for 3 to 5 minutes, until semi-wilted and pliable but not fully cooked.

3. Place a cabbage leaf on a flat surface and spoon about ⅓ cup of the filling onto the center of the leaf. Start rolling away from you, tucking the ends in toward the center over the filling to keep it inside. Roll all the way to the edge, then carefully transfer the egg roll to a platter. Repeat 7 more times until all the rolls are made. Serve immediately. Store leftovers in an airtight container in the refrigerator for up to 5 days.

Note: You can slice the egg rolls in half for a prettier presentation, but they are easier to eat and will hold together a little better if you don't cut them.

CALORIES: 340 **FAT:** 24g **PROTEIN:** 22g **CARBS:** 6g **FIBER:** 2g **NET CARBS:** 4g

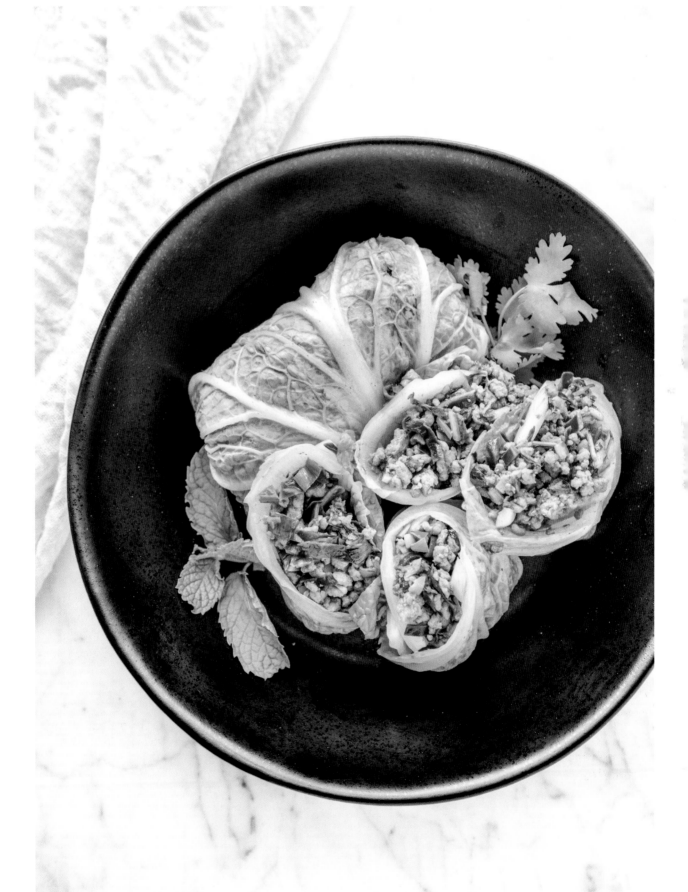

SLOW-ROASTED PORK SHOULDER

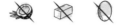

YIELD: 15 servings | SERVING SIZE: 4 ounces cooked pork | PREP TIME: 5 minutes, plus 30 minutes to rest | COOK TIME: 6 hours 20 minutes

I don't know that there is a more enticing smell than a slab of pork roasting in the oven all day. It's torture the entire time, but then comes the big payoff when you get to eat it! This recipe makes about 15 servings, so it's great for gatherings or large families. You can serve this pork roast with a variety of veggie sides to make a complete meal, then use the leftover meat in wraps and salads for lunches during the week.

For the seasoning blend:

2 tablespoons kosher salt

2 tablespoons garlic powder

1 tablespoon dried oregano leaves

1 tablespoon ground black pepper

1 tablespoon ground cumin

1 tablespoon onion powder

1 tablespoon smoked paprika

1 (8-pound) bone-in pork shoulder

1. Preheat the oven to 500°F.

2. Combine the ingredients for the seasoning blend in a small bowl.

3. Make slices just through the layer of fat on the top of the pork roast in a diamond pattern. Rub the seasoning blend all over the roast and into the slices you made in the fat. Place the roast fat side up in a large roasting pan.

4. Roast, uncovered, for 20 minutes. Reduce the oven temperature to 300°F and roast the pork, still uncovered, for an additional 6 hours. Remove the roast from the oven, cover loosely with foil, and let it rest for 30 minutes. Remove the crispy fat cap and break or chop it into chips. Slice or shred the meat and remove any large chunks of fat or gristle before serving. Store leftovers in an airtight container in the refrigerator for up to 5 days or in the freezer for up to 3 months.

CALORIES: 275 | FAT: 15g | PROTEIN: 33g | CARBS: 0g | FIBER: 0g | NET CARBS: 0g

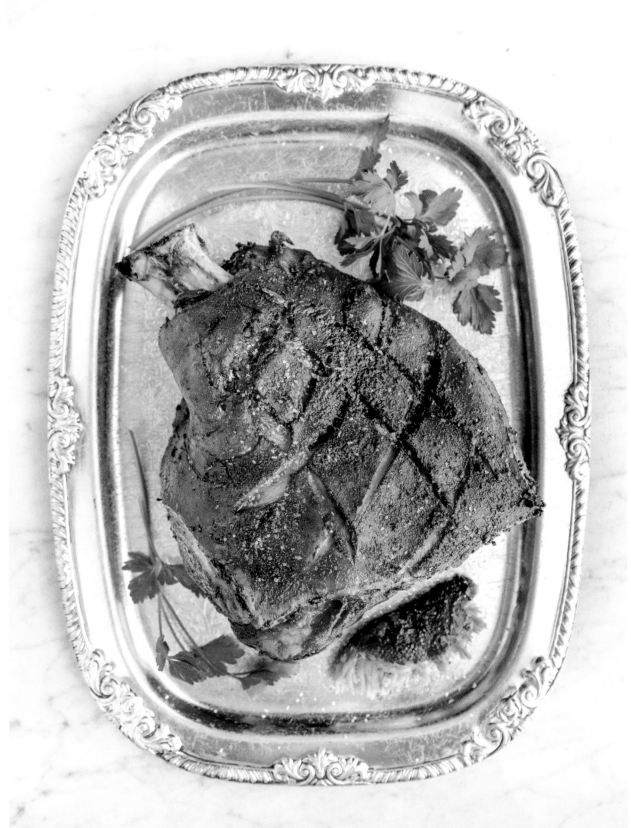

FIVE-SPICE PORK CHOPS

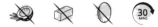

YIELD: 4 chops | SERVING SIZE: 1 chop | PREP TIME: 5 minutes | COOK TIME: 8 minutes

These easy pork chops can be made in just minutes and have a tasty Asian flair from the five-spice powder, which can be purchased in most grocery stores in the spice aisle. I paired them with my Chili-Lime Mayo (page 100), which has a spicy tartness that is a perfect complement to the chops—it's a combination I highly recommend. To make a complete meal, try pairing these chops with Easy Sesame Broccoli (page 294) and Creamy Coconut Cauliflower Rice (page 296).

4 (6-ounce) bone-in pork chops

2 teaspoons Chinese five-spice powder

1 teaspoon kosher salt

1 tablespoon avocado oil or other light-tasting oil

1 teaspoon toasted sesame oil

1. Coat the pork chops in the five-spice powder and salt.

2. Heat the avocado oil and sesame oil in a large skillet over medium-high heat. Add the pork chops to the pan and cook for about 4 minutes per side, until golden brown and cooked through. Remove from the pan and let rest for 5 minutes before serving. Store leftovers in an airtight container in the refrigerator for up to 5 days.

CALORIES: 480 FAT: 33g PROTEIN: 43g CARBS: 0g FIBER: 0g NET CARBS: 0g

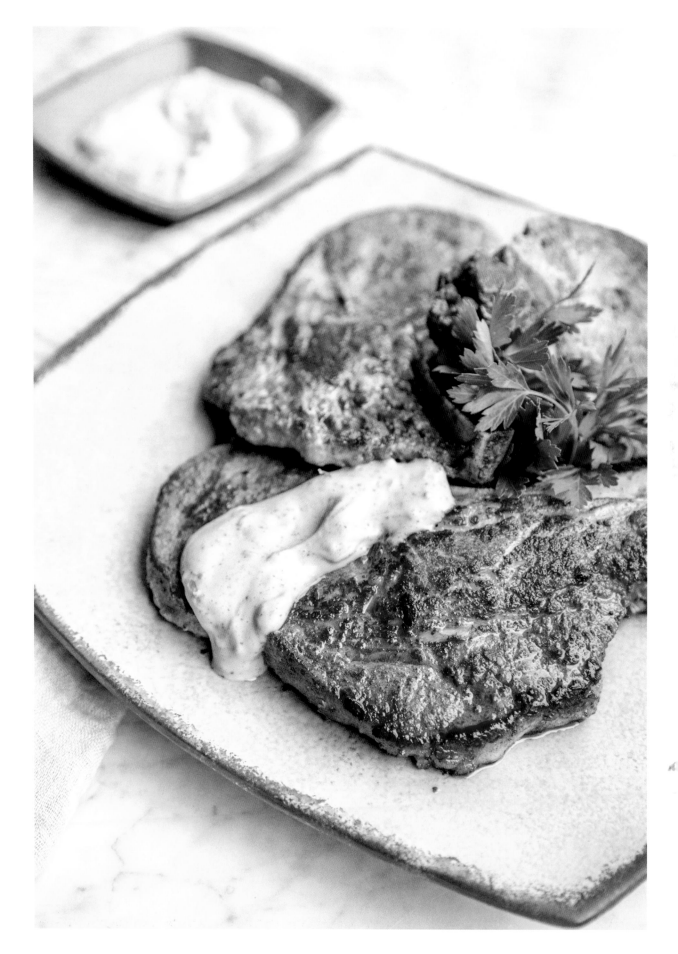

VINDALOO

YIELD: 6 servings | **SERVING SIZE:** ¾ cup | **PREP TIME:** 10 minutes | **COOK TIME:** 20 minutes

---

You've probably noticed that there are a lot of curry recipes in this book. What can I say? I love a good curry! With its spicy tomato base, sweet red peppers, and hint of cloves, this vindaloo might be my favorite curry of them all. You can find vindaloo made with chicken or beef, but pork is the most traditional. I recommend that you serve this dish with cauliflower rice to soak up every last bit of that fiery sauce!

3 tablespoons avocado oil or other light-tasting oil

½ cup chopped red bell peppers

⅓ cup chopped onions

3 cloves garlic, minced

1 tablespoon ground cumin

1 tablespoon red pepper flakes

1 teaspoon ginger powder

1 teaspoon ground cinnamon

1 teaspoon ground coriander

1 teaspoon kosher salt

½ teaspoon ground cardamom

½ teaspoon turmeric powder

¼ teaspoon mustard powder

⅛ teaspoon ground cloves

3 bay leaves

1½ pounds pork loin, cut into bite-sized pieces

½ cup canned crushed tomatoes

½ cup filtered water

2 tablespoons apple cider vinegar

1 tablespoon coconut aminos

1. Heat the oil in a medium-sized saucepan over medium heat. Add the bell peppers, onions, and garlic and cook for 2 to 3 minutes, until soft. Add the cumin, red pepper flakes, ginger powder, cinnamon, coriander, salt, cardamom, turmeric, mustard powder, cloves, and bay leaves to the vegetables. Cook for about 2 minutes, until fragrant.

2. Add the pork pieces to the saucepan and cook, stirring occasionally, for about 5 minutes, until browned. Add the crushed tomatoes, water, vinegar, and coconut aminos and bring to a boil. Reduce the heat and simmer for 10 minutes, or until the pork is cooked through and tender. Remove the bay leaves and serve hot. Store leftovers in an airtight container in the refrigerator for up to 5 days or in the freezer for up to 3 months.

Note: If you don't eat pork, you can substitute the same amount of chicken or beef. The cook time will remain the same. You can also make this recipe with shrimp, but if you do, reduce the final cooking time from 10 minutes to 5 minutes so you don't overcook the shrimp.

CALORIES: 241 | **FAT:** 10g | **PROTEIN:** 27g | **CARBS:** 5g | **FIBER:** 1g | **NET CARBS:** 4g

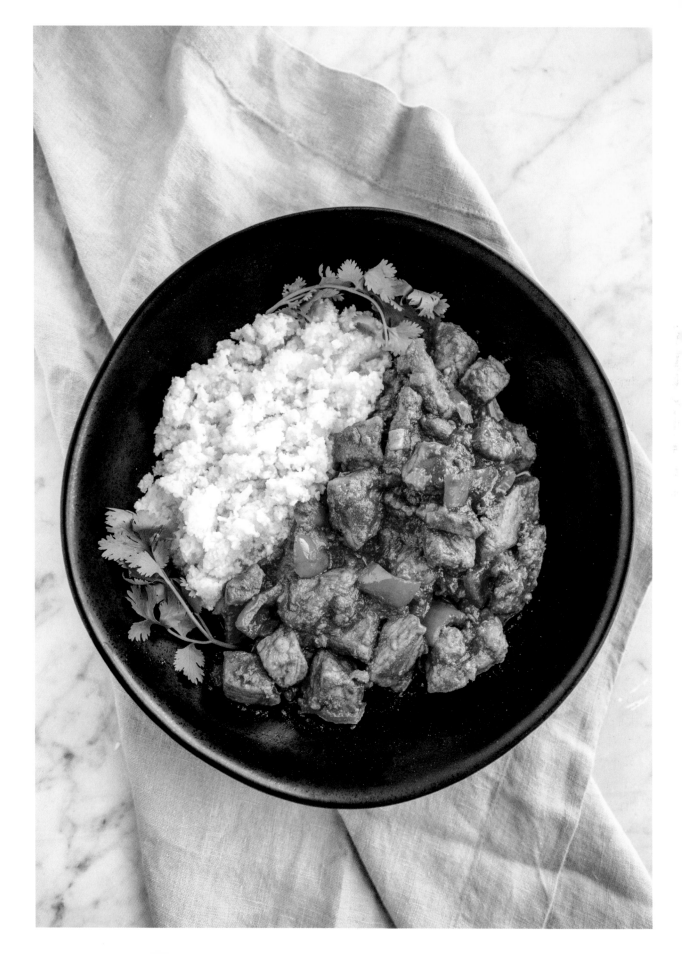

CAJUN PORK TENDERLOIN

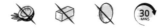

YIELD: 10 servings	**SERVING SIZE:** 4 ounces	**PREP TIME:** 5 minutes	**COOK TIME:** 18 minutes

Just a few ingredients (literally) and less than half an hour are all that are standing between you and this crispy, spicy, juicy Cajun-seasoned pork tenderloin. This flavorful and picky-eater-approved meat can be served alone, but the Creamy Garlic Sauce on page 106 or the addicting All-Purpose Green Sauce on page 98 would make it even more delectable. Perfect for meal prep, this tenderloin can be added to cold wraps or salads all week long.

3 pounds pork tenderloin, silver membrane removed

1 tablespoon avocado oil or other light-tasting oil

2 tablespoons Cajun seasoning

1. Preheat the oven to 400°F.

2. Rub the tenderloin with the oil, then coat it liberally with the Cajun seasoning on all sides.

3. Heat a large cast-iron or other oven-safe heavy-bottomed skillet over high heat. Place the tenderloin in the hot pan and sear for 3 minutes, then turn and sear for an additional 3 minutes on the other side.

4. Transfer the skillet to the hot oven and roast uncovered for 12 minutes, or until a meat thermometer inserted in the thickest part of the tenderloin reads 155°F. (As the meat rests, the temperature will continue to rise due to carryover heat.) Remove the pan from the oven and let the meat rest for 10 minutes before slicing and serving. Store leftovers in an airtight container in the refrigerator for up to 5 days or in the freezer for up to 3 months.

CALORIES: 221   **FAT:** 8g   **PROTEIN:** 35g   **CARBS:** 0g   **FIBER:** 0g   **NET CARBS:** 0g

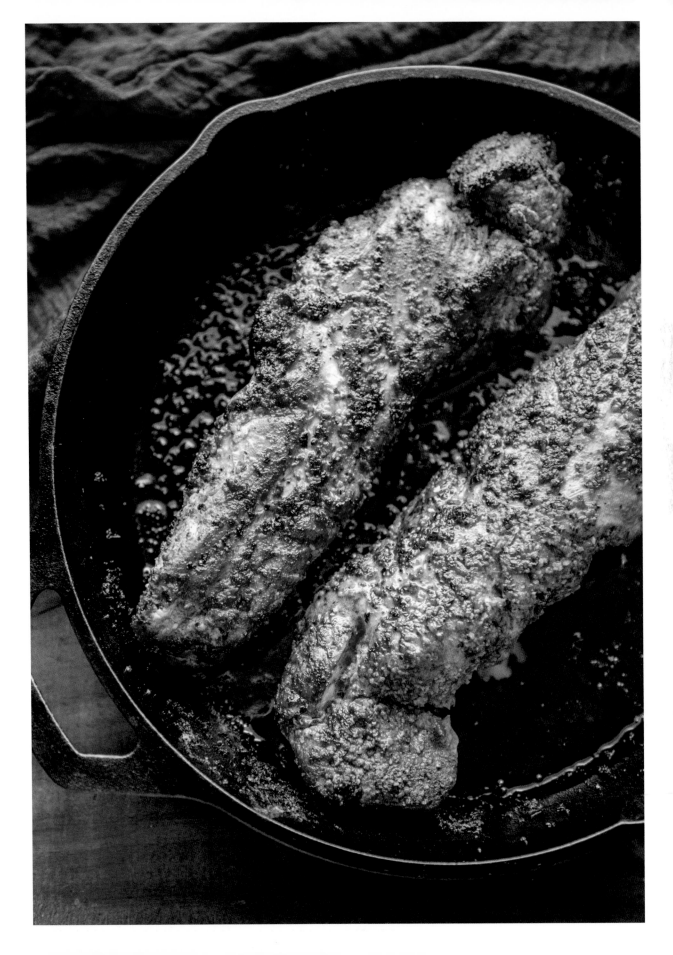

SAUSAGE-STUFFED ONIONS WITH BALSAMIC GLAZE

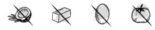

| YIELD: 4 stuffed onions | SERVING SIZE: 1 stuffed onion | PREP TIME: 15 minutes | COOK TIME: 45 minutes |

You can serve these sausage-stuffed onions with a salad and a side for a complete meal, but they also make an impressive first course or appetizer when you're entertaining guests. You can turn this into a two-bite finger food for an appetizer tray by using smaller onions and dividing the pork into 1-inch balls, which should give you around 16 pieces.

1 pound breakfast sausage

4 medium onions (about 6 ounces each)

2 teaspoons Easy Balsamic Glaze (page 86)

1. Preheat the oven to 375°F.

2. Cut the bottom ½ inch and the top inch off of each onion. Peel off the skins. Cut a 1-inch X in the center of each onion with a sharp knife. Using a knife or spoon, remove the cut pieces from the centers of the onions. Peel the remaining layers from the inside by hand and pull them through the top, leaving a ½-inch rim of onion (about 3 layers).

3. Open the sausage and divide it into 4 portions. Pack the center of each onion with a portion of the sausage.

4. Place the stuffed onions on a sheet pan and bake for 45 minutes, or until the onions have softened and browned and the sausage is cooked through. Remove from the oven and drizzle with the glaze before serving. Store leftovers in an airtight container in the refrigerator for up to 5 days.

CALORIES: 367   FAT: 30g   PROTEIN: 17g   CARBS: 6g   FIBER: 1g   NET CARBS: 5g

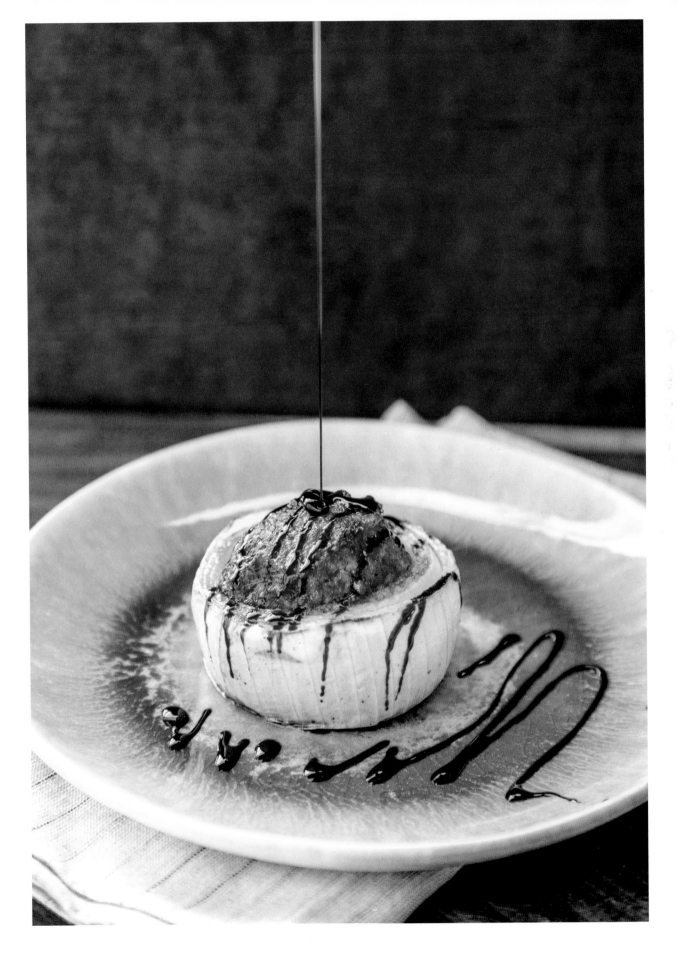

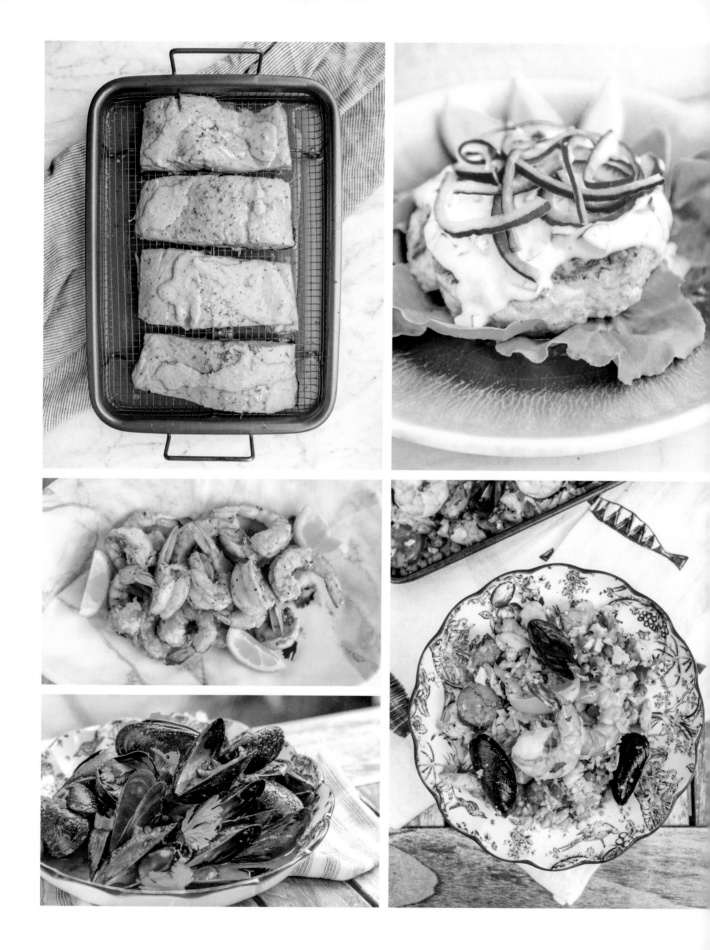

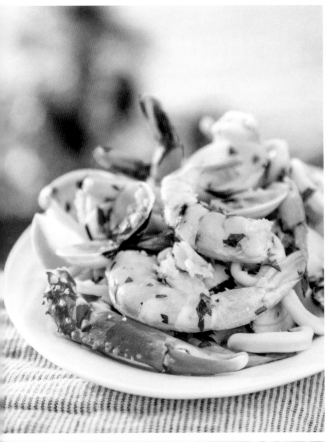

Seafood

Shrimp Piccata with Zoodles / 240

Oven-Roasted Cajun Shrimp / 242

Chilled Seafood Salad / 244

Salmon Burgers / 246

Coriander & Wasabi–Crusted Tuna / 248

Easy Baked Salmon / 250

Fish Curry / 252

Fried Calamari / 254

Brazilian Shrimp Stew (Moqueca de Camarones) / 256

Molcajete Mixto / 258

Mussels in Thai Coconut Broth / 260

Crab Cakes / 262

Sheet Pan Paella / 264

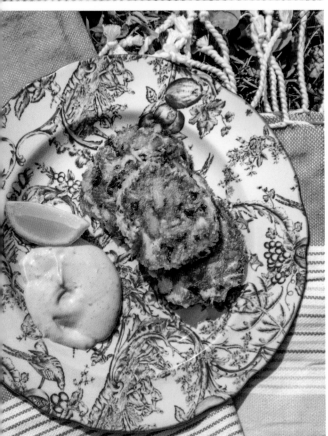

SHRIMP PICCATA WITH ZOODLES

YIELD: 4 servings | **SERVING SIZE:** 2 cups | **PREP TIME:** 5 minutes | **COOK TIME:** 8 minutes

This easy dinner recipe delivers the traditional lemon, caper, and butter flavors of a piccata but substitutes shrimp for the chicken that is typically used. Served on a bed of squeaky clean zoodles, this zesty and delicious one-pot wonder has it all—no sides required.

¼ cup (½ stick) butter

2 tablespoons capers, drained

1 tablespoon grated lemon zest

½ teaspoon kosher salt

¼ teaspoon ground black pepper

1 pound large shrimp, peeled and deveined

4 cups zucchini noodles (about 3 medium zucchini)

2 tablespoons chopped fresh parsley, for garnish

Lemon wedges, for garnish (optional)

Melt the butter in a large skillet over medium-high heat. Add the capers, lemon zest, salt, and pepper and cook for 1 minute, or until fragrant. Add the shrimp to the pan and cook, stirring occasionally, for about 3 minutes, until the shrimp are turning opaque. Add the zucchini noodles and stir. Cook for another 3 minutes, or until the zucchini has softened slightly and the shrimp are fully cooked. Garnish with chopped parsley and serve lemon wedges if desired. Store leftovers in an airtight container in the refrigerator for up to 5 days.

CALORIES: 237 **FAT:** 14g **PROTEIN:** 24g **CARBS:** 4g **FIBER:** 1g **NET CARBS:** 3g

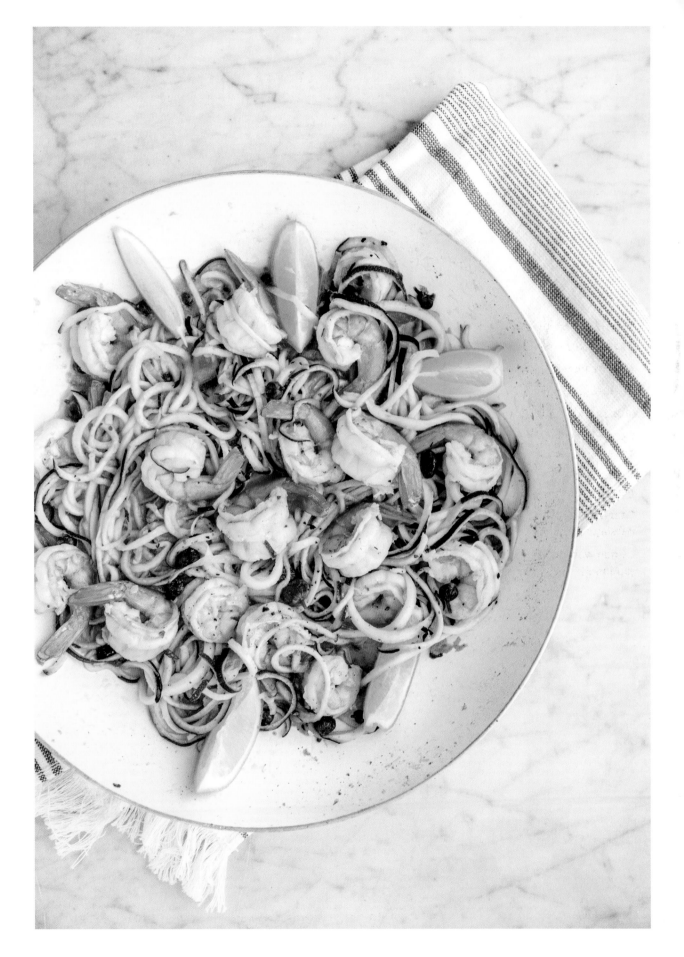

OVEN-ROASTED CAJUN SHRIMP

YIELD: 6 servings | **SERVING SIZE:** 4 ounces | **PREP TIME:** 5 minutes | **COOK TIME:** 5 minutes

It doesn't get much easier than this oven-roasted shrimp recipe. If you haven't tried roasting shrimp, you've been missing out! While boiling leaches flavor out of the shrimp, roasting concentrates the sweetness and gives them a toasty exterior while keeping the interior sweet and juicy—as long as you don't overcook them, that is! These salty and mildly spicy shrimp are made even better by a dunk in my Creamy Garlic Sauce (page 106) or All-Purpose Green Sauce (page 98).

2 pounds jumbo shrimp, peeled and deveined

2½ tablespoons Cajun seasoning

1 tablespoon avocado oil or other light-tasting oil

1 tablespoon fresh lemon juice

1. Preheat the oven to 400°F. Line a sheet pan with parchment paper.

2. Place the shrimp, Cajun seasoning, and oil on the prepared sheet pan. Stir until the shrimp are coated in the oil and seasoning. Spread out the shrimp so they are not touching.

3. Roast for 5 minutes, or until the shrimp are opaque and slightly firm to the touch. Remove from the oven and sprinkle with the lemon juice before serving. Store leftovers in an airtight container in the refrigerator for up to 5 days.

CALORIES: 145 **FAT:** 6g **PROTEIN:** 23g **CARBS:** 1g **FIBER:** 0g **NET CARBS:** 1g

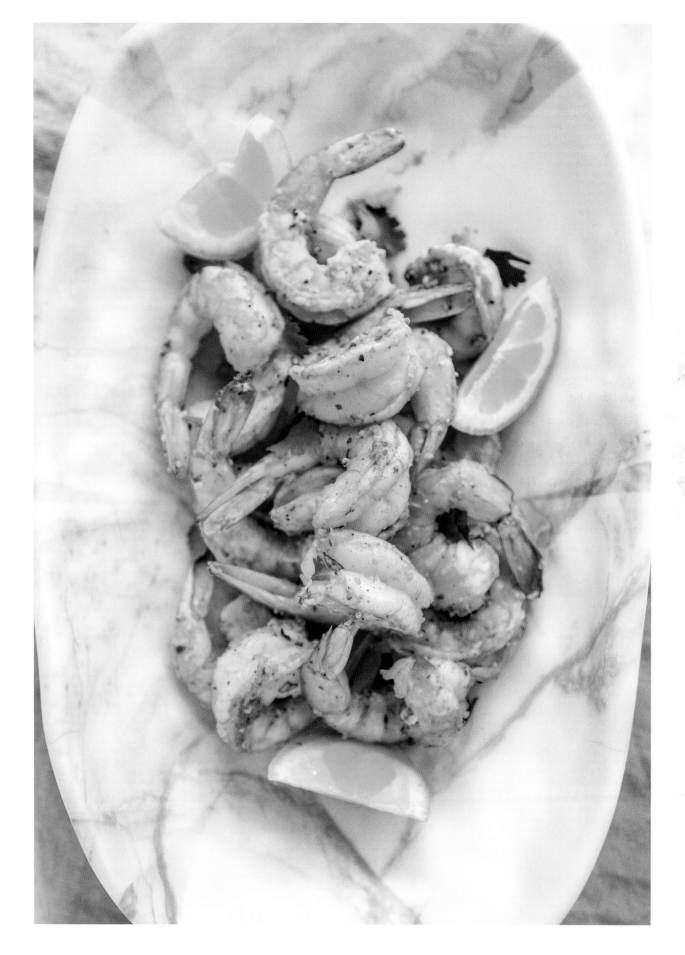

CHILLED SEAFOOD SALAD

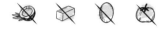

| YIELD: 6 servings | SERVING SIZE: 1 pound prepared salad (with shells) |
| PREP TIME: 10 minutes, plus at least 1 hour to chill | COOK TIME: 9 minutes |

This platter of succulent chilled seafood bathed in a fresh and tangy lemon herb dressing makes for an impressive brunch or first course when entertaining. Or you can just make it and hoard it all to yourself—no judgment here.

2 pounds small clams

2 pounds frozen crab legs, thawed

1 pound jumbo shrimp, peeled and deveined, tails on

1 pound frozen squid rings, thawed

For the dressing:

1 tablespoon grated lemon zest

¼ cup fresh lemon juice

3 tablespoons extra-virgin olive oil

1 teaspoon white vinegar

2 tablespoons chopped fresh parsley

1 teaspoon minced garlic

1 teaspoon kosher salt

¼ teaspoon ground black pepper

1. Bring a large pot of salted water to a boil. Add the clams, crab legs, and shrimp and cook for 7 minutes, or until the clams have opened. Using a slotted spoon, transfer the seafood to a large bowl of ice water to halt the cooking. Add the squid rings to the boiling water and cook for just 2 minutes. Remove with the slotted spoon and add to the ice water.

2. Put the lemon zest, lemon juice, olive oil, vinegar, parsley, garlic, salt, and pepper in a large bowl and whisk to combine.

3. Drain the cooled seafood thoroughly and add it to the bowl with the dressing. Stir well to coat the seafood in the dressing. Place in the refrigerator to chill for at least 1 hour or up to 12 hours. Stir well before serving. Store leftovers in an airtight container in the refrigerator for up to 3 days.

CALORIES: 293 | FAT: 6g | PROTEIN: 43g | CARBS: 4g | FIBER: 0g | NET CARBS: 4g

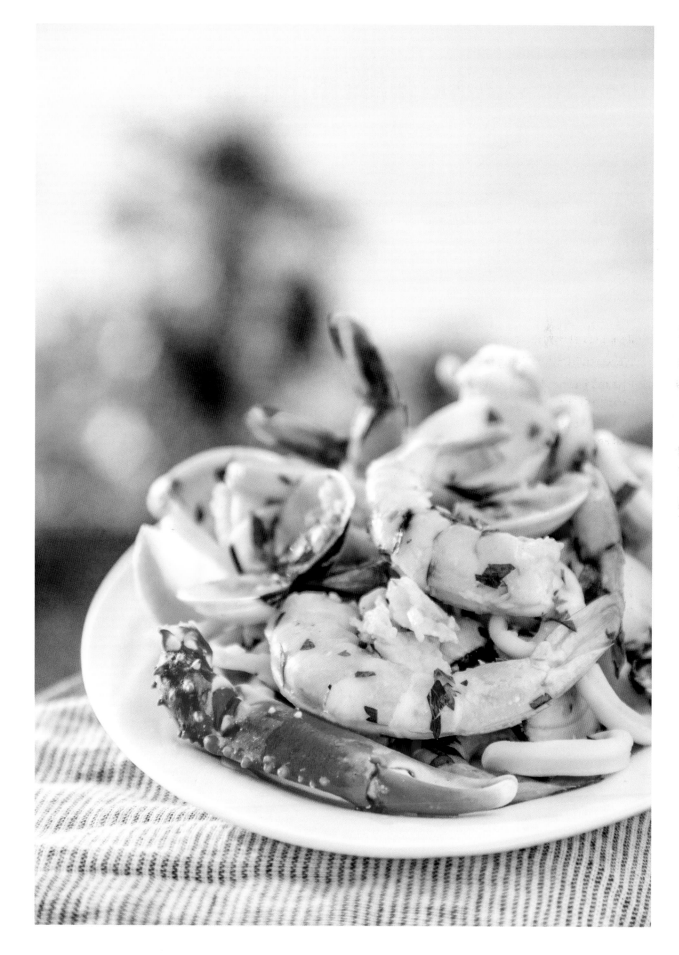

SALMON BURGERS

| YIELD: 4 burgers | SERVING SIZE: 1 burger | PREP TIME: 8 minutes | COOK TIME: 6 minutes |

These juicy salmon burgers are simple to make and a fun departure from the typical beef burger. You can have them made in 15 minutes from start to finish, making this a perfect weeknight meal. As an added bonus, they are equally delicious hot or cold, so you can enjoy them for lunch all week long. I recommend pairing them with my Dill Caper Tartar Sauce (page 104) and Quick-Pickled Red Onions (page 108), as shown here.

1 pound fresh salmon fillets (without skin), chopped

¼ cup mayonnaise

1 tablespoon chopped fresh parsley

1 teaspoon grated lime zest

1 teaspoon fresh lime juice

2 tablespoons coconut flour

½ teaspoon kosher salt

1 tablespoon avocado oil or other light-tasting oil, for frying

Lettuce leaves, for serving

Condiments of your choice, for serving

1. Put the salmon, mayonnaise, parsley, lime zest, lime juice, coconut flour, and salt in a medium-sized bowl. Mix well with your hands and form into 4 equal-size patties about 1 inch thick.

2. Heat the oil in a large nonstick skillet over medium heat until shimmering. Gently place the salmon patties in the pan and cook for about 3 minutes per side, until cooked through. Remove from the pan.

3. Serve on a bed of lettuce with your choice of condiments. Store leftovers in an airtight container in the refrigerator for up to 5 days.

CALORIES: 312 | FAT: 13g | PROTEIN: 23g | CARBS: 2g | FIBER: 1g | NET CARBS: 1g

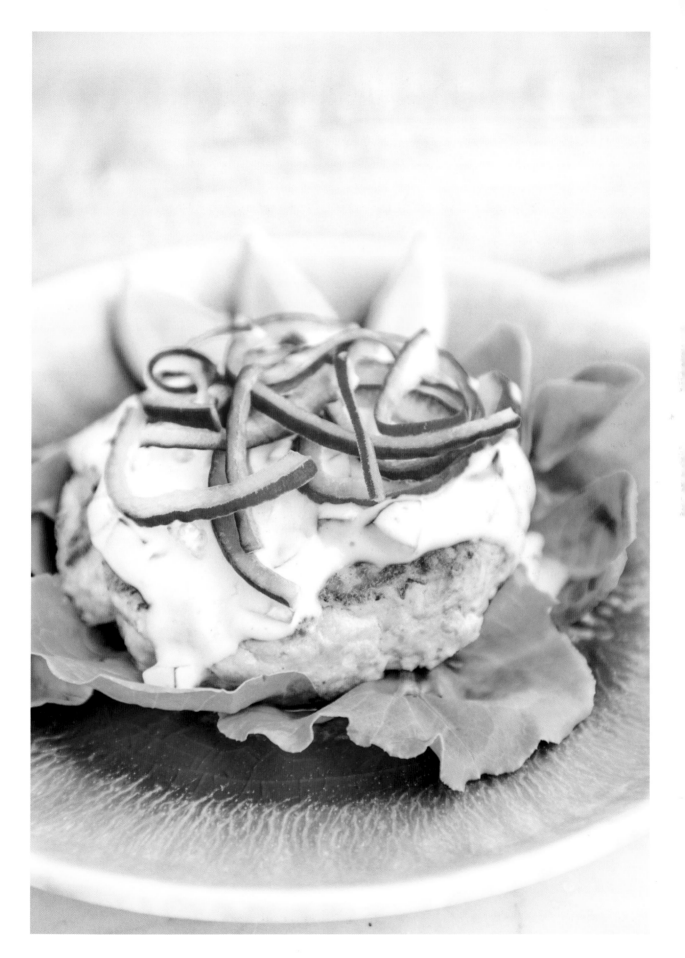

CORIANDER & WASABI-CRUSTED TUNA

  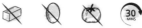

YIELD: 4 servings | **SERVING SIZE:** 4 ounces | **PREP TIME:** 5 minutes | **COOK TIME:** 4 minutes

Don't be intimidated by cooking tuna at home—it's surprisingly easy and takes almost no time at all. Because tuna is a meaty fish, it stands up well to the bold flavors of this spice paste. You can serve it medium-rare as shown here or sashimi style with just a quick sear (about 45 seconds per side) and the center very rare. I recommend pairing it with my Sesame Ginger Dressing (page 90) and cauliflower rice, as pictured.

1 tablespoon coriander seeds

2 teaspoons wasabi powder

1 teaspoon ginger powder

¼ teaspoon kosher salt

1 tablespoon coconut aminos

1 pound ahi tuna steaks

1 tablespoon avocado oil or other light-tasting oil

1. Put the coriander seeds, wasabi, ginger, salt, and coconut aminos in a small blender or food processor and blend into a paste. Coat the tuna steaks completely in the paste, pressing it into the surface.

2. Heat the oil in a medium-sized skillet over high heat until shimmering. Add the tuna steaks and sear for about 2 minutes per side for a medium-rare interior. Remove from the pan and allow to rest for 5 minutes before slicing and serving. Store leftovers in an airtight container in the refrigerator for up to 3 days.

CALORIES: 208 **FAT:** 8g **PROTEIN:** 29g **CARBS:** 1g **FIBER:** 0g **NET CARBS:** 1g

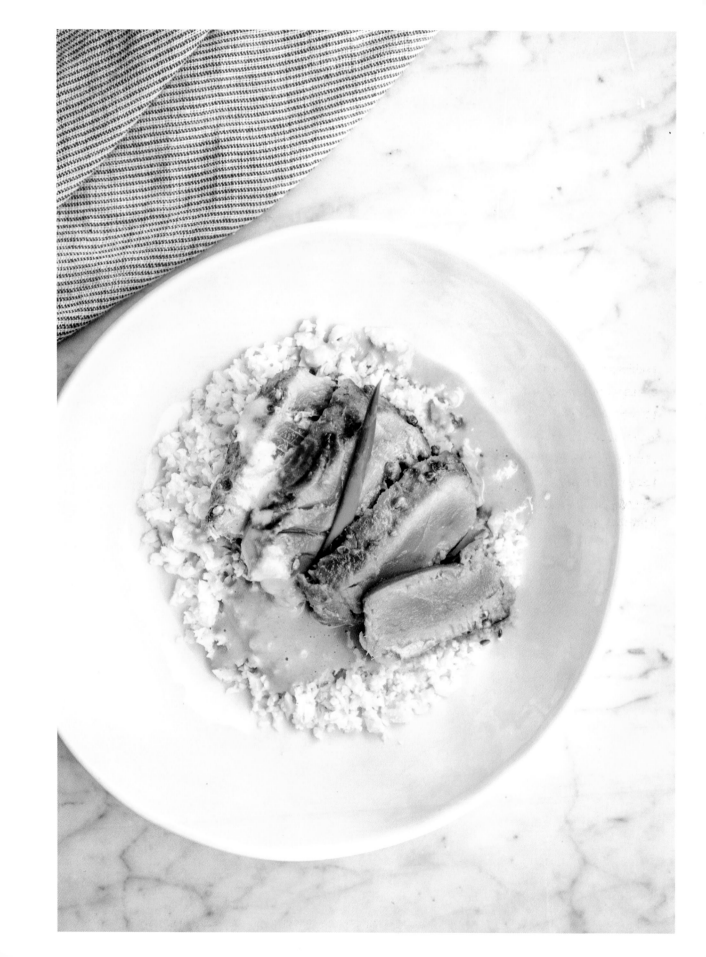

EASY BAKED SALMON

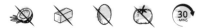

| YIELD: 4 servings | SERVING SIZE: 1 fillet | PREP TIME: 5 minutes | COOK TIME: 18 minutes |

Because of its high fat content, salmon is well suited to baking—as long as you bake it gently at a low heat. This simple preparation is not only easy but allows the flavor and texture of the salmon to shine, without a lot of other ingredients competing for center stage. That being said, I highly recommend introducing this salmon to my All-Purpose Green Sauce (page 98)—I promise they will get along swimmingly. (Sorry, had to.)

4 (6-ounce) salmon fillets, with skin

1 tablespoon extra-virgin olive oil

1 teaspoon kosher salt

¼ teaspoon ground black pepper

½ teaspoon grated lime zest

4 lime wedges

1. Preheat the oven to 325°F.

2. Pat the salmon fillets dry and place them skin side down on a sheet pan. Brush the fillets with the olive oil. Sprinkle with the salt, pepper, and lime zest.

3. Bake for 18 minutes, or until the fillets are light pink in the center and slightly firm to the touch. Remove from the oven and let rest for 5 minutes. Finish with a squeeze of lime juice before serving. Store leftovers in an airtight container in the refrigerator for up to 3 days.

CALORIES: 341 **FAT:** 22g **PROTEIN:** 34g **CARBS:** 0g **FIBER:** 0g **NET CARBS:** 0g

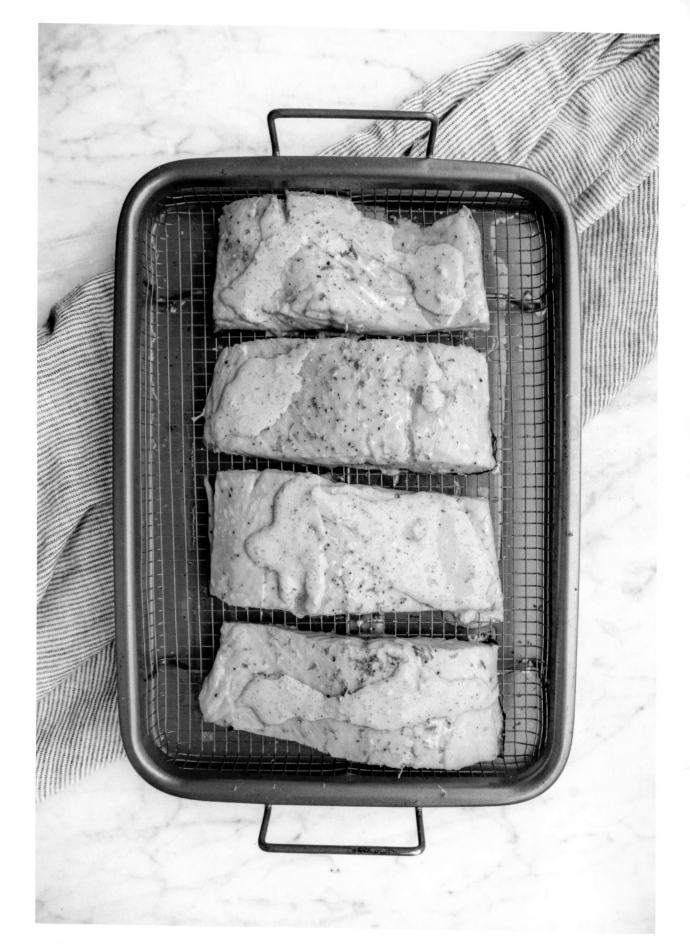

FISH CURRY

YIELD: 4 servings	SERVING SIZE: 1 fillet + ¼ cup sauce	PREP TIME: 10 minutes	COOK TIME: 15 minutes

This fish curry isn't so much a stewed curry as it is fried fish served with a curry sauce. The crunchy texture of the fried fish marries so perfectly with the lush and velvety sauce that it may just bring a tear to your eye. Or maybe that's just me. What can I say, I told you I love a good curry!

For the fish:

1 (1-pound) white fish fillet (without skin), such as snapper, cod, or haddock

⅓ cup Sun-Flour (page 74)

½ teaspoon garlic powder

½ teaspoon smoked paprika

½ teaspoon kosher salt

¼ teaspoon ground black pepper

1 large egg, beaten

¼ cup avocado oil or other light-tasting oil, for frying

For the curry sauce:

1 tablespoon avocado oil

2 tablespoons red curry paste

1 cup canned coconut milk

1 tablespoon fish sauce (no sugar added)

1 teaspoon chopped red chilis, such as bird's eye or ripe serrano

¼ cup chopped fresh cilantro, for garnish

1. **Fry the fish:** Cut the fish into 4 equal-size pieces. Combine the flour, garlic powder, paprika, salt, and pepper in a shallow bowl. Put the beaten egg in another shallow bowl. Heat the oil in a large nonstick skillet over medium heat. Dip the fish pieces in the beaten egg, then coat all sides in the seasoned flour. Place the fish in the hot oil and cook for about 3 minutes per side, until golden brown and firm to the touch. Remove the cooked fish to a paper towel–lined plate. Wipe the skillet with a paper towel.

2. **Make the curry sauce:** Heat the oil in the same skillet over medium heat. Add the curry paste and cook, stirring, for 1 minute, or until fragrant and sizzling. Add the coconut milk, fish sauce, and chopped red chilis. Cook, stirring occasionally, for about 5 minutes, until slightly thickened.

3. Return the fish pieces to the skillet and simmer over low heat for 2 to 3 minutes, or until heated through. Garnish with the cilantro and serve. Store leftovers in an airtight container in the refrigerator for up to 5 days.

Note: I recommend serving this curry with cauliflower rice, both to bulk it up and to soak up all the yummy sauce.

CALORIES: 356	FAT: 26g	PROTEIN: 25g	CARBS: 6g	FIBER: 1g	NET CARBS: 5g

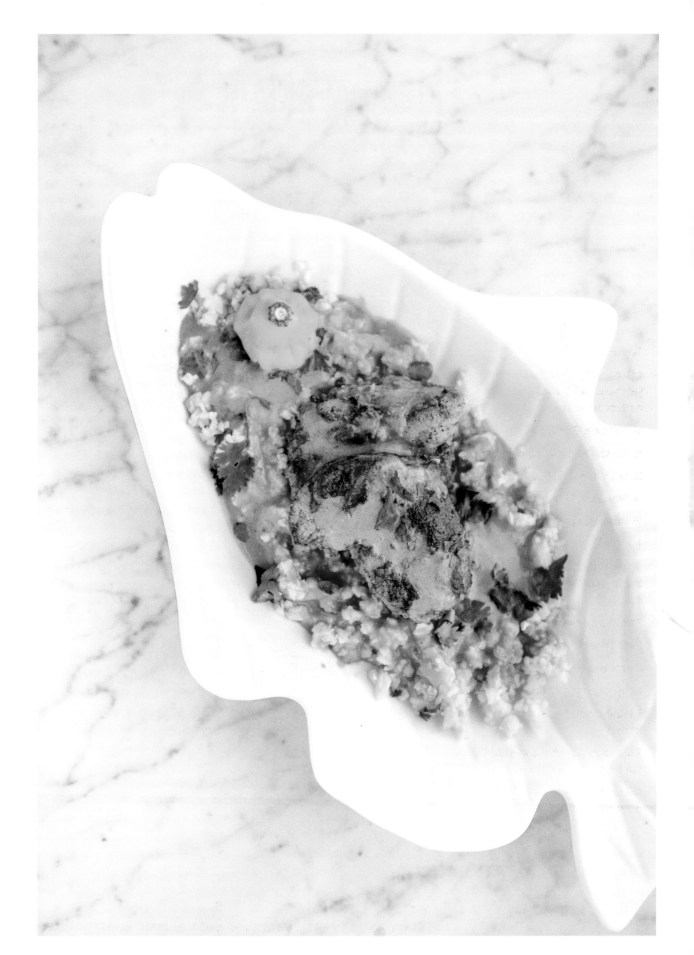

FRIED CALAMARI

| YIELD: 4 servings | SERVING SIZE: 4 ounces | PREP TIME: 10 minutes | COOK TIME: 8 minutes |

No one in my family can resist a plate piled high with crispy fried calamari—and we order it to share at any restaurant we can find it in. I despaired at being able to create a keto-friendly version, let alone a squeaky one, but this recipe is a pretty legit effort. While you simply can't replicate the light crispness of a white flour coating, the psyllium and coconut flour do a decent job of it, and the mayonnaise helps it stay on during frying. Serve this calamari with plenty of lemon wedges and my No-Cook Marinara Sauce (page 84) or Creamy Garlic Sauce (page 106) for dipping.

1 pound frozen calamari rings, thawed

2 tablespoons mayonnaise

⅓ cup coconut flour

1 teaspoon psyllium husk powder

1 teaspoon salt

⅛ teaspoon cayenne pepper

⅛ teaspoon garlic powder

Avocado oil or other light-tasting oil, for frying

4 lemon wedges, for serving

1. Put the calamari and mayonnaise in a medium-sized bowl and stir to coat the rings completely.

2. Put the coconut flour, psyllium husk powder, salt, cayenne, and garlic powder in a medium-sized bowl and stir to combine.

3. Pour oil into a 4-quart saucepan to a depth of about 2 inches. Heat the oil over medium heat until it reaches a temperature of 350°F.

4. Transfer about one-quarter of the calamari rings to the flour mixture and stir to coat. Gently shake off the excess flour, then carefully place the calamari in the hot oil. Fry for about 2 minutes, until golden brown. Remove with a slotted spoon and place on a paper towel–lined plate. Repeat with the remaining calamari until all of it is fried. Serve hot with lemon wedges to squeeze over the top before eating. Store leftovers in an airtight container in the refrigerator for up to 5 days. Reheat on a sheet pan in a preheated 400°F oven for 5 minutes or until crisp and heated through.

| CALORIES: 236 | FAT: 13g | PROTEIN: 18g | CARBS: 7g | FIBER: 3g | NET CARBS: 4g |

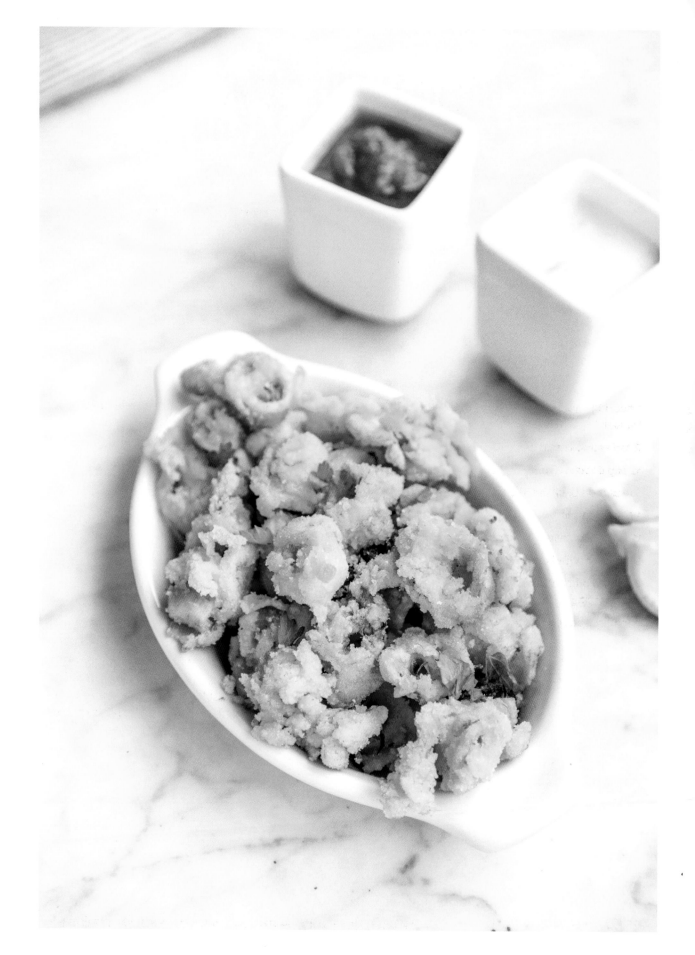

BRAZILIAN SHRIMP STEW (MOQUECA DE CAMARONES)

| YIELD: 4 servings | SERVING SIZE: 1¼ cups | PREP TIME: 10 minutes | COOK TIME: 10 minutes |

This spicy shrimp stew recipe has been popular on my website for years, and it needed no substitutions to be squeaky. Rich and creamy from the coconut milk, this luscious soup also has a hint of sweetness from the tomatoes that perfectly complements the succulent shrimp. Be sure not to overcook the shrimp or it will become rubbery.

¼ cup extra-virgin olive oil

¼ cup diced onions

¼ cup diced roasted red peppers

1 clove garlic, minced

1½ pounds extra-large shrimp, peeled and deveined

1 (14-ounce) can diced tomatoes with chilis

¼ cup chopped fresh cilantro

1 cup canned coconut milk

2 tablespoons Sriracha sauce or sambal oelek

2 tablespoons fresh lime juice

1 teaspoon kosher salt

¼ teaspoon ground black pepper

1. Heat the oil in a medium-sized saucepan over medium heat. Sauté the onions in the oil for several minutes, until translucent, then add the roasted red peppers and garlic and cook for several minutes more, until the vegetables are soft. Add the shrimp, tomatoes with chilis, and cilantro to the pan and simmer gently until the shrimp turn opaque.

2. Pour in the coconut milk and Sriracha sauce and gently cook just until heated through—do not allow it to boil. Remove the pan from the heat and stir in the lime juice, then season the soup with the salt and pepper. Store leftovers in an airtight container in the refrigerator for up to 5 days. Do not freeze.

Note: When reheating leftover stew, remove the shrimp and heat just the broth on the stovetop over medium heat. Once the broth is piping hot, add the shrimp and cook for only 1 minute more. Then remove the pan from the heat and let the stew sit for a minute or two to allow the heat of the broth to gently penetrate the shrimp without overcooking it.

CALORIES: 368 FAT: 24g PROTEIN: 30g CARBS: 7g FIBER: 1g NET CARBS: 6g

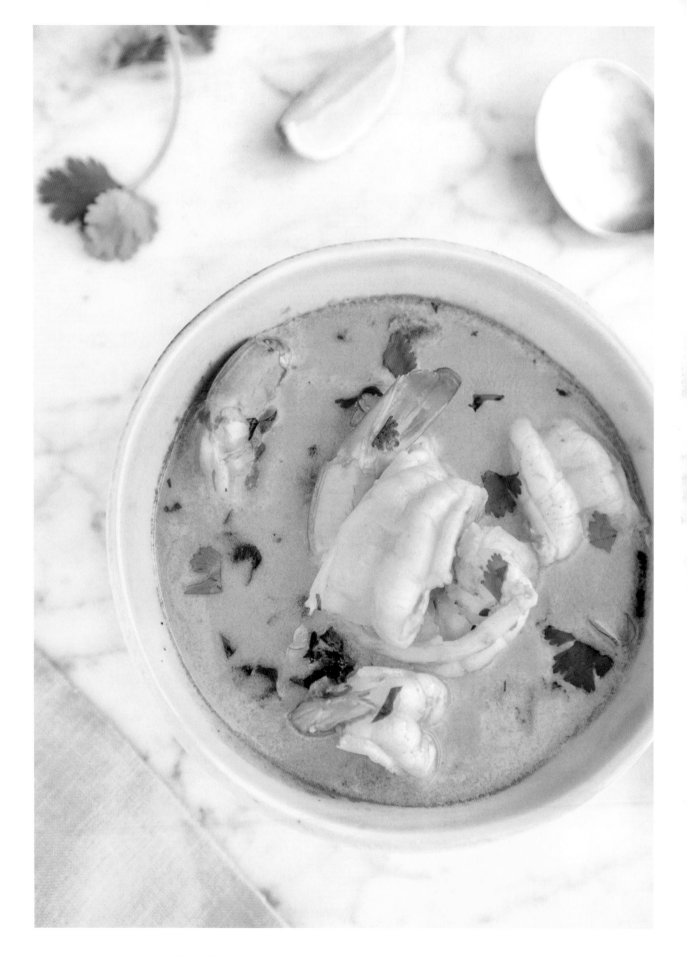

MOLCAJETE MIXTO

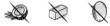

| YIELD: 12 cups | SERVING SIZE: 2 cups | PREP TIME: 8 minutes | COOK TIME: 30 minutes |

This classic Mexican dish is loaded with meat and seafood swimming together in a spicy, tangy green broth made from tomatillos and jalapeños. The first time I had molcajete mixto was at a huge cantina in Orlando—it came to the table audibly sizzling in an impressively large stone molcajete, which is the Mexican version of a mortar. I loved it for the drama initially, and then for the amazing flavors and textures once I tucked into it. I hope you'll love it too, even if you're only serving it in a boring soup bowl like I did here.

1 teaspoon kosher salt

1 tablespoon ground cumin

1 teaspoon smoked paprika

½ teaspoon garlic powder

½ teaspoon ground black pepper

1 pound lean boneless beef steak, such as sirloin or strip, thinly sliced

1 pound large shrimp, peeled and deveined

2 tablespoons extra-virgin olive oil

8 ounces Spanish-style dry-cured chorizo, sliced into ¼-inch discs

⅓ cup chopped red onions

¼ cup finely diced jalapeño peppers

1 teaspoon chopped garlic

2 cups roughly chopped zucchini

1 cup Easy Salsa Verde (page 88)

4 cups chicken broth, store-bought or homemade (page 72)

Fresh cilantro leaves, for garnish

1. Combine the salt and spices in a small bowl. Use half of the spice mixture to season the steak and half to season the shrimp.

2. Heat the oil in a large saucepan over medium-high heat until shimmering. Add the chorizo and cook for 5 minutes, or until golden brown. Using a slotted spoon, transfer the chorizo to a bowl and set aside.

3. Add the seasoned steak to the pan and cook over high heat until seared and browned, about 5 minutes. Remove the steak from the pan and add it to the bowl with the cooked chorizo.

4. Reduce the heat to medium and add the seasoned shrimp to the pan. Cook for 3 minutes, or until golden on the outside and bright white in the center. Remove the shrimp from the pan and add them to the bowl of cooked meats.

5. Add the onions and jalapeños to the pan. Cook, stirring occasionally, for about 5 minutes, until the jalapeños are charred but not burnt. Add the garlic and cook for 1 minute. Add the zucchini, salsa verde, and broth. Bring to a boil and then simmer for about 10 minutes, until the zucchini is fork-tender.

6. To serve, place a few pieces each of steak and chorizo and 3 or 4 shrimp (½ cup of protein altogether) in a bowl. Pour 1½ cups of the soup over the protein. Garnish with cilantro. Store leftovers in an airtight container in the refrigerator for up to 5 days.

CALORIES: 387   FAT: 22g   PROTEIN: 39g   CARBS: 6g   FIBER: 1g   NET CARBS: 5g

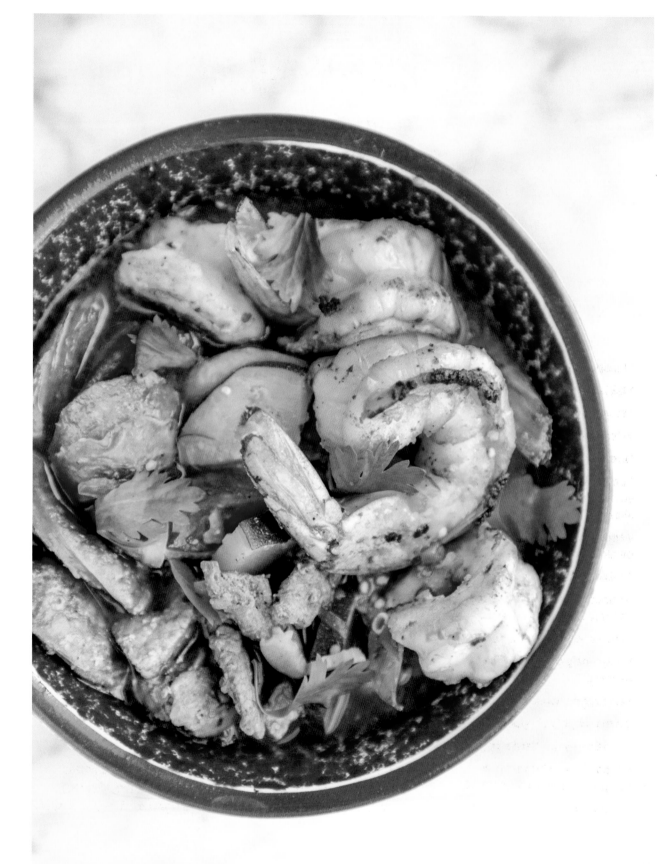

MUSSELS IN THAI COCONUT BROTH

| YIELD: 2 servings | SERVING SIZE: 8 ounces mussels + ⅓ cup broth | PREP TIME: 10 minutes | COOK TIME: 8 minutes |

Mussels are easy to make and one of the less expensive seafood options if you live within a few hours of a coast. High in protein and neutral in flavor, they are pretty much a blank canvas for anything you want to throw at them. This ginger-forward coconut curry broth is only one of the delicious ways to prepare mussels, but it's high on my list of favorites.

1 tablespoon avocado oil or other light-tasting oil

1 tablespoon minced fresh ginger

1 teaspoon minced garlic

1 teaspoon chopped red or green chilis

1 tablespoon red curry paste

⅔ cup canned coconut milk

1 tablespoon coconut aminos

1 pound mussels, scrubbed and debearded (see Notes)

¼ cup sliced scallions

2 tablespoons roughly chopped fresh cilantro

1. Heat the oil in a large skillet over medium-high heat until shimmering. Add the ginger, garlic, and chilis and cook for 2 minutes, or until fragrant. Add the curry paste and cook, stirring constantly, for 1 minute.

2. Add the coconut milk, coconut aminos, and cleaned mussels. Stir well, then cover and cook for 5 to 7 minutes, until the mussels have opened. (Some of the mussels may not open; see Notes below.)

3. Remove the pan from the heat and discard any unopened mussels. Garnish with the scallions and chopped cilantro and serve immediately. Store leftovers in an airtight container in the refrigerator for up to 2 days. To reheat leftovers, place the mussels and broth in a large skillet and heat for 3 to 5 minutes over medium heat, until the broth is steaming and the mussels are hot.

Notes: To clean the mussels, rinse them under cold running water and scrub off any algae or barnacles with a stiff brush. Pull off the hairy "beard" that protrudes from the seam where the two halves of the shell meet. If any of the mussel shells are broken or open (or do not close tightly when handled), discard them; they are already dead and unsafe to eat.

Mussels that remain tightly closed after cooking are also considered unsafe to eat and should be discarded.

CALORIES: 443   FAT: 30g   PROTEIN: 32g   CARBS: 6g   FIBER: 1g   NET CARBS: 5g

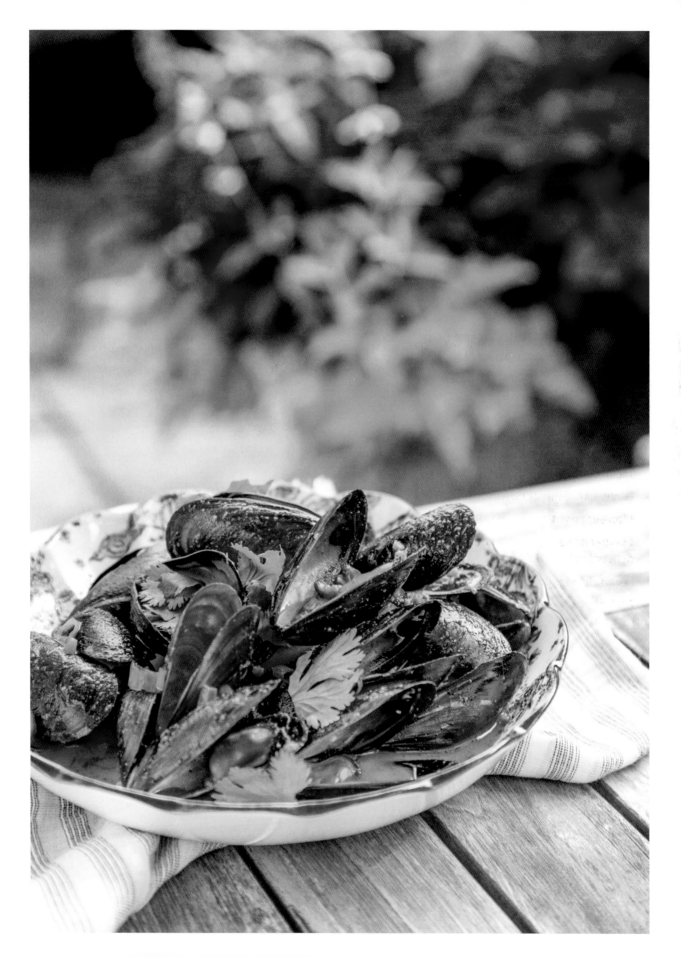

CRAB CAKES

| YIELD: 8 cakes | SERVING SIZE: 2 cakes | PREP TIME: 10 minutes | COOK TIME: 6 minutes |

I'm a sucker for crab cakes, even if they are considered a throwback to the nineties when they were obligatory on every restaurant menu's appetizer section. Let's bring them back, shall we? This recipe keeps it classic, with Old Bay seasoning, lemon juice, Dijon mustard, parsley, and coconut aminos standing in for the traditional Worcestershire sauce. I love to eat these with a squeeze of fresh lemon juice and a dollop of Chili-Lime Mayo (page 100), which adds a spicy kick.

8 ounces lump crab meat

2 tablespoons mayonnaise

1 tablespoon fresh lemon juice

2 teaspoons coconut aminos

1 teaspoon Dijon mustard

2 tablespoons chopped fresh parsley

2 tablespoons coconut flour

2 teaspoons Old Bay seasoning

2 tablespoons avocado oil or other light-tasting oil, for frying

1. Gently pick through the crab to make sure there are no shells or cartilage in the meat, then put the meat in a small bowl.

2. In another small bowl, combine the mayonnaise, lemon juice, coconut aminos, and mustard, mixing until smooth.

3. In a third bowl, combine the parsley, coconut flour, and Old Bay, mixing thoroughly.

4. Gently add the mayonnaise mixture to the crab, folding until combined. Then add the dry ingredients to the crab mixture and gently mix. Try not to break up/shred the pieces of crab too much.

5. Heat the oil in a large nonstick skillet over medium heat. Form the crab mixture into 8 cakes about 2 inches in diameter and carefully place them in the hot oil. Cook for 2 to 3 minutes per side, until golden brown. Remove from the pan to a plate lined with paper towels. Serve hot. Store leftovers in an airtight container in the refrigerator for up to 5 days. Leftovers can be eaten cold or reheated, covered, in the microwave for 1 to 2 minutes.

CALORIES: 130 **FAT:** 8g **PROTEIN:** 12g **CARBS:** 3g **FIBER:** 1g **NET CARBS:** 2g

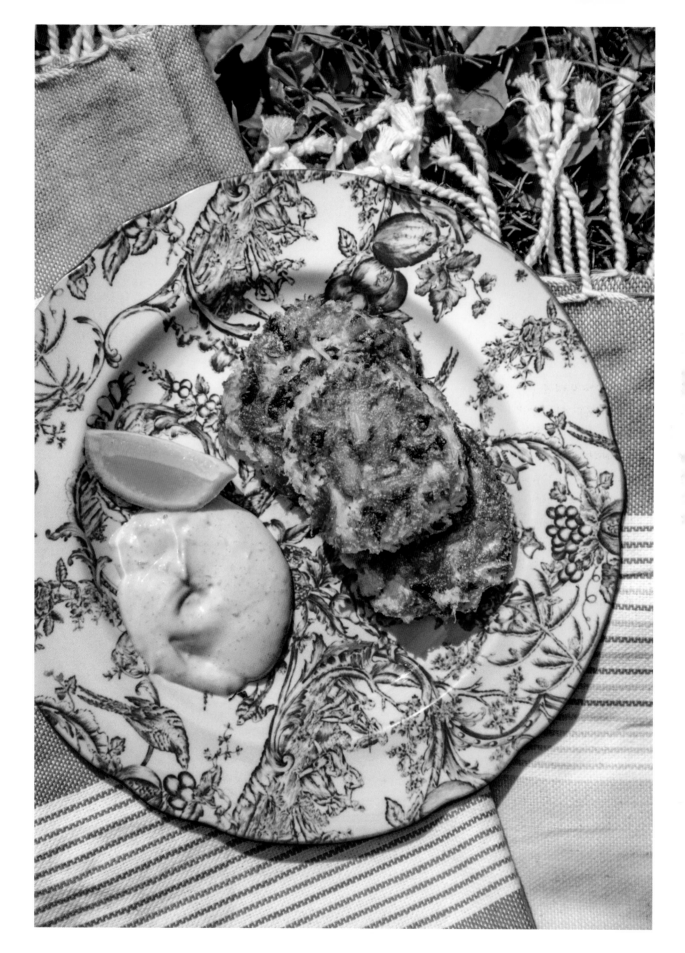

SHEET PAN PAELLA

YIELD: 4 servings | **SERVING SIZE:** 2 cups | **PREP TIME:** 15 minutes | **COOK TIME:** 25 minutes

While classic paella is made with rice, it's easily replaced with riced cauliflower, and most of the other ingredients are keto-friendly already. The peas are a little higher in carbs, but I just couldn't bring myself to leave them out—visually they are so necessary to a real paella, and that little burst of sweetness is a fun break from the other flavors. Making this meal on a sheet pan is the icing on the cake—easy and foolproof, it's going to be a hit every time.

2 tablespoons extra-virgin olive oil

1 pound boneless, skinless chicken breasts, cut into bite-sized pieces

Kosher salt and ground black pepper

8 ounces Spanish-style dry-cured chorizo or andouille sausage, thinly sliced

2 cups riced cauliflower

½ cup chopped onions

⅓ cup chopped red bell peppers

1 teaspoon minced garlic

½ cup canned petite diced tomatoes, drained

⅓ cup frozen peas

¼ cup chicken broth, store-bought or homemade (page 72)

½ teaspoon paprika

Pinch of saffron threads

1 pound jumbo shrimp, peeled and deveined

15 mussels, scrubbed and debearded (see Notes, page 260)

1 teaspoon grated lemon zest

2 tablespoons fresh lemon juice

¼ cup chopped fresh parsley

1. Preheat the oven to 400°F. Spread the olive oil on a sheet pan.

2. Season the chicken pieces with salt and pepper. Arrange on one-quarter of the sheet pan. Spread out the chorizo slices next to the chicken on another quarter of the pan.

3. Put the riced cauliflower, onions, bell peppers, and garlic in a small bowl and stir to combine. Spread over the remaining half of the sheet pan.

4. Bake for 15 minutes. Remove the pan from the oven.

5. Put the tomatoes, peas, broth, paprika, saffron, 1 teaspoon of salt, and ¼ teaspoon of pepper in a medium-sized bowl. Stir well. Pour over the ingredients on the sheet pan and stir well. Spread the mixture evenly over the sheet pan and scatter the shrimp and mussels over the top.

6. Return the pan to the oven and bake for 10 minutes, or until the shrimp are cooked and the mussels have opened. (Some of the mussels may not open) Remove from the oven and discard any unopened mussels. Sprinkle with the lemon zest, lemon juice, and parsley. Serve immediately. Store leftovers in an airtight container in the refrigerator for up to 3 days.

CALORIES: 476 **FAT:** 23g **PROTEIN:** 56g **CARBS:** 10g **FIBER:** 3g **NET CARBS:** 7g

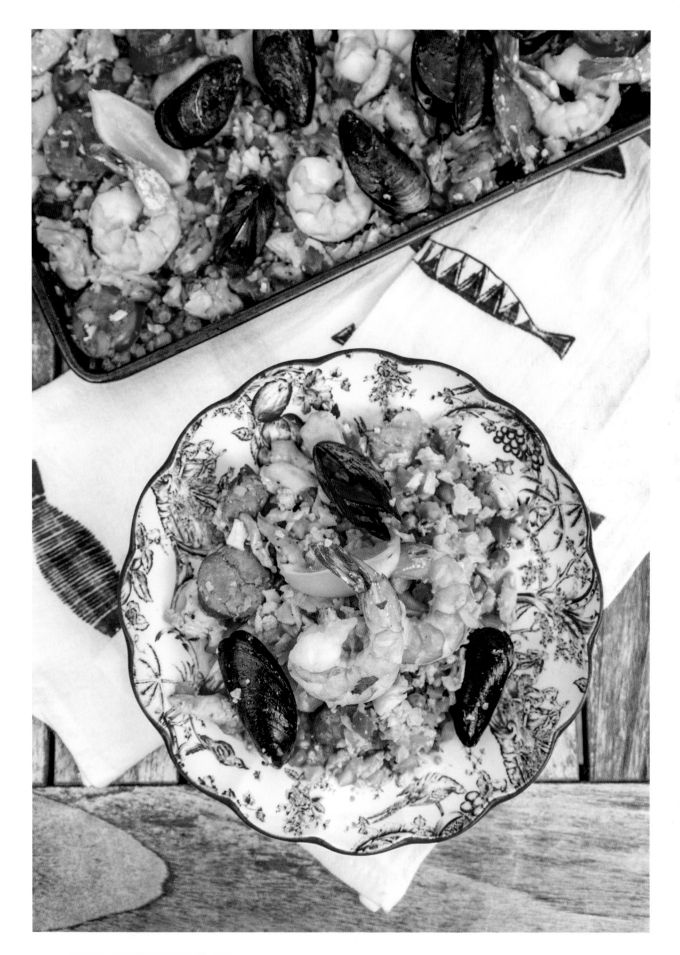

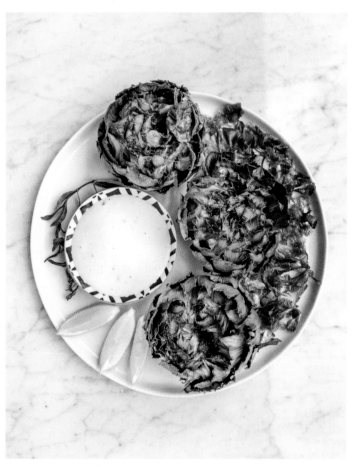

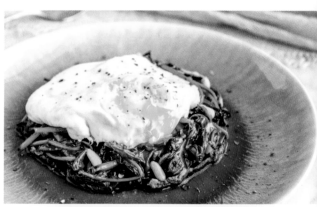

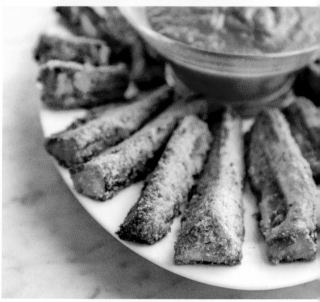

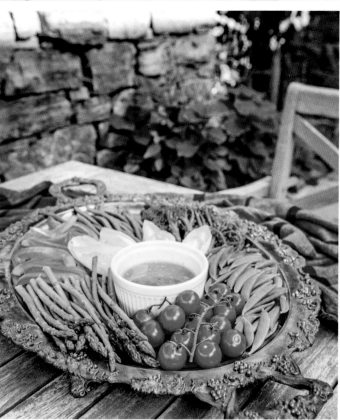

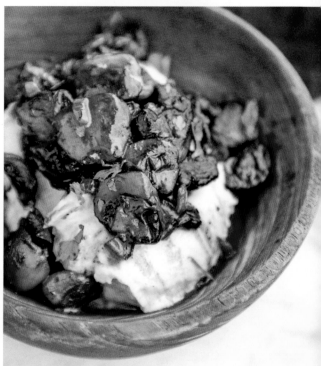

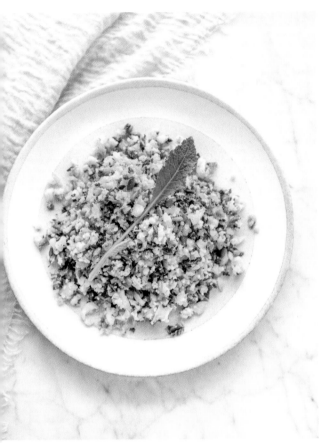

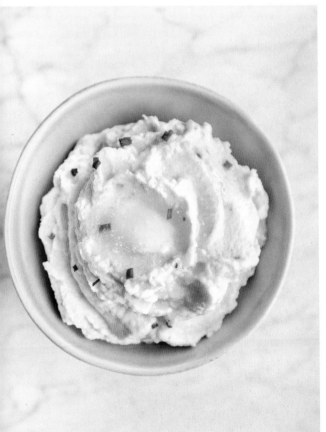

Veggie Mains & Sides

Spinach-Stuffed Portobello Mushrooms / 268

Greek Zucchini Fritters / 270

Eggplant & Cauliflower Fritters / 272

Roman Fried Artichokes / 274

Herbed Mushroom Ragout / 276

Easy Vegetable Curry / 278

Baked Zucchini Fries / 280

Balsamic Roasted Veggies / 282

Cauliflower & Kale Pilaf / 284

Coconut Creamed Spinach / 286

Bagna Cauda / 288

Garlic & Chive Cauliflower Mash / 290

Oven-Roasted Mushrooms / 292

Easy Sesame Broccoli / 294

Creamy Coconut Cauliflower Rice / 296

Sautéed Shredded Brussels Sprouts / 298

Roasted Bacon-Wrapped Cabbage Wedges / 300

Duchess Cauliflower / 302

Everything Roasted Cauliflower Steaks / 304

Sheet Pan Veggie Burgers / 306

Korean Scallion Pancakes (Pajeon) / 308

Spaghetti Squash Puttanesca / 310

SPINACH-STUFFED PORTOBELLO MUSHROOMS

YIELD: 2 mushrooms | **SERVING SIZE:** 1 mushroom | **PREP TIME:** 8 minutes | **COOK TIME:** 20 minutes

Meaty mushrooms, garlicky spinach, creamy pine nuts, and a runny fried egg make for one of the most delicious meat-free dishes I've eaten in a long time! This versatile stuffed mushroom can function as breakfast, a first course to a fancy dinner, or a tasty lunch or dinner when served with a side salad. If you're not opposed to eating meat, some spicy Italian sausage crumbled into the spinach mixture would be a welcome and flavorful addition.

2 large portobello mushroom caps

2 tablespoons extra-virgin olive oil

1 teaspoon minced garlic

4 cups baby spinach

1 tablespoon pine nuts

½ teaspoon kosher salt

⅛ teaspoon ground black pepper

⅛ teaspoon ground nutmeg

1 teaspoon butter

2 large eggs

Note: You may have noticed some pink flecks on the plate and mushroom in this recipe's photo, along with a few others in the book. Just so you're not left wondering, I have a pepper grinder full of a blend of black, white, and pink peppercorns that I often use to garnish a finished dish. You don't need to do that, but I find that the blend adds not just a pretty color, but also a more complex flavor than plain black pepper. Now you know!

1. Preheat the oven to 400°F. Line a sheet pan with parchment paper.

2. Scrape the "ribs" out of the portobellos with a spoon, then place them cavity side up on the prepared sheet pan.

3. Heat the oil in a large skillet over medium heat. Add the garlic and cook for 2 minutes, or until fragrant. Add the spinach, pine nuts, salt, pepper, and nutmeg. Cook, stirring occasionally, for 3 minutes, or until the spinach is wilted and bright green.

4. Divide the hot spinach mixture between the mushroom caps. Bake for 15 minutes, or until the mushrooms are softened and releasing juice onto the pan.

5. Melt the butter in a small skillet over medium heat. Fry the eggs for about 1 minute per side, or until cooked over-medium for still-runny yolks. Top each mushroom with a fried egg and serve immediately. Store leftovers in an airtight container in the refrigerator for up to 5 days. If you are planning to store these, reheat the mushroom(s) in the microwave for 1 to 2 minutes, until hot. Then fry an egg and top the mushroom with it right before eating.

CALORIES: 278 | **FAT:** 14g | **PROTEIN:** 8g | **CARBS:** 9g | **FIBER:** 5g | **NET CARBS:** 4g

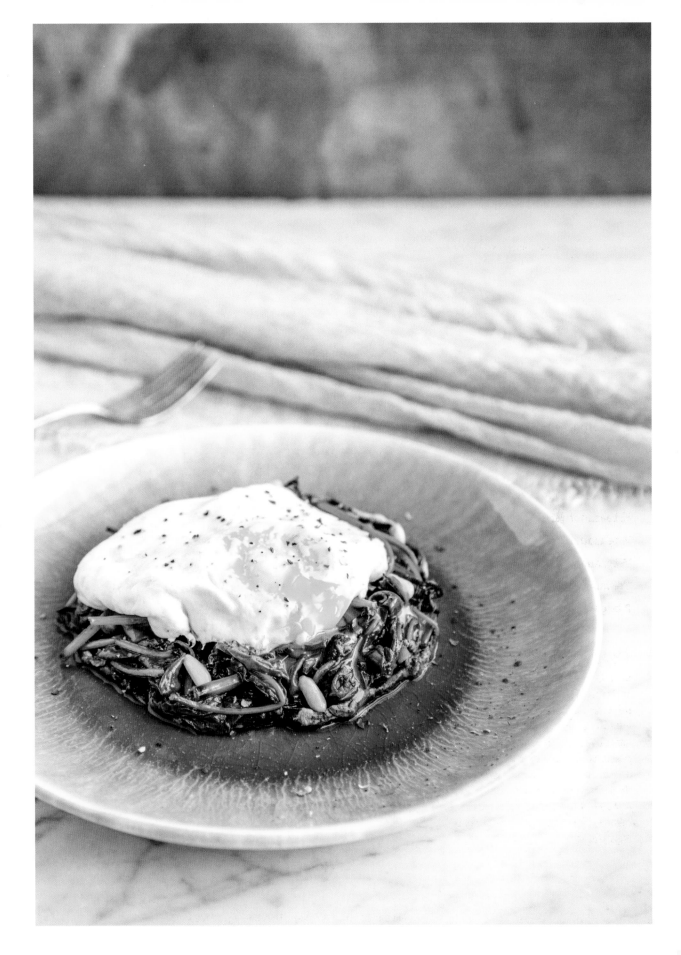

GREEK ZUCCHINI FRITTERS

YIELD: 8 fritters | **SERVING SIZE:** 2 fritters | **PREP TIME:** 10 minutes | **COOK TIME:** 12 minutes

The phrase "fritter away" means to squander or waste, and I think that's a horrible use of the term. Fritters are delicious, and I think to "fritter away" should mean to go forth and make fritters—preferably soon, and often! Let's make this a thing—starting with these delicious Greek-inspired zucchini fritters. Crispy and flavorful, these fritters contain classic Greek ingredients like lemon, dill, oregano, and olives, resulting in a bright and fresh cake that is only made better by a liberal dose of my Dairy-Free Tzatziki (page 96).

2 cups grated zucchini

⅓ cup Sun-Flour (page 74)

1 large egg, beaten

1 tablespoon finely chopped Kalamata olives

1 tablespoon chopped fresh dill

1 teaspoon grated lemon zest

½ teaspoon dried oregano leaves

½ teaspoon kosher salt

¼ teaspoon ground black pepper

2 tablespoons avocado oil or other light-tasting oil, for frying

Lemon wedges, for serving (optional)

1. Place the grated zucchini on a double layer of paper towels and wrap the edges around it to form a loose ball. Squeeze the ball tightly over the sink to get out as much of the liquid as possible. Shake the zucchini out of the paper towels into a large bowl.

2. To the bowl with the zucchini, add the flour, egg, olives, dill, lemon zest, oregano, salt, and pepper. Stir with a fork until fully combined.

3. Heat the oil in a large nonstick skillet over medium heat until shimmering. Drop large spoonfuls of the zucchini mixture into the hot oil, about ¼ cup each. Press down with a fork to form a ½-inch-thick patty. Cook for 2 to 3 minutes per side, until golden brown and firm in the center. Remove to a paper towel–lined plate to drain. Serve hot with lemon wedges if desired. Store leftovers in an airtight container in the refrigerator for up to 5 days.

Note: If not fully squeaky and avoiding dairy, add ⅓ cup chopped feta cheese to the zucchini mixture before frying. Use sheep's milk feta if you can get it; most people with lactose intolerance issues respond much better to sheep's milk cheeses than cow milk. Also, the taste is far superior, in my opinion.

CALORIES: 185 **FAT:** 8g **PROTEIN:** 4g **CARBS:** 4g **FIBER:** 1g **NET CARBS:** 3g

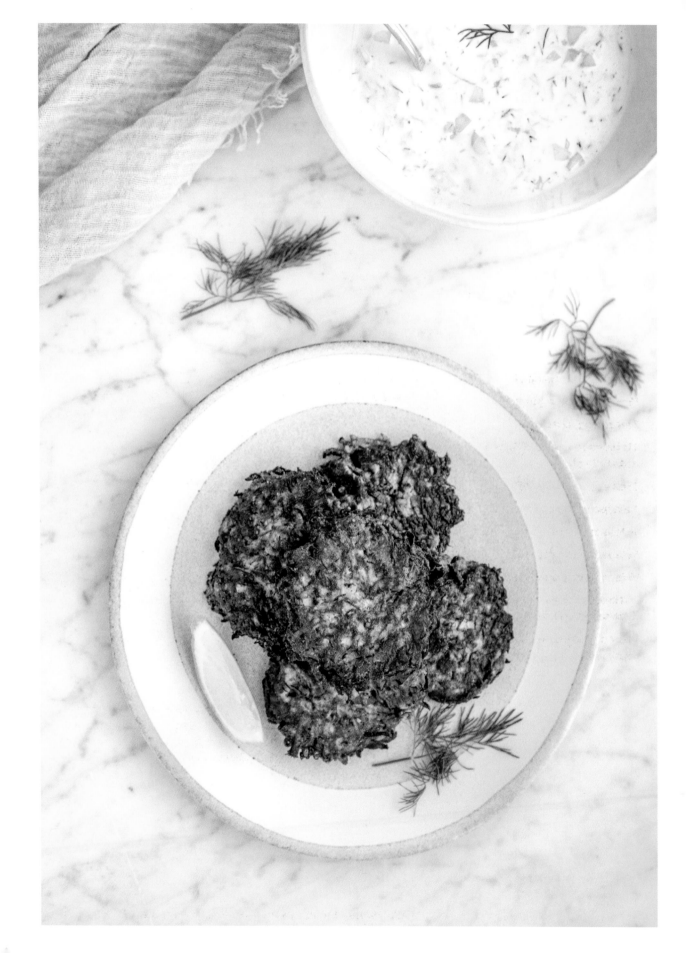

EGGPLANT & CAULIFLOWER FRITTERS

YIELD: 9 fritters | **SERVING SIZE:** 3 fritters | **PREP TIME:** 10 minutes | **COOK TIME:** 6 minutes

Creamy eggplant, toothsome cauliflower—we've got all the best textures in these mouth-watering fritters. Smoky paprika, bright lemon zest, sweet red bell pepper, and a fresh blast of basil and parsley make these tasty cakes both flavorful and nutrient dense. When served on a bed of No-Cook Marinara Sauce (page 84) and topped with a drizzle of Easy Balsamic Glaze (page 86) for sweetness, your biggest challenge will be to avoid eating them all in one sitting!

2 cups peeled and finely chopped eggplant

2 cups riced cauliflower

¼ cup finely chopped red bell peppers

2 tablespoons chopped fresh basil

2 tablespoons chopped fresh parsley

1 teaspoon grated lemon zest

⅓ cup mayonnaise

1 teaspoon coconut aminos

½ cup Sun-Flour (page 74)

2 tablespoons coconut flour

1 teaspoon psyllium husk powder

1¼ teaspoons kosher salt

1 teaspoon garlic powder

1 teaspoon onion powder

1 teaspoon smoked paprika

¼ teaspoon ground nutmeg

¼ teaspoon ground black pepper

2 tablespoons extra-virgin olive oil, for the pan

1. Put all the ingredients, except the oil, in a medium-sized bowl and mix well. Using your hands, form into round patties about 2 inches wide and ½ inch thick.

2. Heat the oil in a large nonstick skillet over medium heat until shimmering. Carefully place the fritters in the hot oil. Cook for 3 minutes per side, or until golden brown and slightly firm in the center. Remove to a paper towel–lined plate to drain before serving. Store leftovers in an airtight container in the refrigerator for up to 5 days.

CALORIES: 244 | **FAT:** 7g | **PROTEIN:** 6g | **CARBS:** 6g | **FIBER:** 2g | **NET CARBS:** 4g

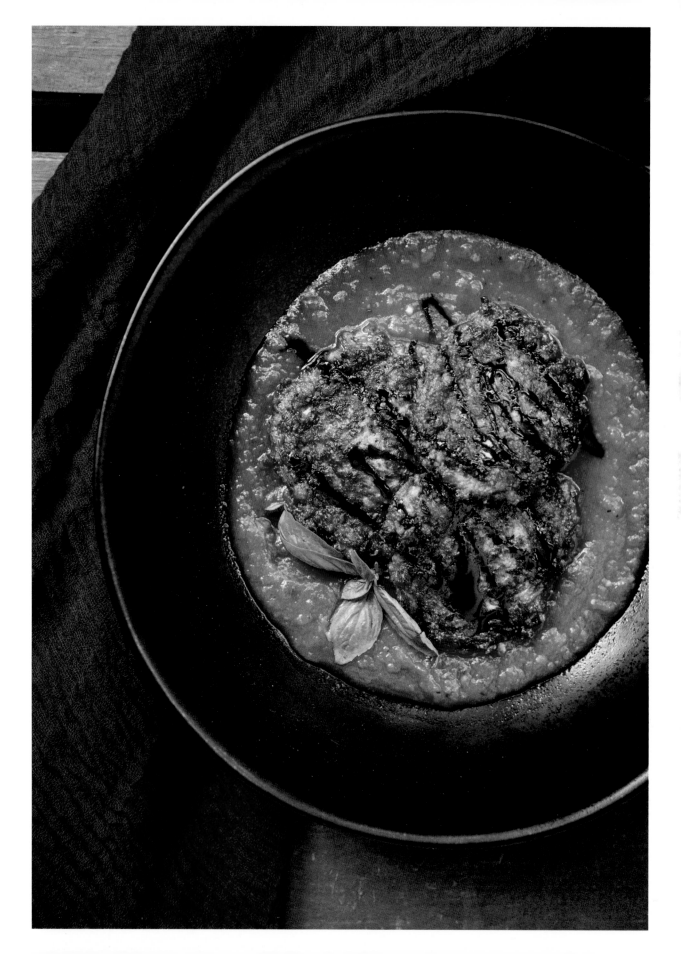

ROMAN FRIED ARTICHOKES

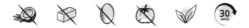

YIELD: 4 artichokes	SERVING SIZE: 1 artichoke	PREP TIME: 12 minutes	COOK TIME: 13 minutes

The first time I tried fried artichokes was in Italy, the summer before I began writing this book. I've always loved artichokes, but this deep-fried, super crispy Roman preparation immediately became my hands-down favorite way to eat them. I just couldn't believe how much the crispy thin inner leaves resembled potato chips! Since crispy textures are hard to come by on keto, and even more so on Squeaky Clean Keto, I knew I had to include this recipe in the book. It's a little labor-intensive, but once that first salty leaf shatters on your tongue, you'll know it's worth it. Make sure you eat the heart as well, which is at least as good if not better than the delicious leaves. Serve these with lemon wedges and my Garlicky Lemon & Tarragon Dressing (page 91) for a fun and impressive first course.

4 large globe artichokes

Peanut oil or other light-tasting oil, for frying

1 teaspoon kosher salt

Notes: Never put artichoke leaves or trimmings in the garbage disposal—their woody leaves can jam it and burn out the motor.

Typically, you would place trimmed artichokes in lemon water to prevent oxidization and browning, but you don't need to do so for this recipe because the chokes turn brown when fried anyway, and the water would cause the oil to pop.

1. Pour oil about 5 inches deep into a 4-quart saucepan and bring it to 350°F over medium heat—this will take about 8 minutes.

2. Meanwhile, snip off the thorns or sharp tips from the artichoke leaves with scissors. Cut off the top one-third of each artichoke with a serrated knife, which will make it easier to saw through the woody leaves. Cut off all but ½ inch of the base stem.

3. Gently place the artichokes in the hot oil and fry for 8 minutes. Remove the artichokes from the oil with a slotted spoon to a paper towel–lined plate. When cool enough to handle, pull out the thin center leaves with your fingers or a spoon. Use a spoon to scoop out all the hairy "choke" in the center, being careful not to scoop out the edible heart. Smash the artichokes from the top to flatten them slightly.

4. Return the artichokes to the hot oil and fry for an additional 5 minutes, or until the leaves are golden and crisp. Remove from the oil and sprinkle liberally with the salt. Serve immediately. Store leftovers in an airtight container in the refrigerator for up to 5 days. Reheat on a baking sheet in a preheated 400°F oven for 12 to 15 minutes, until heated through.

CALORIES: 164	FAT: 10g	PROTEIN: 4g	CARBS: 14g	FIBER: 10g	NET CARBS: 4g

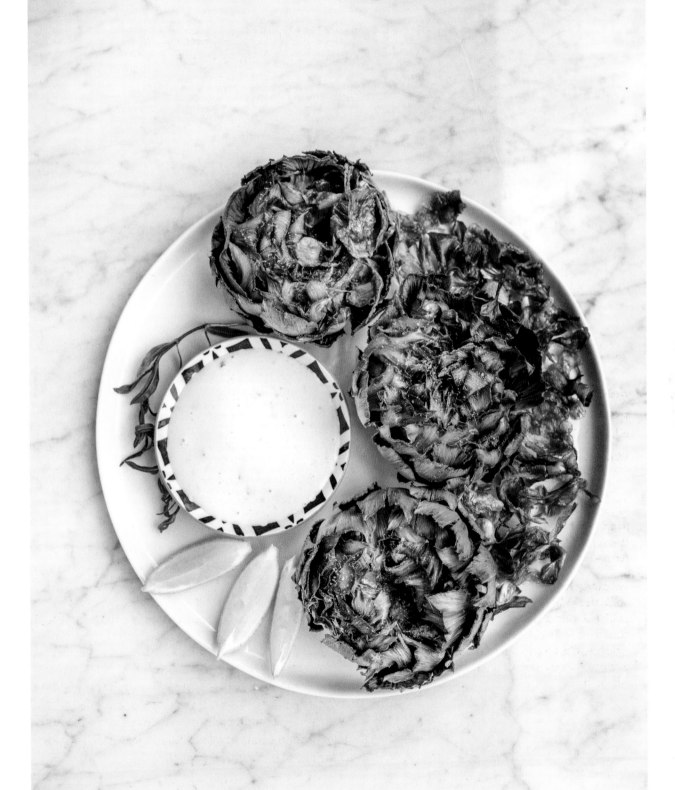

HERBED MUSHROOM RAGOUT

YIELD: 4 servings	**SERVING SIZE:** ⅔ cup	**PREP TIME:** 10 minutes	**COOK TIME:** 15 minutes

Delicious as a side dish, this earthy mushroom ragout becomes a substantial main dish when served over Garlic & Chive Cauliflower Mash (page 290), spaghetti squash, or zucchini noodles. You'll never miss the meat in this flavorful and hearty recipe.

½ cup (1 stick) butter

1 pound white mushrooms, quartered

¼ cup dried porcini mushrooms, rinsed

1 teaspoon kosher salt

½ teaspoon ground black pepper

½ cup chopped onions

1 teaspoon minced garlic

½ cup filtered water

⅓ cup canned coconut milk

1 teaspoon coconut aminos

2 tablespoons chopped fresh parsley

1 teaspoon chopped fresh tarragon

Melt the butter in a large skillet over medium heat. Add the mushrooms, salt, and pepper. Cook for about 8 minutes, stirring occasionally, until golden brown. Add the onions and garlic and cook for about 3 minutes, until the onions are translucent. Pour in the water, coconut milk, and coconut aminos. Cook, stirring occasionally, for about 3 minutes, until the liquid is reduced and thickened enough to coat a spoon. Remove the pan from the heat and stir in the parsley and tarragon. Store leftovers in an airtight container in the refrigerator for up to 5 days.

CALORIES: 217	**FAT:** 22g	**PROTEIN:** 3g	**CARBS:** 5g	**FIBER:** 1g	**NET CARBS:** 4g

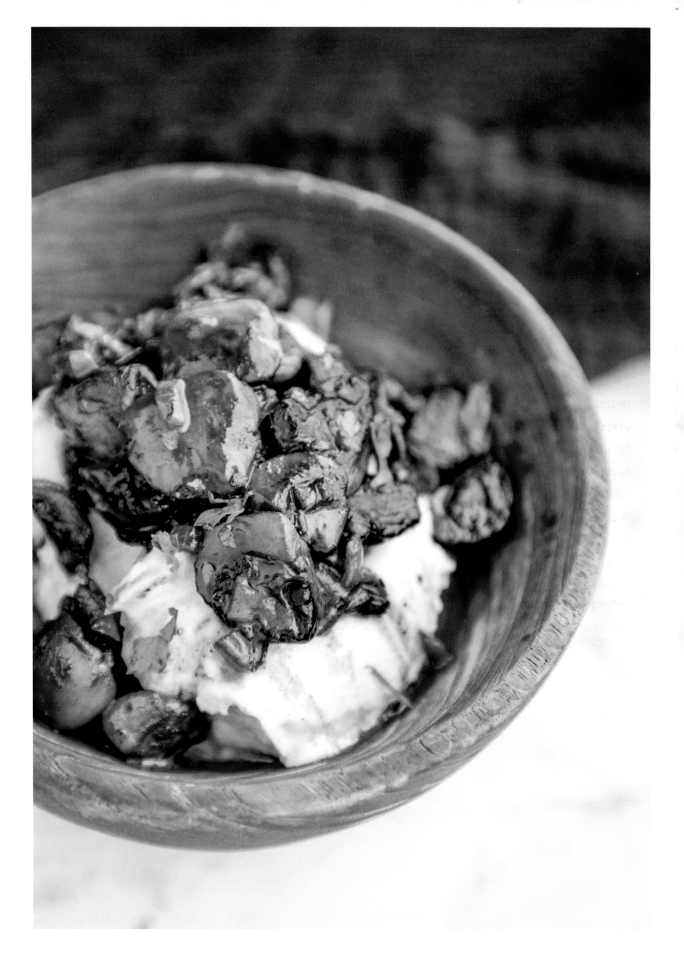

EASY VEGETABLE CURRY

YIELD: 4 servings | **SERVING SIZE:** 2 cups | **PREP TIME:** 15 minutes | **COOK TIME:** 15 minutes

If you're on the hunt for more meatless main dishes, then this hearty and delicious curry is for you. Loaded with flavor and swimming in a rich and creamy sauce, vegetables never tasted so good! Only moderately spicy as is, you can kick up the heat by adding more jalapeño or red pepper flakes when serving.

2 tablespoons avocado oil

1 tablespoon chopped jalapeño peppers

1 teaspoon minced garlic

3 cups peeled and roughly chopped eggplant

3 cups roughly chopped zucchini

2 cups roughly chopped green beans

1 teaspoon coconut aminos

1½ tablespoons yellow curry powder

1 teaspoon kosher salt

¼ teaspoon ground black pepper

¼ teaspoon red pepper flakes

½ cup canned coconut milk

1. Heat the oil in a large skillet over medium-high heat. Add the jalapeños and garlic and cook until fragrant, about 2 minutes. Add the eggplant, zucchini, and green beans and cook, stirring occasionally, for about 5 minutes, until browned and slightly softened.

2. Add the coconut aminos, curry powder, salt, black pepper, and red pepper flakes and stir well to coat. Cook, stirring occasionally, for 3 minutes, or until the curry powder has dissolved. Pour in the coconut milk and stir well until smooth. Cook for an additional 5 minutes, or until the liquid is reduced and thickened enough to coat a spoon. Serve hot. Store leftovers in an airtight container in the refrigerator for up to 1 week.

Note: You can customize this recipe with other keto-friendly veggies such as bell peppers, broccoli, cauliflower, and onions. Be sure to adjust the nutrition info to account for any substitutions.

CALORIES: 164 | **FAT:** 12g | **PROTEIN:** 3g | **CARBS:** 12g | **FIBER:** 5g | **NET CARBS:** 7g

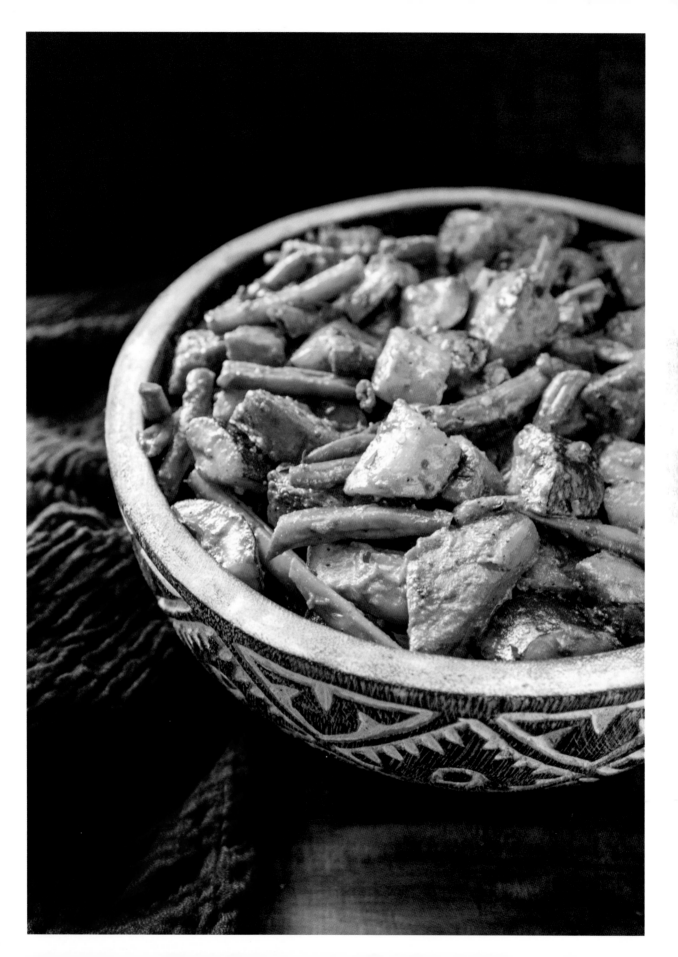

BAKED ZUCCHINI FRIES

YIELD: 6 servings	SERVING SIZE: 10 fries	PREP TIME: 10 minutes	COOK TIME: 30 minutes

Ah, the versatile zucchini. While I love it as noodles, in a gratin, or stuffed with tasty fillings, these crunchy zucchini fries might be my favorite preparation yet. Baking keeps it easy, and the mayonnaise prevents the coating from falling off and makes the fries super crunchy. These fries are guaranteed to be a hit with the kids, especially when dipped in my No-Cook Marinara Sauce (page 84) or, for a change, Creamy Garlic Sauce (page 106), Roasted Red Pepper Sauce (page 94), or Chili-Lime Mayo (page 100) if you like a spicy kick!

2 tablespoons extra-virgin olive oil

3 medium zucchini

3 tablespoons mayonnaise

⅔ cup Sun-Flour (page 74)

⅓ cup coconut flour

1 teaspoon kosher salt

½ teaspoon garlic powder

½ teaspoon onion powder

½ teaspoon paprika

¼ teaspoon dried oregano leaves

1. Preheat the oven to 400°F. Grease a sheet pan with the olive oil.

2. Cut the zucchini in half lengthwise, then cut each half into about 10 sticks or wedges. Put the zucchini in a large bowl and add the mayonnaise. Stir to coat all the zucchini pieces in the mayonnaise.

3. Put the flours, salt, garlic powder, onion powder, paprika, and oregano in a small bowl. Stir well. Carefully roll the zucchini pieces in the flour coating one at a time, then place on the prepared sheet pan.

4. Bake the fries for 20 minutes. Remove from the oven and carefully turn the fries over with tongs or a fork. Bake for an additional 10 minutes, until golden brown. Serve hot. Store leftovers in an airtight container in the refrigerator for up to 1 week. Reheat leftovers on a sheet pan in a 400°F oven for 8 to 10 minutes, until crisp and heated through.

CALORIES: 185	FAT: 15g	PROTEIN: 5g	CARBS: 10g	FIBER: 5g	NET CARBS: 5g

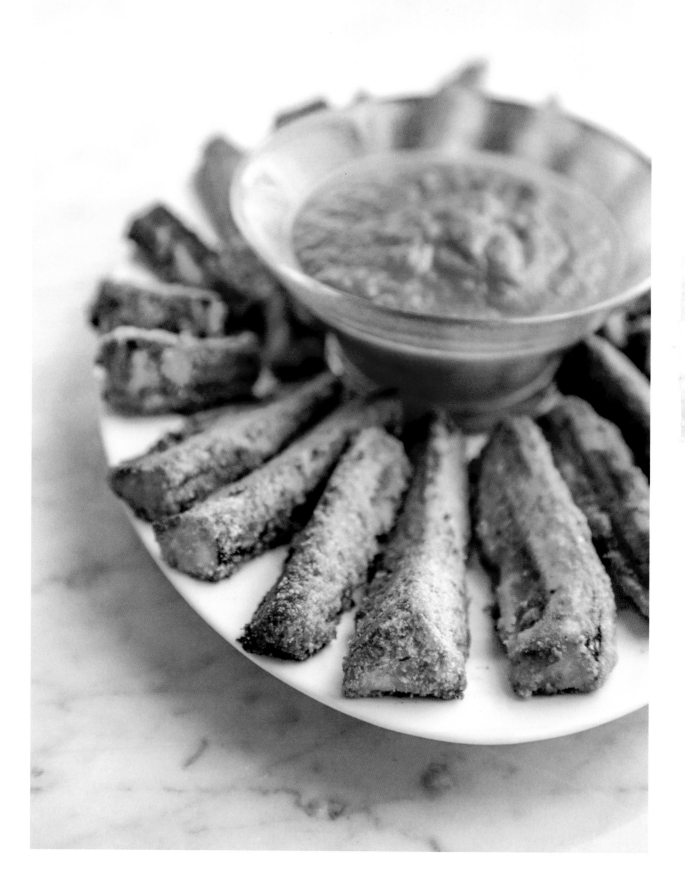

BALSAMIC ROASTED VEGGIES

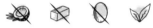

| YIELD: 4 servings | SERVING SIZE: 1 cup | PREP TIME: 10 minutes | COOK TIME: 40 minutes |

Low in calories but big on flavor, these toasty veggies are soft and luscious from roasting and slightly sweet and tangy from the balsamic vinegar—a perfect side to roasted or grilled meats. The leftovers are delicious chilled and added to a salad or wrap.

2 cups roughly chopped eggplant

2 cups roughly chopped zucchini

1 cup roughly chopped red bell peppers

½ cup red onion slices

3 tablespoons extra-virgin olive oil

2 tablespoons balsamic vinegar (no sugar added)

1 teaspoon kosher salt

¼ teaspoon ground black pepper

Preheat the oven to 400°F. Place all the ingredients on a sheet pan. Stir well to coat the vegetables with the oil, vinegar, and seasonings. Bake for 40 minutes, or until the vegetables are soft and starting to brown. Serve hot or chilled. Store leftovers in an airtight container in the refrigerator for up to 5 days.

CALORIES: 156 FAT: 10g PROTEIN: 2g CARBS: 10g FIBER: 3g NET CARBS: 7g

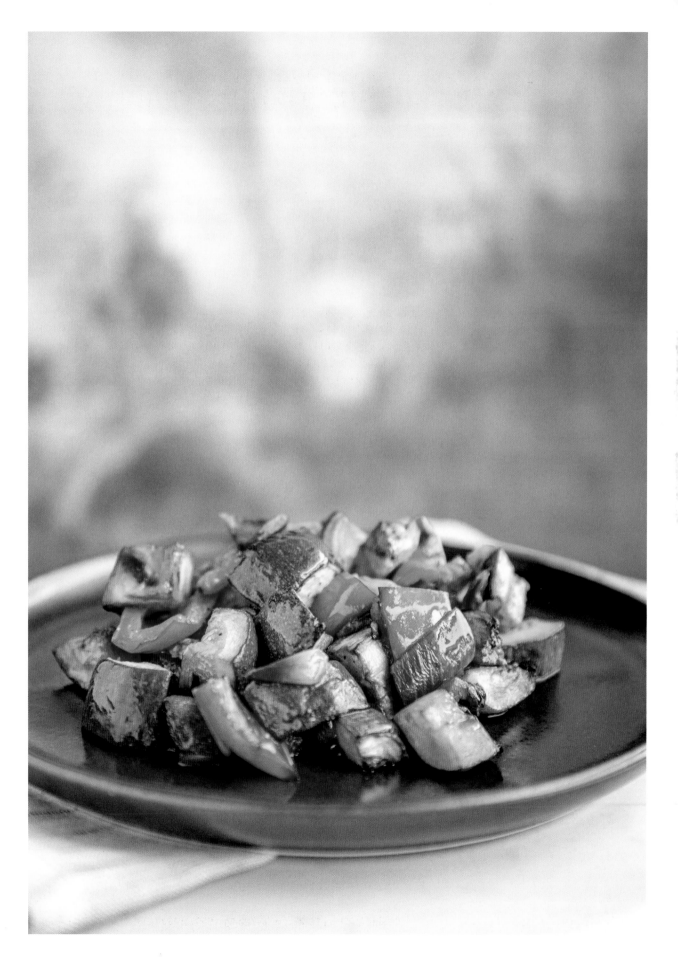

CAULIFLOWER & KALE PILAF

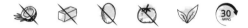

| YIELD: 4 servings | SERVING SIZE: 1 cup | PREP TIME: 8 minutes | COOK TIME: 8 minutes |

Quick, simple, beautiful, delicious—all words that easily describe this fun pilaf made with toasty sunflower seeds and super healthy kale. Incredibly hearty and loaded with flavor and texture, this yummy pilaf can be served with a fried egg for added protein, which makes for a satisfying vegetarian main dish. One of my favorites!

3 tablespoons extra-virgin olive oil

½ cup shelled raw sunflower seeds

1 teaspoon minced garlic

1 teaspoon kosher salt

¼ teaspoon ground black pepper

⅛ teaspoon ground nutmeg

3 cups riced cauliflower

1 cup finely chopped kale

Heat the oil in a large skillet over medium heat. Add the sunflower seeds, garlic, salt, pepper, and nutmeg and stir well. Cook for 2 minutes, or until fragrant and sizzling. Add the riced cauliflower and kale and stir well. Cook for about 5 minutes, until the cauliflower has softened and the kale has wilted. Serve warm or chilled. Store leftovers in an airtight container in the refrigerator for up to 5 days.

| CALORIES: 248 | FAT: 15g | PROTEIN: 5g | CARBS: 7g | FIBER: 3g | NET CARBS: 4g |

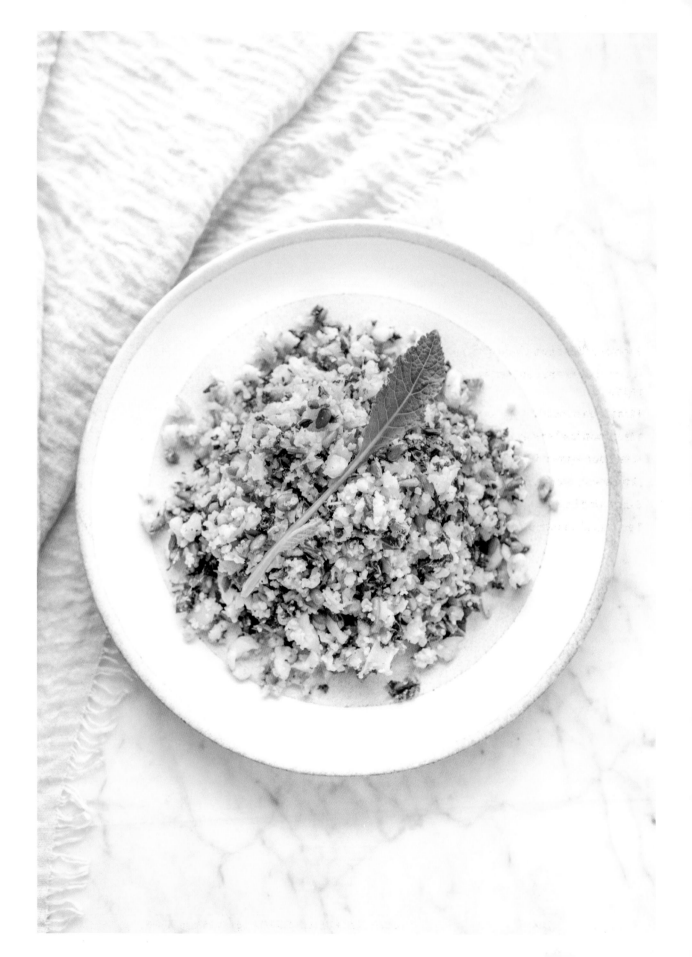

COCONUT CREAMED SPINACH

YIELD: 2 servings | **SERVING SIZE:** ⅔ cup | **PREP TIME:** 2 minutes | **COOK TIME:** 5 minutes

---

It doesn't get much easier than this creamed spinach when you need a side dish, and quick! It is creamy and slightly sweet from the coconut milk, and the nutmeg adds an earthy taste that perfectly complements the "green" flavor of the spinach. The small amount of cayenne pepper gives this dish a little heat that I really enjoy, but you can leave out the cayenne if you prefer or reduce it to just a pinch. Simple and delicious, this is a nutrient-dense recipe that you'll want to make over and over again!

⅓ cup canned coconut milk

4 cups baby spinach

½ teaspoon kosher salt

⅛ teaspoon cayenne pepper

⅛ teaspoon ground nutmeg

Heat the coconut milk in a medium-sized saucepan over medium heat until bubbling, about 2 minutes. Add the spinach and cook, stirring occasionally, for about 3 minutes, until wilted and bright green. Stir in the salt, cayenne pepper, and nutmeg. Serve hot. Store leftovers in an airtight container in the refrigerator for up to 5 days.

CALORIES: 78 **FAT:** 8g **PROTEIN:** 2g **CARBS:** 4g **FIBER:** 2g **NET CARBS:** 2g

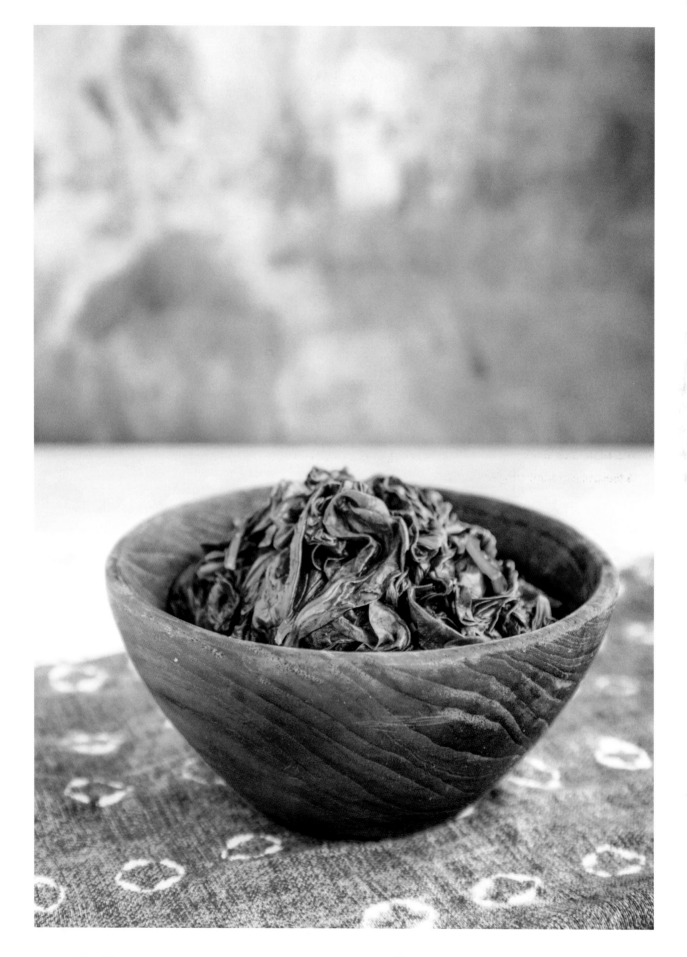

BAGNA CAUDA

YIELD: 1½ cups | **SERVING SIZE:** 2 tablespoons | **PREP TIME:** 5 minutes | **COOK TIME:** 5 minutes

Bagna cauda, which translates to "warm bath," is a rich, garlicky dip that originated in Piedmont, Italy. Traditionally served with a variety of fresh vegetables for dipping (or bread, if you're serving it to non-keto guests), the garlic and anchovies make it pungent and surprisingly addicting. Though it's not what it's meant for originally, I have found it to be a delicious sauce for grilled chicken and shrimp, as well as a bold salad dressing. This dip is perfect for entertaining! You can enjoy it warm or at room temperature; if you prefer it warm, you can serve it in a small slow cooker or fondue pot, or just pop it into the microwave for 30 seconds to reheat as necessary.

⅔ cup extra-virgin olive oil

½ cup (1 stick) unsalted butter

12 anchovy fillets, roughly chopped

2 tablespoons roughly chopped garlic

Put all the ingredients in a small blender or food processor and blend for 10 seconds, or until mostly smooth. Pour the mixture into a small saucepan and cook over medium heat for 5 minutes, or until hot and steaming. Transfer to a serving dish and serve with a variety of raw vegetables for dipping. Store leftovers in an airtight container in the refrigerator for up to 5 days. Reheat in the microwave for 1 to 2 minutes, until liquefied and very warm.

Note: The nutrition info does not include any vegetables you dip in the sauce, so be sure to calculate your macros on those separately.

CALORIES: 184   **FAT:** 21g   **PROTEIN:** 1g   **CARBS:** 0g   **FIBER:** 0g   **NET CARBS:** 0g

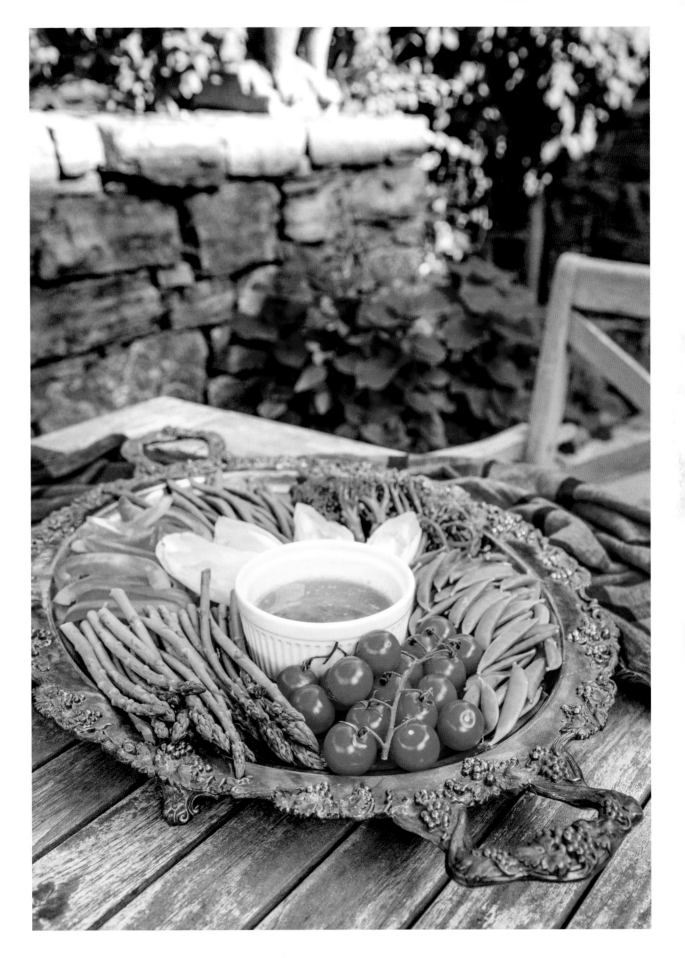

GARLIC & CHIVE CAULIFLOWER MASH

YIELD: 4 servings | **SERVING SIZE:** ½ cup | **PREP TIME:** 8 minutes | **COOK TIME:** 12 minutes

---

This decadent mash is so creamy and delicious that nobody will guess it doesn't contain any cream or cheese. Shhhhhh—I won't tell if you don't! Serve it with a generous pat of salted butter to make it even more luscious.

5 cups cauliflower florets (about 1 large head)

⅓ cup mayonnaise

1 clove garlic, peeled

1 tablespoon filtered water

½ teaspoon kosher salt

⅛ teaspoon ground black pepper

½ teaspoon grated lemon zest

¼ teaspoon fresh lemon juice

1 tablespoon chopped fresh chives, plus more for garnish if desired

Combine the cauliflower, mayonnaise, garlic, water, salt, and pepper in a large microwave-safe bowl, stirring until the cauliflower is evenly coated. Microwave on high, uncovered, for 12 minutes, or until the cauliflower is fork-tender. Transfer the cauliflower mixture to a blender or food processor and puree until smooth. Add the lemon zest, lemon juice, and chives and pulse until combined. Serve warm, garnish with extra chives if desired. Store leftovers in an airtight container in the refrigerator for up to 5 days.

CALORIES: 184 **FAT:** 18g **PROTEIN:** 2g **CARBS:** 5g **FIBER:** 2g **NET CARBS:** 3g

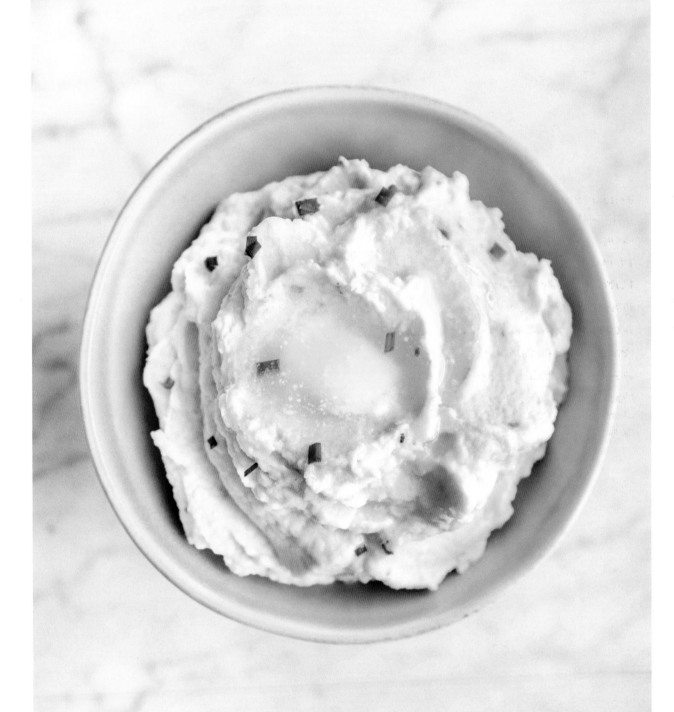

OVEN-ROASTED MUSHROOMS

| YIELD: 4 servings | SERVING SIZE: ⅓ cup | PREP TIME: 5 minutes | COOK TIME: 20 minutes |

This easy recipe involves very little hands-on time but results in the tastiest and toastiest roasted mushrooms ever. This is one of Hungry Jr.'s favorite recipes in this book, and we eat these delicious mushrooms often alongside a juicy steak, with potatoes for the guys and a fluffy pile of Garlic & Chive Cauliflower Mash (page 290) for me. Everybody wins!

8 ounces white mushrooms, halved or quartered if large

2 tablespoons extra-virgin olive oil

¼ cup (½ stick) butter, melted

½ teaspoon dried thyme leaves

1 teaspoon kosher salt

¼ teaspoon ground black pepper

Preheat the oven to 400°F. Place the mushrooms on a sheet pan and add the oil, melted butter, thyme, salt, and pepper. Mix together until the mushrooms are coated, then spread the mushrooms evenly over the sheet pan. Bake for 20 minutes, or until golden brown. Serve hot. Store leftovers in an airtight container in the refrigerator for up to 5 days.

CALORIES: 175   FAT: 19g   PROTEIN: 2g   CARBS: 2g   FIBER: 1g   NET CARBS: 1g

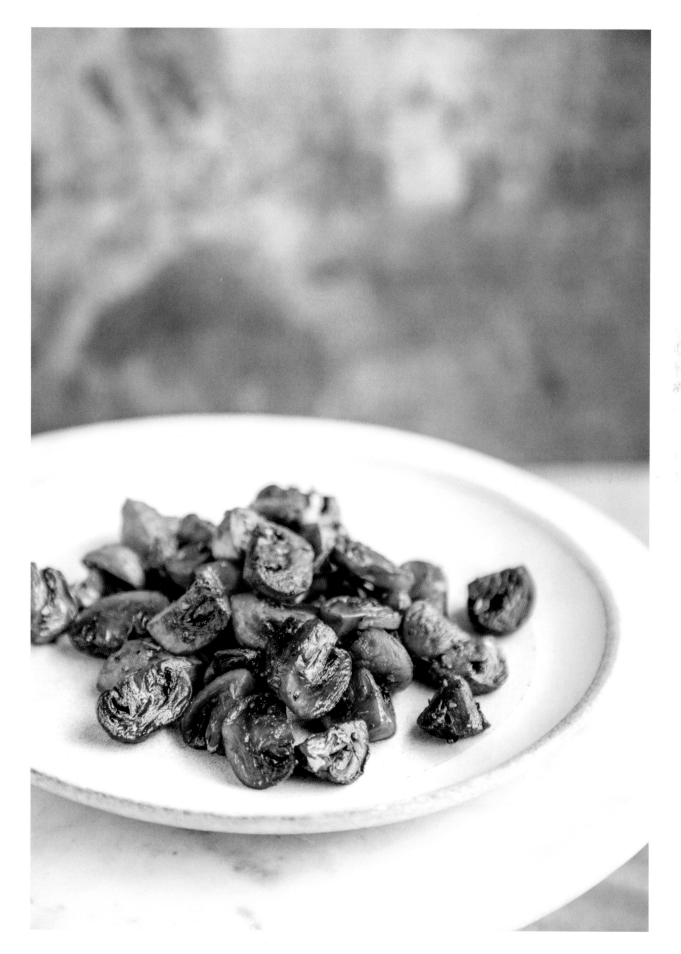

EASY SESAME BROCCOLI

  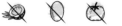

YIELD: 4 servings | **SERVING SIZE:** 1 cup | **PREP TIME:** 5 minutes | **COOK TIME:** 8 minutes

You can have this easy and healthy side dish on the table in less than 15 minutes, and you won't believe how much flavor such a simple preparation of broccoli can deliver! Sesame and broccoli—who knew? It is one of my new favorite ways to eat this keto superfood; if you're a broccoli fan, you're going to love this one.

4 cups fresh or frozen broccoli florets (1 large head or 2 [10-ounce] packages)

¼ cup filtered water

2 tablespoons butter

1 teaspoon toasted sesame oil

½ teaspoon kosher salt

1 tablespoon sesame seeds

Place the broccoli and water in a microwave-safe dish. Cook on high, uncovered, for 8 minutes, or until fork-tender. Remove from the microwave and drain any remaining water. Add the butter, sesame oil, salt, and sesame seeds to the dish and stir until the butter is melted and the florets are coated. Serve hot. Store leftovers in an airtight container in the refrigerator for up to 1 week.

CALORIES: 108 **FAT:** 8g **PROTEIN:** 2g **CARBS:** 6g **FIBER:** 3g **NET CARBS:** 3g

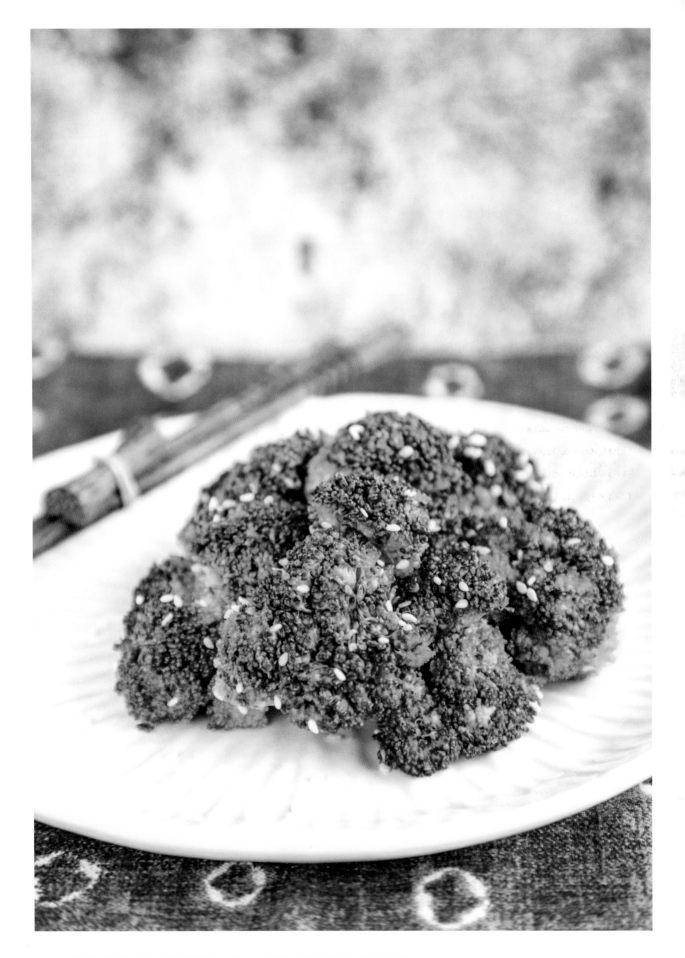

CREAMY COCONUT CAULIFLOWER RICE

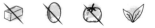

YIELD: 5 servings	**SERVING SIZE:** ½ cup	**PREP TIME:** 5 minutes	**COOK TIME:** 7 minutes

This super simple cauliflower rice is tasty on its own but works especially well as a side to curries and Asian-inspired dishes.

3 cups riced cauliflower

½ cup canned coconut milk

1 teaspoon coconut aminos

Put the riced cauliflower, coconut milk, and coconut aminos in a microwave-safe bowl. Microwave on high, uncovered, for 4 minutes. Stir and microwave for an additional 3 minutes, or until the cauliflower is tender but not mushy. Stir and serve hot. Store leftovers in an airtight container in the refrigerator for up to 1 week.

CALORIES: 74 | **FAT:** 3g | **PROTEIN:** 2g | **CARBS:** 3g | **FIBER:** 1g | **NET CARBS:** 2g

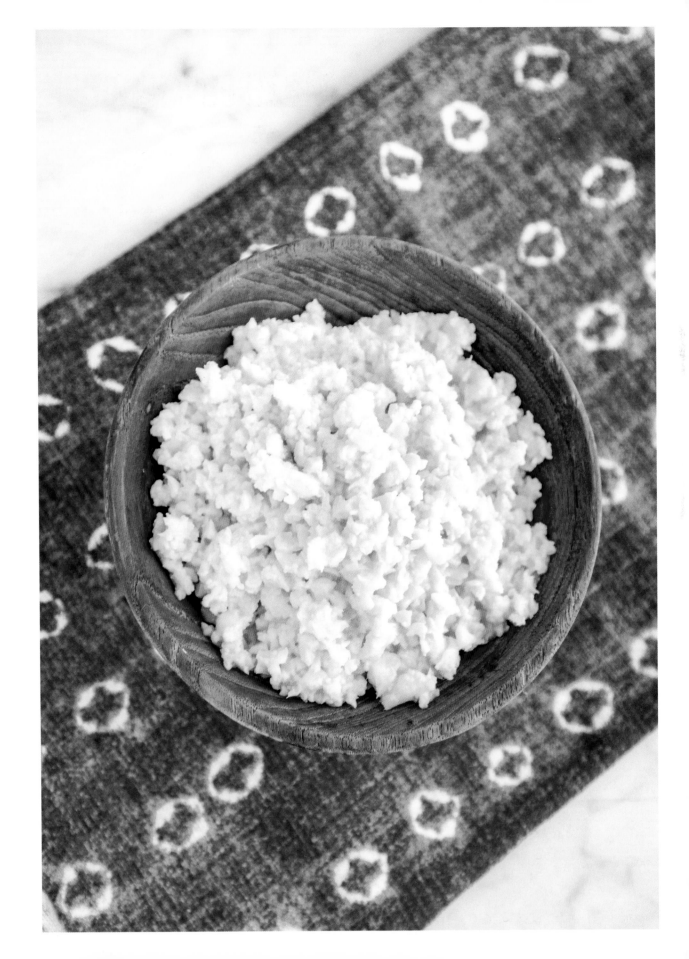

SAUTÉED SHREDDED BRUSSELS SPROUTS

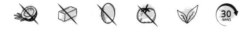

YIELD: 4 servings | **SERVING SIZE:** 1 cup | **PREP TIME:** 10 minutes | **COOK TIME:** 10 minutes

Light, fresh, and slightly sweet equals side dish perfection in my book. Often, people who think they don't like Brussels sprouts just haven't had them prepared correctly. If your experience has been underwhelming in the past, it could be because you were eating whole sprouts where all the seasoning is on the outside layer, leaving the center bland and unappealing. Shredding or thinly slicing eliminates that problem, allowing the seasonings to flavor the entire dish—and it cuts down on the cooking time. This version, flavored with plenty of garlic and lemon zest, will not disappoint!

3 tablespoons extra-virgin olive oil

6 cups trimmed and thinly sliced Brussels sprouts (about 1½ pounds whole sprouts) (see Note)

1 tablespoon grated lemon zest

1 teaspoon minced garlic

¾ teaspoon kosher salt

¼ teaspoon ground black pepper

½ teaspoon red wine vinegar

Heat the oil in a large skillet over medium-high heat until shimmering. Add the Brussels sprouts and cook for about 5 minutes, stirring occasionally, until wilted, bright green, and beginning to caramelize. Stir in the lemon zest, garlic, salt, and pepper. Turn the heat down to low and cook for another 3 to 5 minutes, until the Brussels sprouts are tender but not mushy. Remove the pan from the heat and stir in the vinegar. Serve warm. Store leftovers in an airtight container in the refrigerator for up to 5 days.

Note: Sometimes you can find bags of presliced (aka preshaved or preshredded) Brussels sprouts in the grocery store produce department. These prepped bags will save you time but can be more expensive than buying whole sprouts and prepping them yourself. If purchasing preprepped Brussels sprouts, ensure that the package contains at least 6 cups, or about 18 ounces by weight.

CALORIES: 118 **FAT:** 9g **PROTEIN:** 2g **CARBS:** 11g **FIBER:** 5g **NET CARBS:** 6g

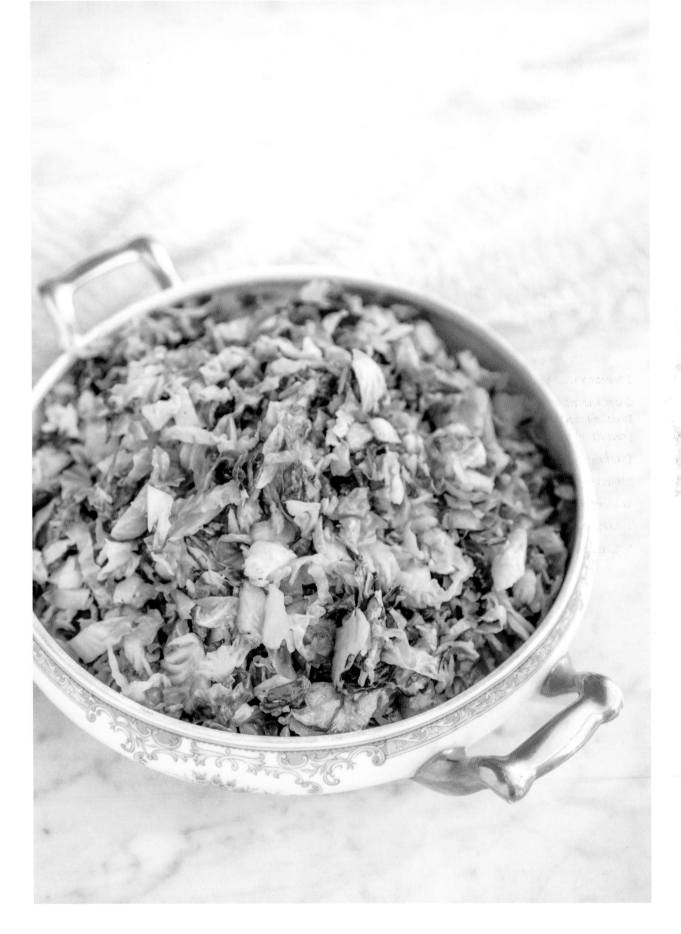

ROASTED BACON-WRAPPED CABBAGE WEDGES

 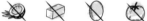

| YIELD: 6 wedges | SERVING SIZE: 1 wedge | PREP TIME: 8 minutes | COOK TIME: 45 minutes |

For such a simple dish, these oven-roasted cabbage wedges bring a ton of flavor to your plate. Roasting sweetens the cabbage, while the bacon fat melts into it and gives it a luxurious texture. This is my new go-to side dish when I don't have a lot of time to prep. If you're feeding a crowd, this is an easy recipe to double, and it can be made a couple of hours ahead and reheated in the microwave just before serving.

1 medium head green cabbage (about 2 pounds)

6 slices bacon

1 tablespoon extra-virgin olive oil

½ teaspoon kosher salt

¼ teaspoon ground black pepper

1. Preheat the oven to 375°F.

2. Cut the cabbage head in half, then cut each half into 3 wedges. Wrap a slice of bacon around each wedge. Place the wedges on a sheet pan. Brush with the oil and sprinkle with the salt and pepper.

3. Bake for 45 minutes, or until the cabbage is tender and the bacon is golden brown. Serve immediately. Store leftovers in an airtight container in the refrigerator for up to 5 days.

| CALORIES: 123 | FAT: 8g | PROTEIN: 5g | CARBS: 6g | FIBER: 2g | NET CARBS: 4g |

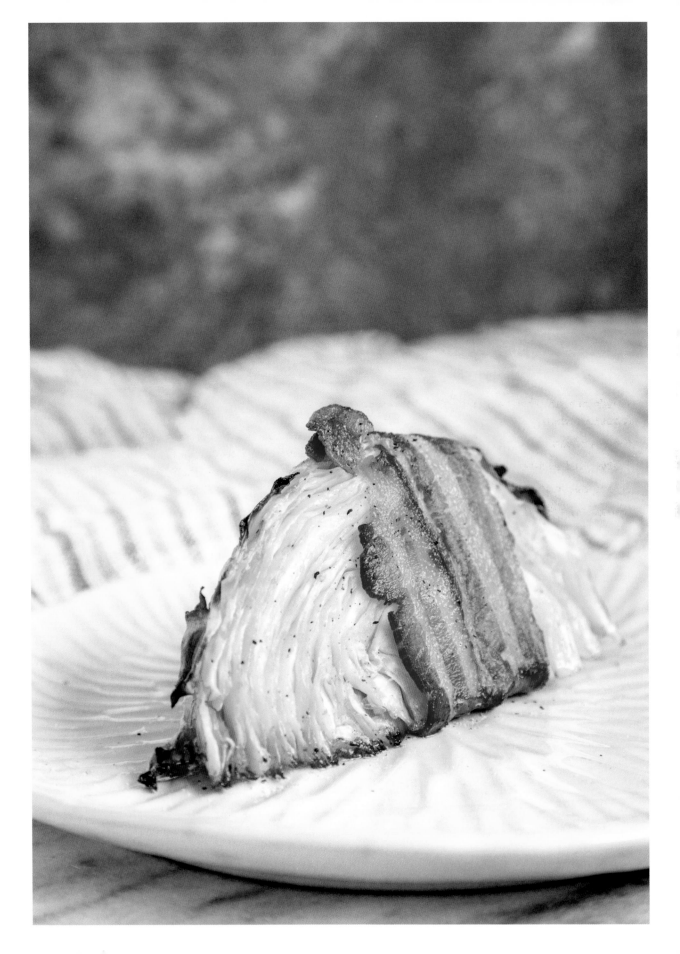

DUCHESS CAULIFLOWER

| YIELD: 12 pieces | SERVING SIZE: 2 pieces | PREP TIME: 10 minutes | COOK TIME: 30 minutes |

Duchess potatoes is a classic French preparation of mashed potatoes mixed with cream, flour, butter, and seasonings that is then piped into a swirl and baked. In this Squeaky Clean Keto version, cauliflower stands in for the potatoes and mayonnaise makes it creamy and luscious. While preparing this dish takes a little more work than your basic cauliflower mash, the crispy tops and creamy interior are well worth the effort. These make the perfect caps to the Meatloaf Cupcakes on page 210.

6 cups fresh cauliflower florets (about 2 medium heads)

¼ cup (½ stick) butter

¼ cup mayonnaise

1 tablespoon coconut flour

1 teaspoon kosher salt

¼ teaspoon ground black pepper

½ teaspoon garlic powder

½ teaspoon onion powder

⅛ teaspoon ground nutmeg

1. Preheat the oven to 375°F. Line a sheet pan with parchment paper.

2. Put the cauliflower in a large microwave-safe bowl and microwave, uncovered, for 12 minutes, or until fork-tender.

3. Put the cauliflower in a blender or food processor (see Notes). Add the butter, mayonnaise, coconut flour, salt, pepper, garlic powder, onion powder, and nutmeg and blend until smooth.

4. Spoon or pipe the cauliflower onto the prepared sheet pan. Bake for 15 to 18 minutes, until puffed and golden brown. Serve immediately. Store leftovers in an airtight container in the refrigerator for up to 5 days.

Notes: For a cauliflower puree with a thick consistency that will stand up to piping, I prefer the microwave method above because it is fast and allows liquid to evaporate. If you don't have a microwave, you can roast the cauliflower in a 400°F oven for 30 minutes or until tender before blending. Another method is to steam or boil the cauliflower until tender—but in order to get a thick consistency, you must drain the cauliflower in a colander for at least 10 minutes before blending, or it will be too watery to work in this recipe.

If you're not using a high-powered blender, stop the blender frequently and scrape down the sides with a rubber spatula to facilitate even blending.

CALORIES: 210   FAT: 12g   PROTEIN: 1g   CARBS: 5g   FIBER: 3g   NET CARBS: 3g

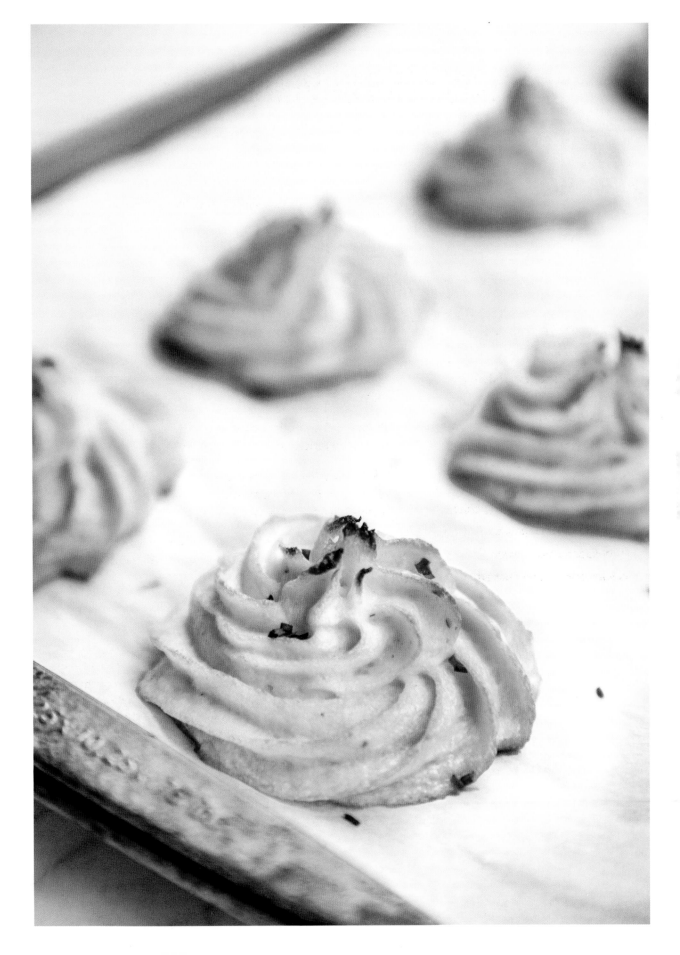

EVERYTHING ROASTED CAULIFLOWER STEAKS

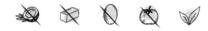

YIELD: 4 servings | **SERVING SIZE:** 4 ounces | **PREP TIME:** 5 minutes | **COOK TIME:** 35 minutes

---

This everything roasted cauliflower is simple and surprisingly addictive. Roasty, sweet cauliflower married with the garlicky crunch of everything bagel seasoning is the perfect combination! No worries if you can't get the steaks to hold together—it tastes just as good made with florets.

1 medium head cauliflower (about 2 pounds)

2 tablespoons avocado oil

2 tablespoons Everything Bagel Seasoning (page 80)

1. Preheat the oven to 375°F.

2. Trim the cauliflower head of any leaves and brown spots, then slice it into 1-inch steaks or break it into florets. Brush with the oil and sprinkle with the everything bagel seasoning. Spread out on a sheet pan.

3. Roast the cauliflower for 35 minutes, or until golden brown and fork-tender. Serve hot. Store leftovers in an airtight container in the refrigerator for up to 1 week.

CALORIES: 117 **FAT:** 9g **PROTEIN:** 4g **CARBS:** 8g **FIBER:** 4g **NET CARBS:** 4g

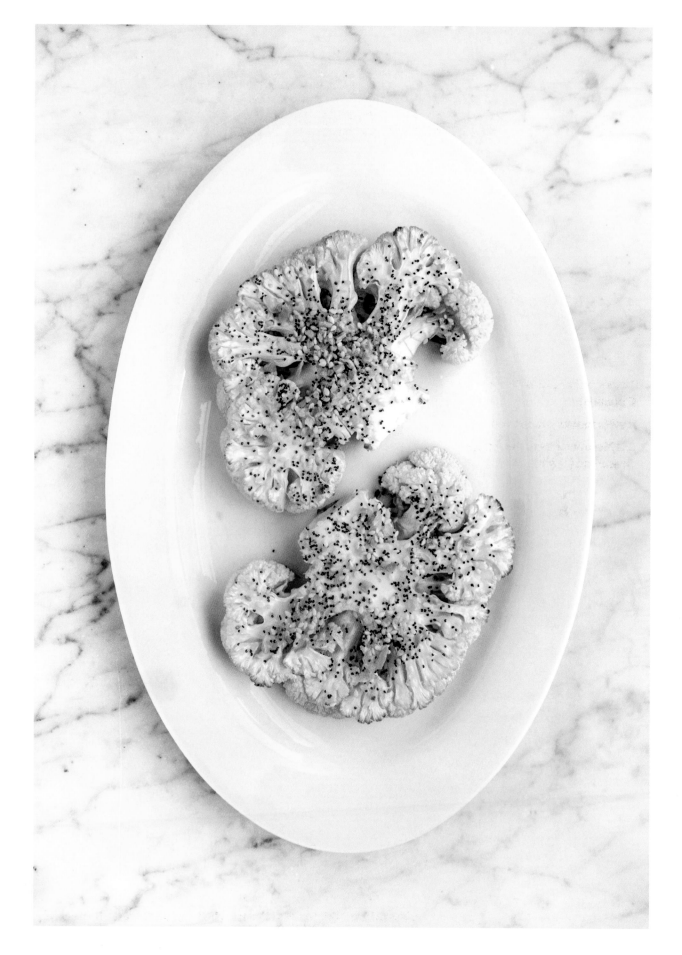

SHEET PAN VEGGIE BURGERS

| YIELD: 4 burgers | SERVING SIZE: 1 burger | PREP TIME: 15 minutes | COOK TIME: 25 minutes |

These surprisingly hearty patties, with just enough texture, go so well with my spicy Chili-Lime Mayo (page 100) and tangy Quick-Pickled Red Onions (page 108). Throw on some smooth and creamy avocado slices and you've got the perfect veggie bite. Not quite as chewy as meat-based burgers, these are still incredibly satisfying—even for a bacon cheeseburger lover like me! One of my favorite recipes in this book.

2 cups roughly chopped fresh broccoli florets (see Note)

2 cups roughly chopped fresh cauliflower florets (see Note)

½ cup roughly chopped white mushrooms

1 clove garlic, peeled

½ cup shelled hemp seeds (hemp hearts)

½ cup unsweetened shredded coconut

1 teaspoon psyllium husk powder

½ cup mayonnaise

1 teaspoon coconut aminos

1½ teaspoons kosher salt

1 teaspoon ground cumin

1 teaspoon smoked paprika

½ teaspoon ground black pepper

½ teaspoon onion powder

⅛ teaspoon ground nutmeg

1. Preheat the oven to 375°F. Line a sheet pan with parchment paper.

2. Put the broccoli, cauliflower, mushrooms, and garlic in a food processor. Pulse until the mixture resembles coarse crumbs. Add the shelled hemp seeds, shredded coconut, psyllium powder, mayonnaise, coconut aminos, salt, and spices. Pulse until the mixture is fully combined and uniform looking but not smooth or liquefied.

3. Form the mixture into 4 patties about 5 inches in diameter and 1 inch thick and place on the prepared sheet pan.

4. Bake the patties for 25 minutes, or until golden brown and firm to the touch in the center. Store leftovers in an airtight container in the refrigerator for up to 5 days.

Note: While either fresh or frozen broccoli or cauliflower can be used in other recipes in this book, in this case fresh is best because it blends better and provides the right texture. Since frozen vegetables are blanched first, they will be softer and are not ideal for use in this recipe.

| CALORIES: 370 | FAT: 33g | PROTEIN: 9g | CARBS: 11g | FIBER: 6g | NET CARBS: 5g |

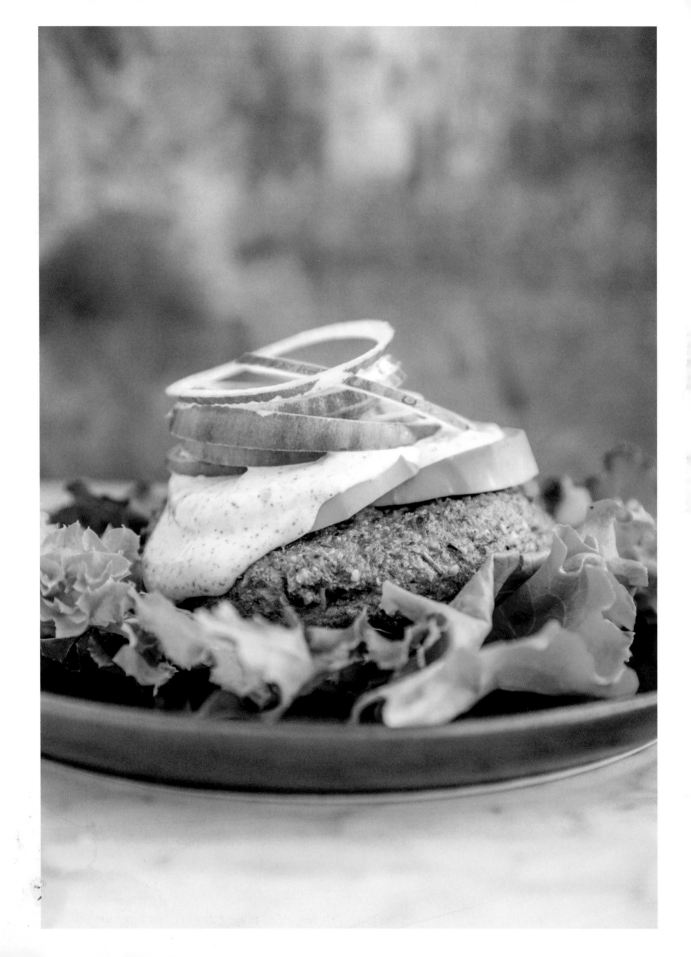

KOREAN SCALLION PANCAKES (PAJEON)

YIELD: 6 pancakes | SERVING SIZE: 1 pancake + 1 tablespoon sauce | PREP TIME: 8 minutes | COOK TIME: 24 minutes

A staple of Korean cuisine, scallion pancakes are usually made with a combination of tempura flour, rice flour, and white flour, making them very soft and pliable, with a chewy texture you don't find in what most Americans think of as a pancake. My keto version uses coconut flour and psyllium husk powder, which gives the pancakes a similar, slightly gummy texture that makes them surprisingly authentic. Pajeon can contain other veggies (I like to add sliced chilis for heat) and even seafood for a main course, but in this recipe we are sticking to the classic scallion version, which is typically served as a side dish or first course. Once you get it down, feel free to experiment with your own variations!

For the pancakes:

6 large eggs

3 tablespoons coconut flour

1 teaspoon psyllium husk powder

Pinch of kosher salt

¾ cup filtered water

1 teaspoon toasted sesame oil

3 tablespoons avocado oil, divided

1½ cups chopped scallions, green parts only

For the dipping sauce:

¼ cup filtered water

1 tablespoon coconut aminos

1 teaspoon fish sauce (no sugar added)

1 teaspoon toasted sesame oil

1 teaspoon sesame seeds, for garnish

1. *Make the pancakes:* Put the eggs, coconut flour, psyllium powder, salt, water, sesame oil, and 1 tablespoon of the avocado oil in a blender and blend until smooth. Heat 1 teaspoon of the avocado oil in a 12-inch or larger nonstick skillet over medium heat and add ¼ cup of the scallions to the oil. Cook for about 1 minute, until bright green. Pour in ¼ cup of the batter and spread it over the scallions with a rubber spatula, forming a circular pancake about 10 inches in diameter. Cook for about 2 minutes, until firm in the center. Carefully flip and cook for an additional 1 minute, or until firm to the touch. Remove and set aside on a serving plate. Repeat with the remaining scallions and batter, adding more avocado oil to the pan after every second pancake, or as needed.

2. *Make the dipping sauce:* Put the water, coconut aminos, fish sauce, and sesame oil in a small bowl. Stir with a fork until combined. Garnish with the sesame seeds. Dip pieces of the pancake into the sauce before eating. Store leftovers in an airtight container in the refrigerator for up to 5 days. Reheat the pancakes in the microwave, uncovered, for 30 seconds to 1 minute, until hot.

PANCAKES:	CALORIES: 155	FAT: 13g	PROTEIN: 7g	CARBS: 4g	FIBER: 2g	NET CARBS: 2g
SAUCE:	CALORIES: 10	FAT: 1g	PROTEIN: 0g	CARBS: 1g	FIBER: 0g	NET CARBS: 1g

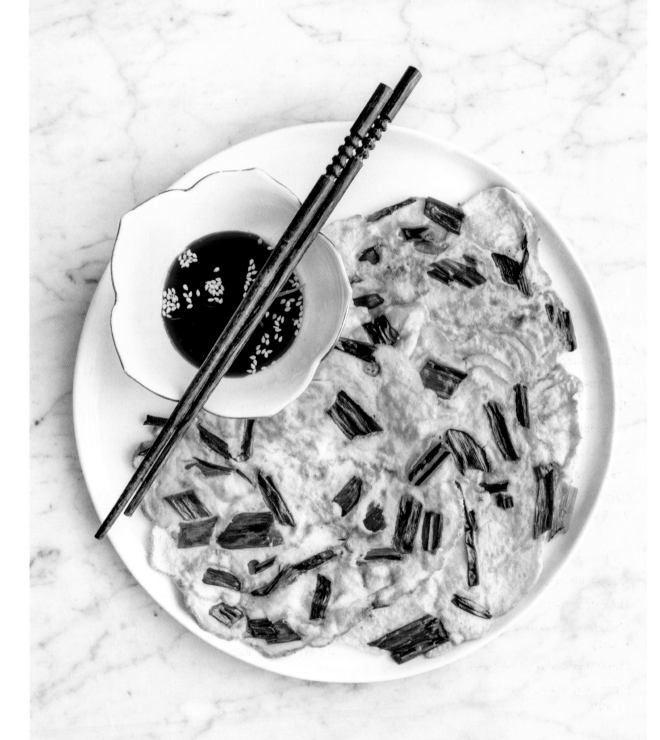

SPAGHETTI SQUASH PUTTANESCA

YIELD: 4 servings | **SERVING SIZE:** 1½ cups | **PREP TIME:** 5 minutes | **COOK TIME:** 7 minutes

This keto spaghetti squash puttanesca is rich, tangy, and ultra-satisfying! It's also very easy to throw together at a moment's notice with ingredients you probably already have in your pantry. Not a fan of spaghetti squash? This sauce can easily be served over zucchini noodles instead.

¼ cup extra-virgin olive oil

15 green olives, pitted and roughly chopped

2 cloves garlic, chopped

1 tablespoon capers, drained and roughly chopped

1 teaspoon anchovy paste (optional)

1 cup canned crushed tomatoes

1 teaspoon red pepper flakes

3 cups cooked spaghetti squash (1 medium squash)

Chopped fresh parsley, for garnish

Heat the oil in a large skillet over medium heat. Add the olives, garlic, capers, and anchovy paste (if using) and cook for 2 minutes, or until fragrant. Add the tomatoes and red pepper flakes and simmer, stirring occasionally, for 5 minutes. Stir in the cooked spaghetti squash and remove the pan from the heat. Garnish with fresh parsley and serve immediately. Store leftovers in an airtight container in the refrigerator for up to 5 days.

CALORIES: 193 | **FAT:** 16g | **PROTEIN:** 3g | **CARBS:** 11g | **FIBER:** 3g | **NET CARBS:** 8g

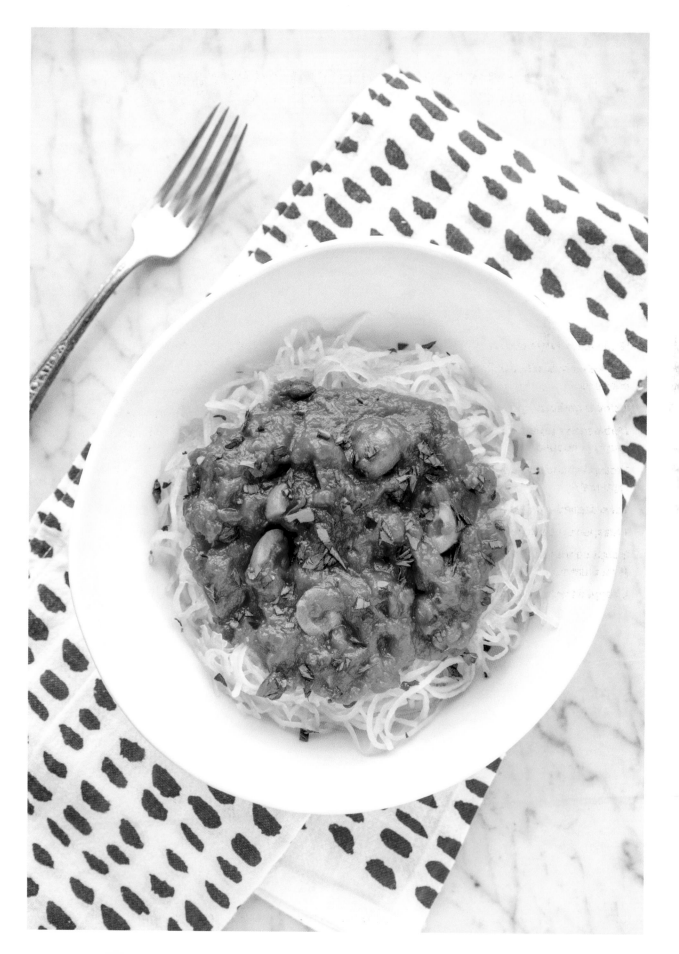

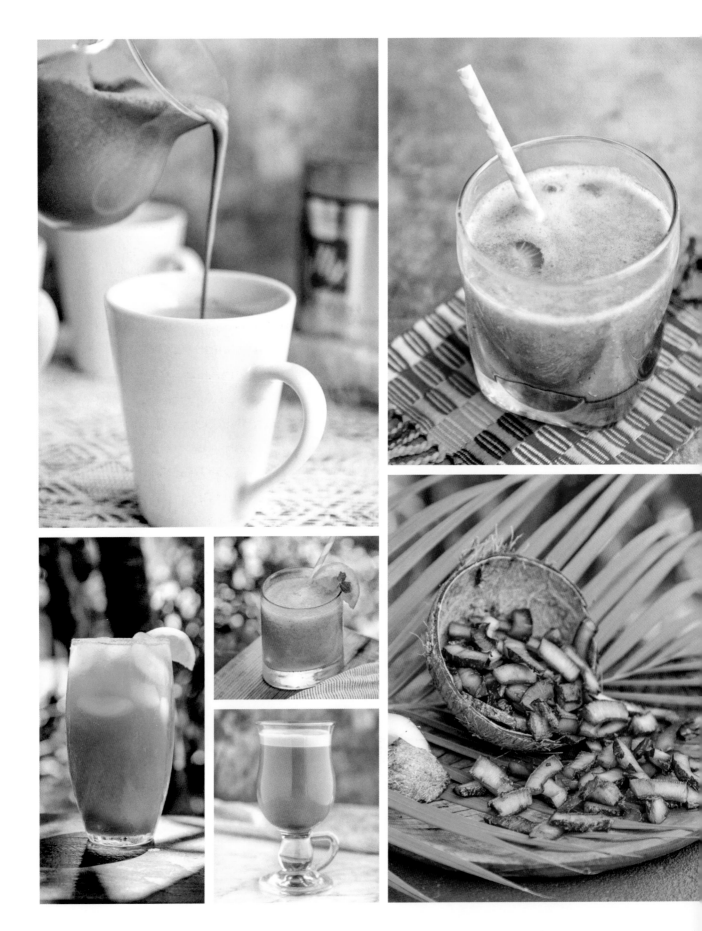

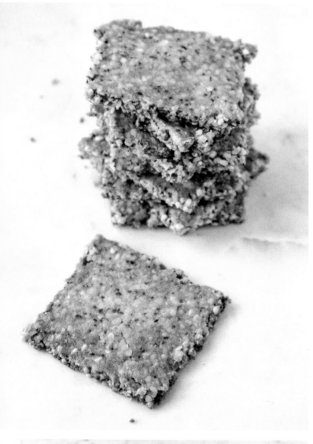

Drinks & Snacks

Hibiscus Elderberry Tea / 314

Cucumber Mint Cooler / 316

Strawberry Lime Refresher / 318

Raspberry Green Tea / 320

Vanilla Mocha Coconut Creamer / 322

Basic Bulletproof Coffee / 324

Bulletproof Chai Latte / 326

Vanilla Hemp Milk / 328

Hemp Milk Cappuccino / 330

Green Lemonade / 332

Ginger Lemon Detox Drink / 334

Sweet Sesame Coconut Chips / 336

Salty Wasabi Coconut Chips / 338

Baba Ghanoush / 340

Everything Hemp Crackers / 342

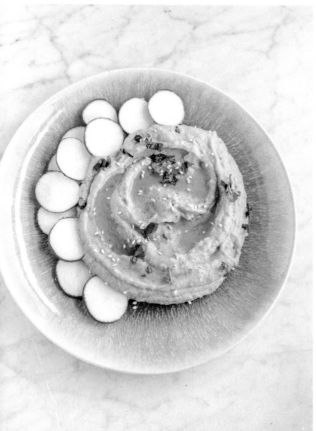

HIBISCUS ELDERBERRY TEA

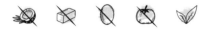

YIELD: 5 cups concentrate	SERVING SIZE: ½ cup concentrate + 1½ cups water or seltzer	PREP TIME: 2 minutes

COOK TIME: 8 minutes, plus 1 hour to infuse

This tasty zero-carb tea is not only super refreshing but also insanely good for you. Hibiscus and elderberries are both high in vitamin C and rich in antioxidant compounds rumored to fight infection (including UTIs), reduce inflammation, boost overall immunity, improve liver health, and even lower blood pressure. All those potential benefits—and the fact that it's delicious too—make this one of my favorite drinks in this book.

6 cups filtered water

2 tablespoons dried elderberries

½ cup dried hibiscus flower petals

2 cinnamon sticks

2 strips lemon zest, about 1 inch wide

1. Put all the ingredients in a medium-sized saucepan. Bring to a boil over high heat, then simmer, uncovered, for 5 minutes. Turn off the heat and let the mixture cool on the stovetop for 1 hour.

2. Pour the cooled mixture through a fine-mesh sieve to remove the solids. Store the concentrate in an airtight container in the refrigerator for up to 1 week or in the freezer for up to 6 months.

3. To serve, use ½ cup concentrate to 1½ cups of water. It can be served hot or chilled over ice, as shown, to make a hibiscus-elderberry cooler. The chilled concentrate can also be mixed with seltzer instead of water.

Notes: You can purchase organic dried elderberries (Sambucus nigra) and dried hibiscus petals from Amazon at very reasonable prices.

If you are prone to food allergies, test a small amount of this tea to be sure you won't react to it before you make it a regular part of your diet.

You can freeze the concentrate into ice cubes to flavor water.

CALORIES: 5	FAT: 0g	PROTEIN: 0g	CARBS: 0g	FIBER: 0g	NET CARBS: 0g

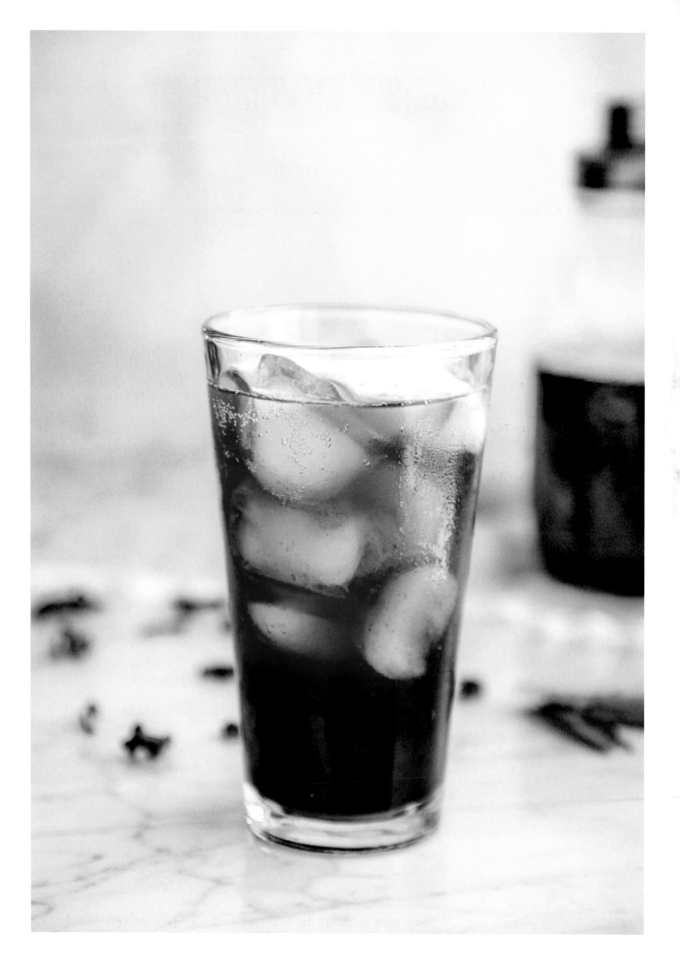

CUCUMBER MINT COOLER

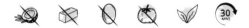

YIELD: 1 serving | **SERVING SIZE:** 12 ounces | **PREP TIME:** 5 minutes

Fresh mint gives this super healthy and refreshing tonic a mojito vibe that feels party ready. Ultra-hydrating, the cucumbers in this bevvie deliver a lot of nutrients, including potassium, which is especially important on a keto diet. You'll want to stock up on cucumbers and mint once you taste this one—it's a delicious way to boost your electrolytes naturally!

1 cup peeled and sliced cucumbers

2 tablespoons fresh mint leaves

2 teaspoons fresh lemon juice

Pinch of ground Himalayan pink salt

½ cup filtered water

5 ice cubes

Place all the ingredients in a blender and blend until smooth. Serve immediately.

CALORIES: 19 **FAT:** 0g **PROTEIN:** 1g **CARBS:** 3g **FIBER:** 1g **NET CARBS:** 2g

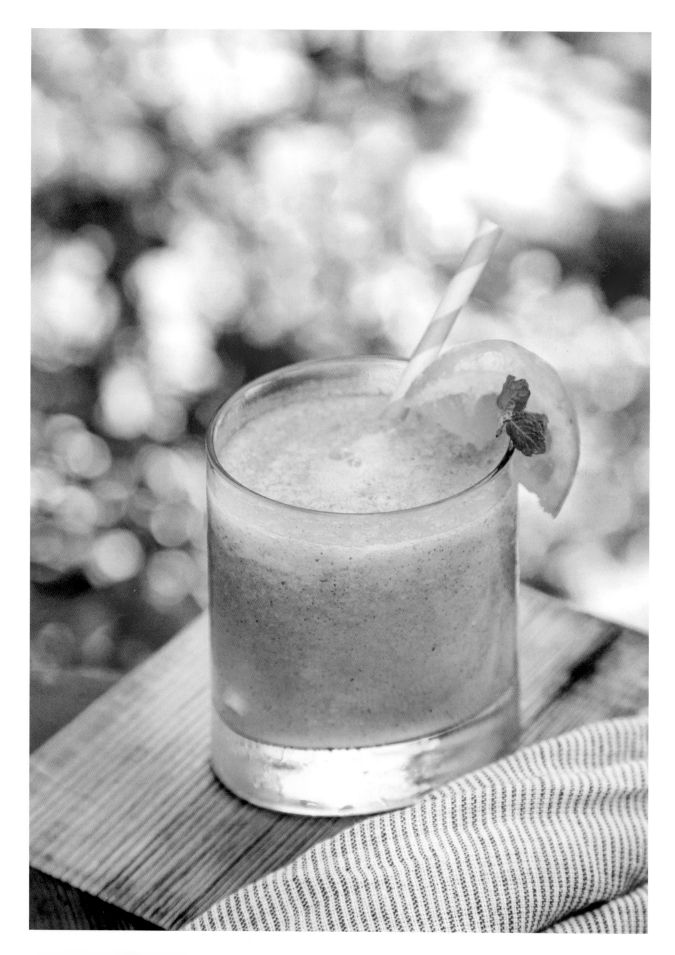

STRAWBERRY LIME REFRESHER

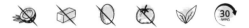

| YIELD: 1 serving | SERVING SIZE: 8 ounces | PREP TIME: 5 minutes |

Refreshing and slightly sweet, this is the perfect drink for when everyone around you is having a cocktail and you're keeping it squeaky. The acid of the lime juice balances out the sweetness of the strawberries, while the club soda adds a pleasant fizz. Loaded with vitamin C and phytonutrients, this pretty tonic is super healthy for you, and worth the few extra carbs.

½ cup sliced strawberries (fresh or frozen)

1 teaspoon fresh lime juice

4 or 5 ice cubes

4 ounces club soda or lime-flavored seltzer

Blend the strawberries and lime juice in a small blender until smooth. Pour into a 12-ounce glass. Add the ice cubes and club soda. Stir and serve immediately.

Notes: *If not squeaky, you can add 1 teaspoon of powdered erythritol to sweeten this drink.*

If you want a smoother drink with no seeds, press the strawberry and lime juice mixture through a fine-mesh sieve after blending.

CALORIES: 31   FAT: 0g   PROTEIN: 0g   CARBS: 6g   FIBER: 2g   NET CARBS: 4g

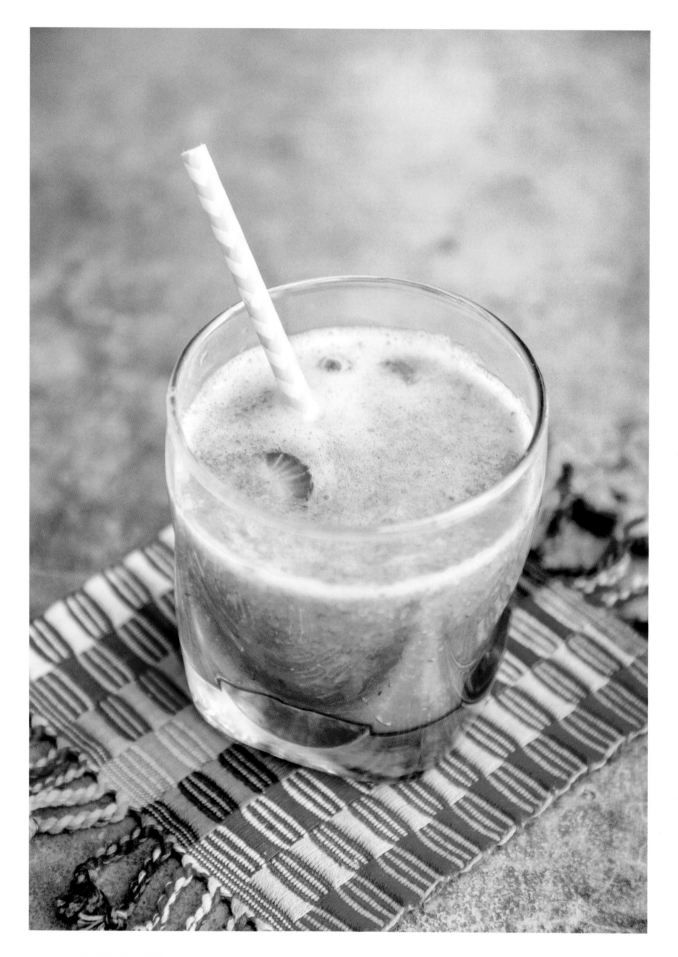

RASPBERRY GREEN TEA

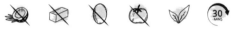

YIELD: 2 servings | **SERVING SIZE:** 14 ounces | **PREP TIME:** 5 minutes, plus 20 minutes to steep and cool

---

A tasty departure from your water drinking routine, this raspberry green tea contains a bounty of antioxidants and polyphenols that are said to prevent cancer, boost metabolism, and even make you smarter. I don't know if all that's true, but this tea is delicious, and the small hit of caffeine will give you a boost of energy to get you through the afternoon.

4 cups filtered water

2 green tea bags

10 raspberries, plus more for garnish if desired

¼ cup packed fresh mint leaves, plus 2 sprigs for garnish if desired

Bring the water to a boil in a medium-sized saucepan, then remove the pan from the heat. Add the tea bags, raspberries, and mint leaves to the hot water. Let steep for 5 minutes, then remove the tea bags. Let cool for 15 minutes, then blend in a blender for 10 seconds. Pour the liquid through a fine-mesh sieve to remove the solids. Serve hot or iced, garnished with additional raspberries and mint sprigs if desired.

Note: If not squeaky, feel free to sweeten the tea as desired.

CALORIES: 7   **FAT:** 0g   **PROTEIN:** 0g   **CARBS:** 1g   **FIBER:** 0g   **NET CARBS:** 1g

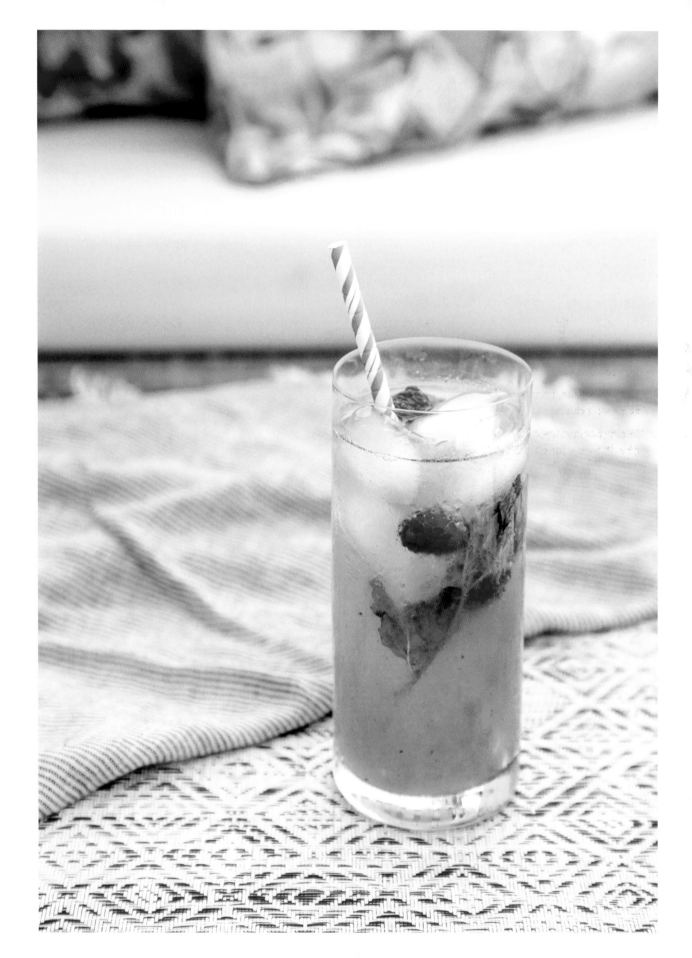

VANILLA MOCHA COCONUT CREAMER

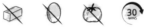

YIELD: 2 cups | **SERVING SIZE:** 2 tablespoons | **PREP TIME:** 5 minutes

---

If you're a mocha lover, then this cocoa-flavored creamer is going to be right up your alley. Super rich and creamy, your morning coffee just got a little more exciting. I've used this creamer in hot and iced coffee, and both are great.

1 (14-ounce) can coconut milk

1 (2-ounce) packet coconut milk powder

¼ cup collagen peptides (aka hydrolysate)

1 tablespoon cocoa powder

1 teaspoon pure vanilla extract

Put all the ingredients in a blender and blend for 15 seconds, or until smooth. Store in an airtight container in the refrigerator for up to 1 week.

Note: If not squeaky, feel free to sweeten the creamer as desired.

CALORIES: 66 | **FAT:** 6g | **PROTEIN:** 1g | **CARBS:** 1g | **FIBER:** 0g | **NET CARBS:** 1g

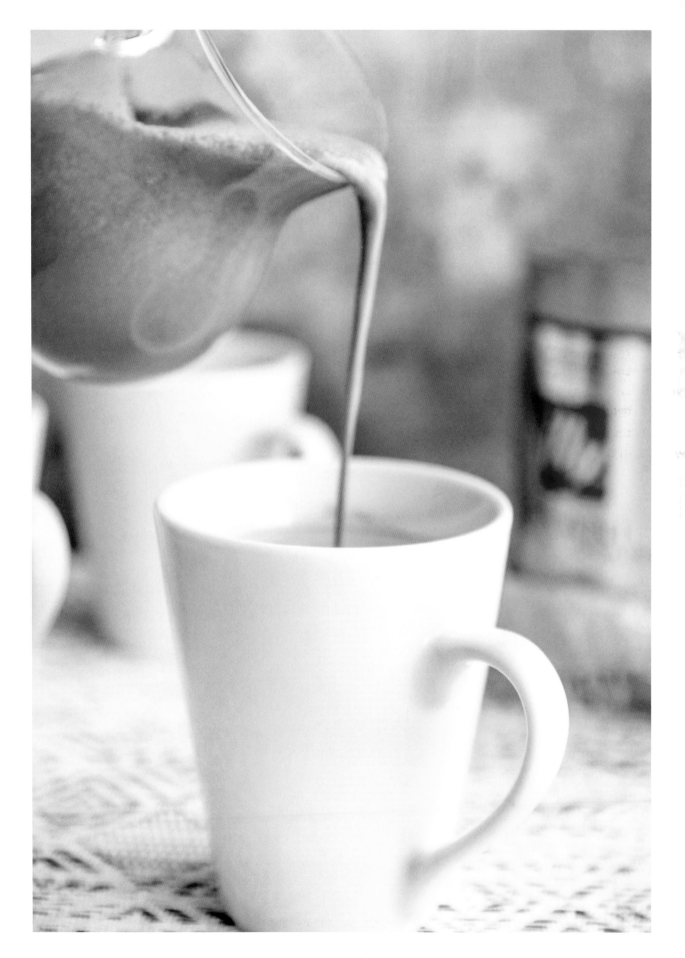

BASIC BULLETPROOF COFFEE

YIELD: 1 serving | **SERVING SIZE:** 10 ounces | **PREP TIME:** 2 minutes

This is a simple "bulletproof" coffee recipe that can be customized in a variety of ways according to your preferences. The powdered collagen peptides are optional but recommended for texture and to keep the fats from separating—not to mention that they're a great source of protein and reported to be excellent for bone, skin, hair, and gut health.

8 ounces brewed coffee

1 tablespoon unrefined coconut oil or MCT oil (see page 35)

1 tablespoon unsalted butter

1 tablespoon collagen peptides (aka hydrolysate) (optional)

Place all the ingredients in a blender and blend for 10 seconds, or until frothy. Pour into a 12-ounce coffee mug and serve immediately.

Note: If not squeaky, feel free to sweeten the drink as desired.

CALORIES: 232   **FAT:** 26g   **PROTEIN:** 0g   **CARBS:** 0g   **FIBER:** 0g   **NET CARBS:** 0g

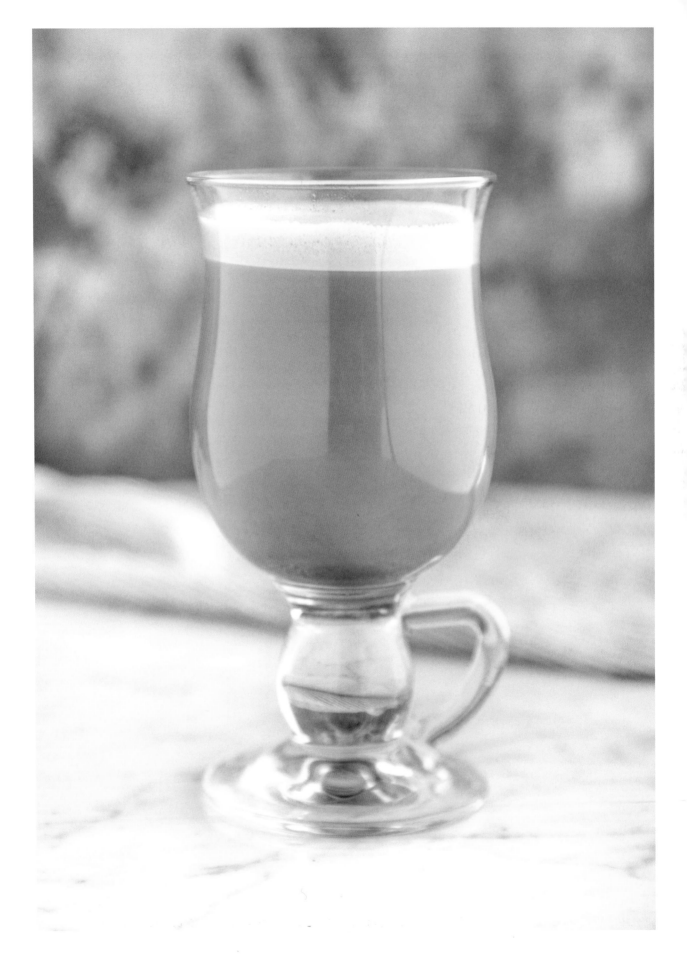

BULLETPROOF CHAI LATTE

YIELD: 1 serving | **SERVING SIZE:** 10 ounces | **PREP TIME:** 2 minutes

If you're not a coffee drinker (it's okay, we can still be friends), or you just like to change it up every once in a while, then you're going to love the warm and spicy flavors of this chai latte. As in the Basic Bulletproof Coffee recipe on page 324, the powdered collagen peptides are optional but recommended for the texture and also the health benefits. If you're using a bulletproof beverage as your morning meal, the collagen powder also makes it more filling, allowing you to go hours before your first solid meal of the day.

8 ounces brewed chai tea

1 tablespoon unrefined coconut oil or MCT oil (see page 35)

1 tablespoon unsalted butter

1 tablespoon collagen peptides (aka hydrolysate) (optional)

⅛ teaspoon ground cinnamon, for garnish

Put the brewed tea, coconut oil, butter, and collagen, if using, in a blender. Blend for 10 seconds, or until frothy. Pour into a 12-ounce coffee mug. Sprinkle with the cinnamon and serve immediately.

Note: *If not squeaky, feel free to sweeten the drink as desired.*

WITHOUT COLLAGEN: **CALORIES:** 235 **FAT:** 26g **PROTEIN:** 0g **CARBS:** 0g **FIBER:** 0g **NET CARBS:** 0g

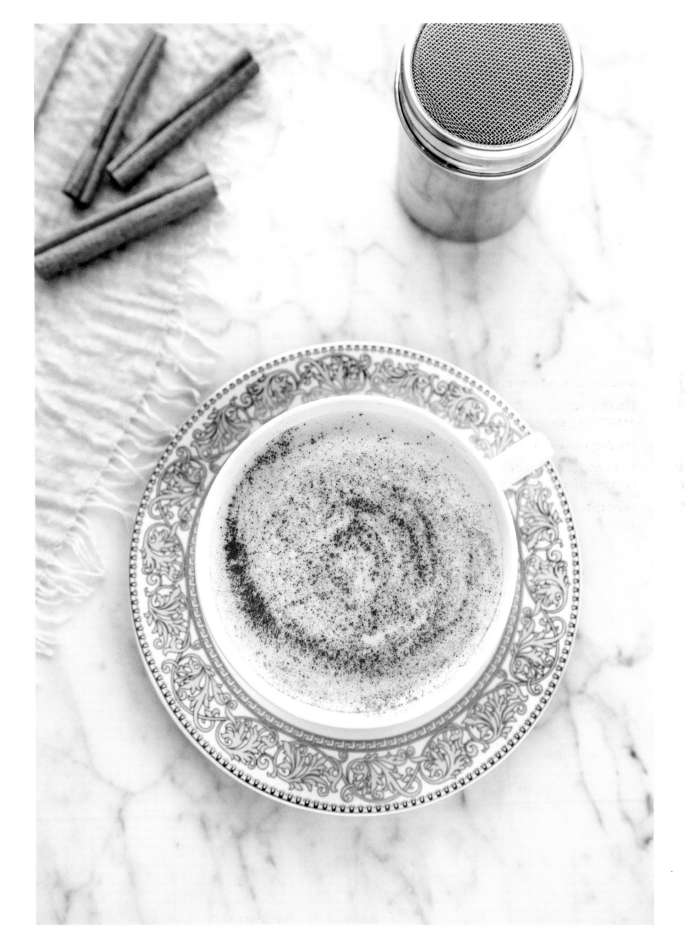

VANILLA HEMP MILK

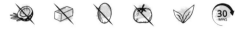

YIELD: 4 cups | **SERVING SIZE:** ½ cup | **PREP TIME:** 8 minutes

---

Nut and seed milks are expensive to buy and can be labor-intensive to make because they usually require hours of soaking prior to blending. This hemp seed milk can be made in just minutes—no soaking required—and it's the most delicious plant-based milk I've ever tried. Loaded with potassium, magnesium, and heart-healthy fats, this milk is a fantastic addition to your entire family's diet—even if they aren't eating keto.

4 cups filtered water

⅔ cup shelled hemp seeds (hemp hearts)

1 teaspoon vanilla extract

Pinch of kosher salt

Put all the ingredients in a high-powered blender and blend until completely smooth. Line a large-mesh sieve with a clean white T-shirt and set it over a large bowl. Pour the milk into it. Allow to drain completely, then squeeze the pulp tightly in the T-shirt to extract any remaining milk. Discard the pulp. Store in an airtight container in the refrigerator for up to 1 week.

Variations: **Strawberry Hemp Milk.** *Add 5 ripe strawberries to the blender before blending.*

Chocolate Hemp Milk. *Add 2 tablespoons of cocoa powder to the blender before blending.*

Note: *If not squeaky, feel free to sweeten the milk as desired.*

CALORIES: 72 **FAT:** 6g **PROTEIN:** 3g **CARBS:** 0g **FIBER:** 0g **NET CARBS:** 0g

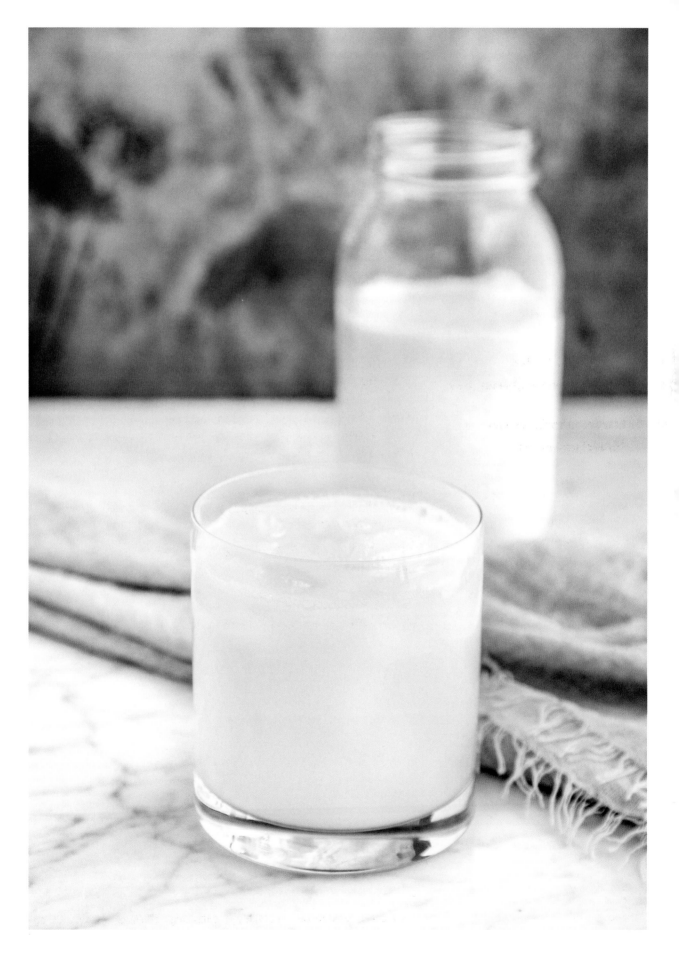

HEMP MILK CAPPUCCINO

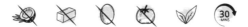

YIELD: 1 serving | **SERVING SIZE:** 6 ounces | **PREP TIME:** 2 minutes

I stumbled on this recipe accidentally when I was whipping up a batch of hemp milk and a mound of foam was left behind in the blender. It reminded me of the foam from my cappuccino maker, so I brewed some espresso and experimented with it. It was so good that I immediately snapped some photos and added this recipe to the book. The best part is that no tedious steaming is required: you simply add the already-prepared hemp milk to a blender and it foams up perfectly in seconds!

2 ounces brewed espresso

½ cup Vanilla Hemp Milk (page 328)

¼ teaspoon ground cinnamon or cocoa powder, for garnish (optional)

Pour the espresso into an 8-ounce mug. Pour the hemp milk into a blender and blend for 30 seconds, or until foamy. Pour the liquid into the coffee and spoon the foam onto the top. Sprinkle with the cinnamon or cocoa powder if desired.

Notes: When I make this drink for myself, I use hemp milk right from the fridge, and the result is a warm to hot cappuccino. If you prefer your coffee piping hot, you can warm the hemp milk in the microwave for 20 to 30 seconds before blending.

If not squeaky, feel free to sweeten the drink as desired.

CALORIES: 72 | **FAT:** 6g | **PROTEIN:** 3g | **CARBS:** 0g | **FIBER:** 0g | **NET CARBS:** 0g

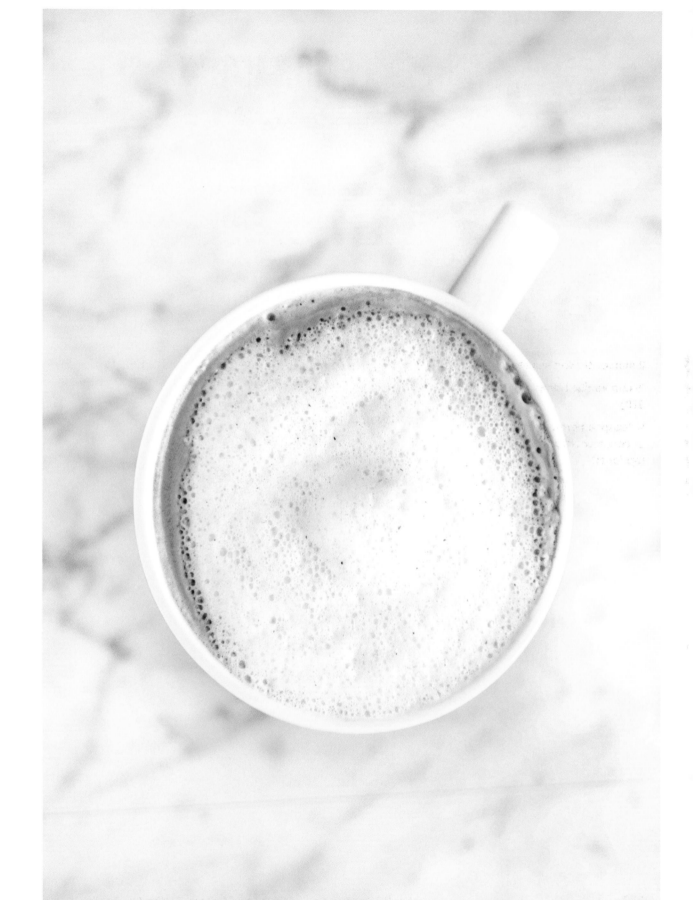

GREEN LEMONADE

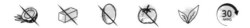

YIELD: 2 servings | **SERVING SIZE:** 12 ounces | **PREP TIME:** 10 minutes

Once you embrace the "green" flavor and your mouth gets used to the fact that this is not a sweet drink, you'll find that you can't get enough of it! It's a little higher in carbs, so you'll have to limit this one to occasional use, but when you do drink it, you'll get a huge boost in nutrients and electrolytes.

1 cup roughly chopped romaine lettuce

½ cup chopped celery

½ cup chopped cucumbers

¼ cup chopped Granny Smith apples

1 (1-inch) piece fresh ginger, peeled and minced

1 teaspoon grated lemon zest

1 teaspoon fresh lemon juice

⅛ teaspoon coarse Himalayan pink salt

2 cups cold filtered water

2 lemon wedges, for garnish (optional)

Put all the ingredients, except the lemon wedges, in a blender and blend until smooth. Strain and serve over ice. Garnish with a lemon wedge if desired. While best consumed right away, this lemonade will keep for up to 2 days in the refrigerator.

Note: If not squeaky, feel free to sweeten the lemonade as desired.

CALORIES: 25 | **FAT:** 0g | **PROTEIN:** 0g | **CARBS:** 4g | **FIBER:** 1g | **NET CARBS:** 3g

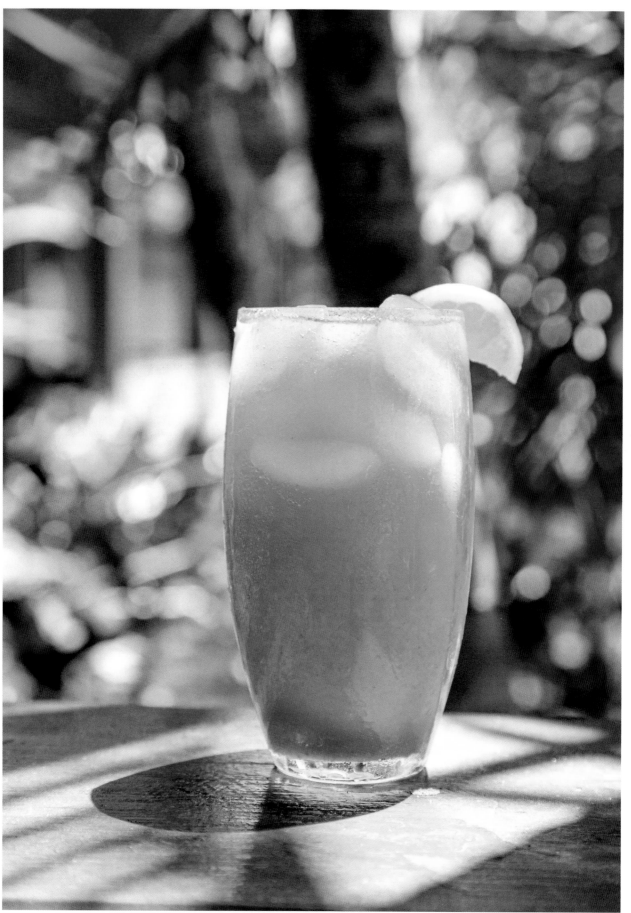

GINGER LEMON DETOX DRINK

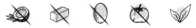

YIELD: 6 servings | SERVING SIZE: 10 ounces | PREP TIME: 8 minutes, plus 4 hours to steep | COOK TIME: 5 minutes

It's well documented that ginger is a potent anti-inflammatory agent, so this drink is doubly effective when it comes to reducing inflammation. Since Squeaky Clean Keto is already designed to reduce inflammation, adding a couple of servings of this ginger lemon drink to your day can boost your results even further. Enjoy it hot or iced—it's equally delicious and refreshing both ways!

2 quarts filtered water

¼ cup peeled lemon zest strips

¼ cup chopped fresh ginger

2 tablespoons fresh lemon juice

Put the water, lemon zest, and ginger in a large stainless-steel saucepan. Bring to a boil, then remove the pan from the heat. Cover and let steep for 4 hours. Strain the liquid into a large container or pitcher and discard the solids. Stir in the lemon juice. Serve hot or iced. Store in an airtight container in the refrigerator for up to 1 week.

Notes: I call for a stainless-steel saucepan here because of the long steeping time and acidic lemon, which can cause nonstick or aluminum pans to leach chemicals or heavy metal into your liquid. If you don't have stainless steel, you can boil the ingredients as directed and then transfer the mixture to another container to steep before straining.

If not squeaky, feel free to sweeten the drink as desired.

CALORIES: 6 | FAT: 0g | PROTEIN: 0g | CARBS: 1g | FIBER: 0g | NET CARBS: 1g

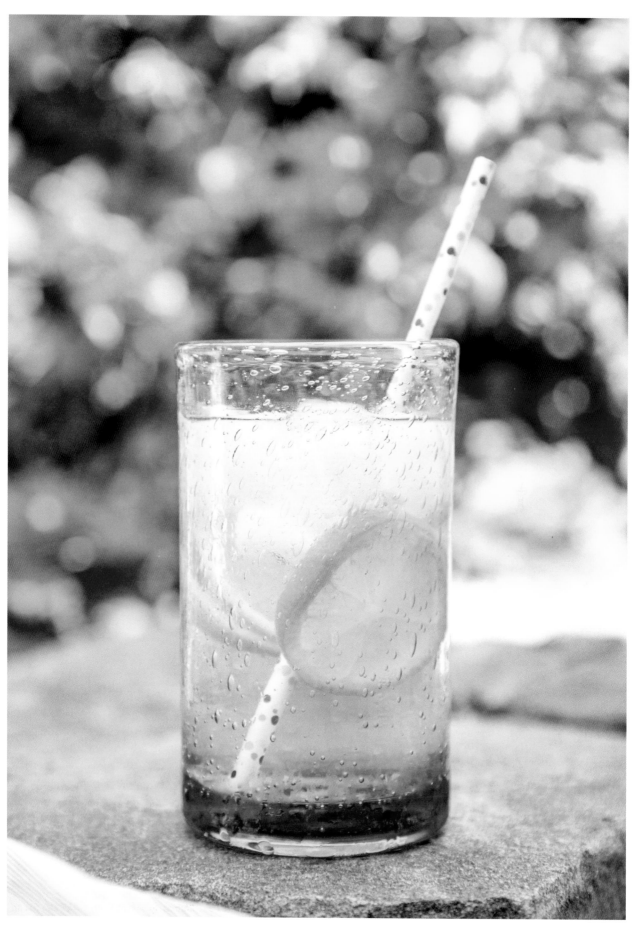

SWEET SESAME COCONUT CHIPS

  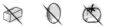

YIELD: 3 cups | **SERVING SIZE:** ⅓ cup | **PREP TIME:** 15 minutes | **COOK TIME:** 30 minutes

While snacking can be a slippery slope (read my thoughts on page 21), sometimes you need a treat, and these sweet coconut chips definitely fit the bill. The coconut aminos bake on and create a sticky-sweet coating that is lightly flavored by the sesame oil. While these chips aren't really crispy, they do have a crunchy/chewy texture that is very satisfying. Maybe too satisfying, if you know what I mean. Getting the coconut meat out of the shell is a little labor-intensive, but it's probably the only deterrent to your eating these chips by the truckful, so it's not necessarily a bad thing.

1 ripe brown coconut

1 teaspoon coconut aminos

1 teaspoon toasted sesame oil

1. Preheat the oven to 325°F. Line a sheet pan with parchment paper.

2. Break open the coconut with a couple of hammer strikes to the middle and drain the liquid. Carefully pry all the meat loose from the shell with a metal spatula or butter knife. Slice the coconut into thin pieces to make "chips."

3. Put the coconut chips, coconut aminos, and sesame oil in a medium-sized bowl and stir well to coat. Spread out the chips on the prepared sheet pan.

4. Bake the chips for 30 minutes, stirring every 10 minutes, until dry and slightly crisp. Remove and let cool before eating. Store in an airtight container in the refrigerator for up to 1 week.

CALORIES: 161 **FAT:** 15g **PROTEIN:** 2g **CARBS:** 7g **FIBER:** 4g **NET CARBS:** 3g

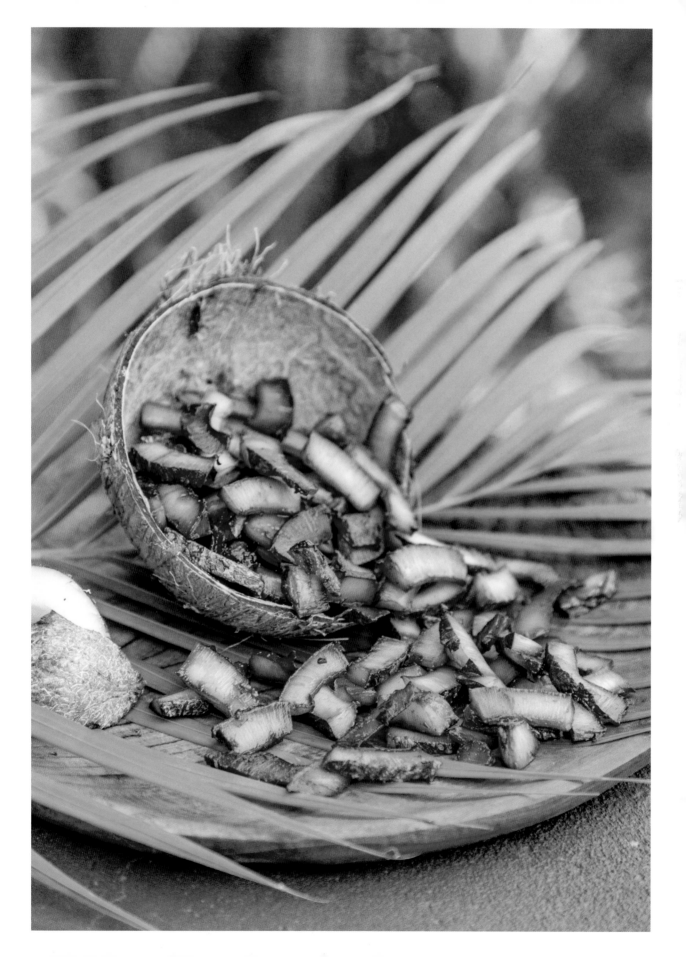

SALTY WASABI COCONUT CHIPS

  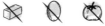

YIELD: 3 cups | SERVING SIZE: ⅓ cup | PREP TIME: 15 minutes | COOK TIME: 30 minutes

I love the nose-clearing punch that wasabi delivers, and it works really well with these lightly sweet and salty coconut chips. Like the Sweet Sesame Coconut Chips on page 336, these are almost too delicious, and therefore easy to overeat, which can stall your progress. I recommend portioning them out in advance to avoid deluding yourself about how much you really ate when you suddenly reach into the bowl and it's impossibly empty. Not that I would know from experience or anything...

1 ripe brown coconut

1 tablespoon avocado oil

1 teaspoon fish sauce (no sugar added)

1 teaspoon wasabi powder

½ teaspoon coconut aminos

1. Preheat the oven to 325°F. Line a sheet pan with parchment paper.

2. Break open the coconut with a couple of hammer strikes to the middle and drain the liquid. Carefully pry all the meat loose from the shell with a metal spatula or butter knife. Slice the coconut into thin pieces to make "chips."

3. Put the coconut chips, oil, fish sauce, wasabi powder, and coconut aminos in a medium-sized bowl and stir well to coat. Spread out the chips on the prepared sheet pan.

4. Bake the chips for 30 minutes, stirring every 10 minutes, until dry and crisp. Store leftovers in an airtight container in the refrigerator for up to 1 week.

CALORIES: 172 | FAT: 16g | PROTEIN: 2g | CARBS: 7g | FIBER: 4g | NET CARBS: 3g

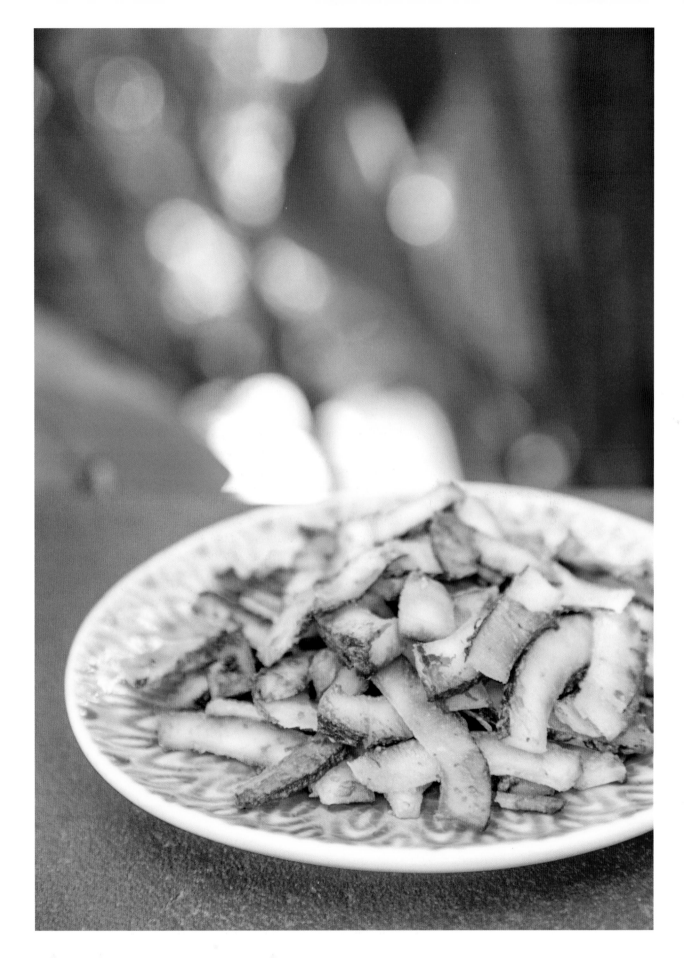

BABA GHANOUSH

YIELD: 9 servings | **SERVING SIZE:** ¼ cup | **PREP TIME:** 10 minutes | **COOK TIME:** 25 minutes

Baba ghanoush (pronounced "BAH-bah gah-NOOSH") is almost as delicious to eat as it is satisfying to say—especially when yelled after you stub your toe on the edge of a kitchen cabinet. True story. Try it and you'll see what I mean—the yelling, not the stubbing. Anyway, I digress. Similar to hummus in texture, baba ghanoush is a Middle Eastern dip made with roasted eggplant as a base. Lots of garlic, lemon, tahini, and smoked paprika make this smoky ambrosia a delight to eat. I recommend serving it with a combination of radish chips, bell pepper strips, pork rinds, and/or Everything Hemp Crackers (page 342).

3 medium eggplants

1½ tablespoons extra-virgin olive oil, divided

½ teaspoon smoked paprika

¼ cup tahini

2 tablespoons fresh lemon juice

1 tablespoon minced garlic

1 teaspoon kosher salt, plus more to taste

¼ teaspoon red pepper flakes

1 tablespoon chopped fresh parsley, for garnish

1 teaspoon sesame seeds, for garnish (optional)

1. Preheat the oven to 425°F.

2. Cut the eggplants in half lengthwise and rub the cut sides with ½ tablespoon of the olive oil. Sprinkle liberally with the paprika and place cut side down on a sheet pan. Roast the eggplants for 20 to 25 minutes, until soft. Remove from the oven and let cool slightly.

3. Scoop out the eggplant flesh with a spoon and measure 2 cups (reserve any extra for another use). Put the 2 cups of cooked eggplant in a food processor or blender.

4. To the food processor, add the tahini, lemon juice, garlic, salt, and red pepper flakes. Process for about 20 seconds, until mostly smooth but not liquid. Transfer the mixture to a bowl or serving platter and garnish with the remaining tablespoon of olive oil, the chopped parsley, and sesame seeds if desired. Store leftovers in an airtight container in the refrigerator for up to 5 days.

CALORIES: 89   **FAT:** 5g   **PROTEIN:** 3g   **CARBS:** 8g   **FIBER:** 4g   **NET CARBS:** 3g

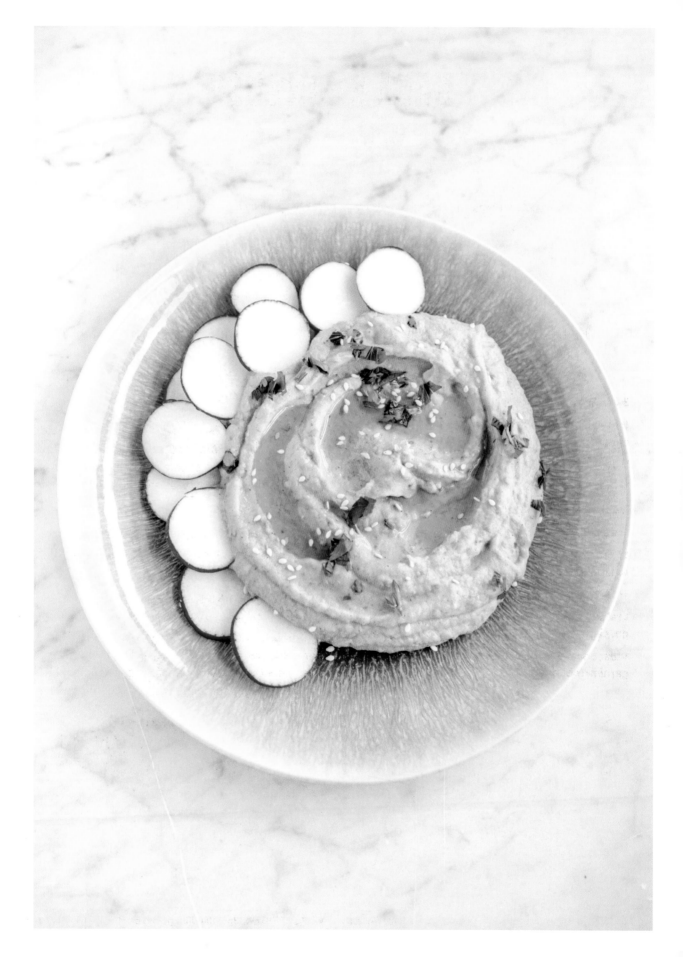

EVERYTHING HEMP CRACKERS

YIELD: 50 (2-inch) crackers | **SERVING SIZE:** 5 crackers | **PREP TIME:** 15 minutes | **COOK TIME:** 15 minutes

Crisp and ethereal, these lightweight crackers are laced with your favorite everything bagel flavors. Delicious on their own, these crackers are also fantastic schmeared with Baba Ghanoush (page 340), crumbled over Curried Turnip & Cauliflower Soup (page 142), or even crushed and used as a tasty breading for oven-baked chicken or fish. If you're not squeaky, of course they are also delicious with cheese.

½ cup (1 stick) butter, melted (see Note)

¾ cup Sun-Flour (page 74)

¾ cup shelled hemp seeds (hemp hearts)

¼ cup coconut flour

1 large egg white

2 tablespoons Everything Bagel Seasoning (page 80)

1. Preheat the oven to 350°F.

2. Put all the ingredients in a medium-sized bowl and mix well. Form the mixture into a ball of dough and place in the center of a large sheet of parchment paper. Top with another large sheet of parchment. Use a rolling pin to roll the dough into a rectangle about ⅛ inch thick. Transfer to a sheet pan and carefully peel off the top layer of parchment.

3. Cut through the dough in lines 2 inches apart to create cracker shapes—diamonds or squares according to your preference. Bake for 14 to 16 minutes, until golden and crisp. Remove from the oven and let cool. Break apart carefully and store in an airtight container for up to 1 week or in the freezer for up to 3 months.

Note: As in most of my cooking, I use salted butter for this recipe. If you use unsalted butter, you will need to add ¼ teaspoon of salt. Otherwise, the crackers will be bland.

CALORIES: 205 **FAT:** 19g **PROTEIN:** 3g **CARBS:** 4g **FIBER:** 2g **NET CARBS:** 2g

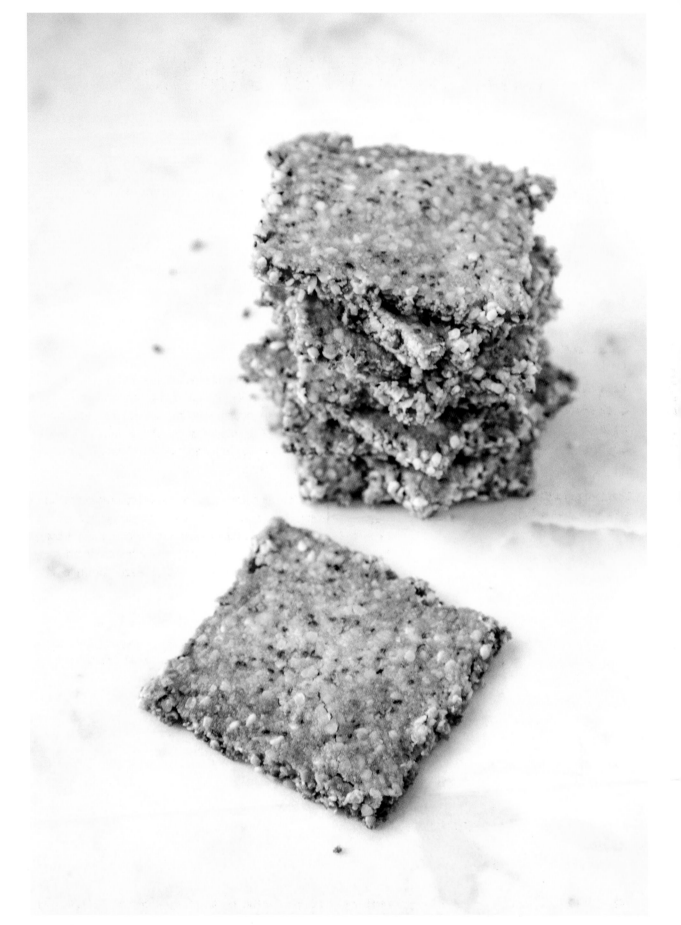

RESOURCE Guide

When you follow a Squeaky Clean Keto diet, you have to be a little more diligent when checking the ingredients in store-bought items than when you're on regular keto. The SCK guidelines allow for up to 1 gram of sugar in purchased items because it's cost-prohibitive and almost impossible to find brands that use no sugar at all. You can go the extra mile to purchase more expensive "clean" brands like Primal Kitchen, but if that's going to make the difference between "going squeaky" and not bothering to try it because it's too hard or expensive, then I'd rather have you go for it even when a product contains trace amounts of sugar or other non-squeaky ingredients.

With that in mind, I'm giving you a list of my favorite brands to use on this plan, but bear in mind that while these are the best I know of at the time of writing this book, things can change; by the time this book is in your hands, the ingredients used in some brands may have changed, and some brands may not even be available. For that reason, I suggest that you read labels and check ingredients before you make a purchase.

While you can find a lot of the following brands in stores, online retailers like Amazon.com and Thrive Market usually offer the best prices. Thrive is a membership-based site that costs around $60 per year, but it has a great selection and excellent prices, and it's constantly running deals that make the subscription fee completely worth it, in my opinion. That being said, sometimes you can't beat a brick-and-mortar store sale, so keep your eyes open and stock up when you find something on the cheap!

BONE BROTH:

Bare Bones

Epic

Imagine

Kettle & Fire

Kitchen Basics

Pacific Foods

CACAO/COCOA BUTTER:

Anthony's Goods

Healthworks

Navitas Organics

Nuvia Organics

Sunfood

Terrasoul Superfoods

COCONUT AMINOS:

BetterBody Foods

Bragg

Coconut Secret

Thrive Brand

COCONUT MILK:

Aroy-D

Native Forest

Parrot

Thai Kitchen

365 Everyday Value Organic

Thrive Market

COCONUT MILK POWDER:

Grace

Micro Ingredients Organic Coconut Milk
  Powder

HEMP MILK:

Living Harvest Tempt Unsweetened
  Original Hemp Milk

Pacific Foods Unsweetened Hemp
  Plant-Based Beverage

HEMP SEEDS:

Healthworks

Manitoba Harvest

Mighty Seed Hemp Co.

Navitas Organics

Nutiva

MARINARA SAUCE:

Cucina Antica

Mezzetta Italian Plum Tomato Marinara

Organico Bello

Rao's Marinara

365 Everyday Value Organic Marinara

MAYONNAISE:

Duke's Mayonnaise

Hellmann's Mayonnaise

Primal Kitchen Avocado Oil Mayonnaise

PSYLLIUM HUSK POWDER:

Healthworks

Kate Naturals

Viva Naturals

PUMPKIN SEEDS:

Anthony's Goods

Go Raw

Oh! Nuts

Sunbest Natural

We Got Nuts

SALSA:

Amy's Organic

Kirkland Organic Signature Salsa
  (contains trace amounts of sugar)

Pace

365 Everyday Value

SUNFLOWER SEED BUTTER:

Gopal's Sprouted Organic Raw Unsalted
  Sunflower Seed Butter

Laurel's Butter

SunButter No Sugar Added

Trader Joe's Unsweetened Sunflower Seed
  Spread

VOR Pure Sunflower Seed Butter

SUNFLOWER SEED FLOUR:

Gerbs

Think.Eat.Live Sunflour

SUNFLOWER SEED KERNELS:

Food to Live

Sincerely Nuts

Terrasoul Superfoods

365 Everyday Value Organic

We Got Nuts

RECIPE	PAGE	🦐	📦	🌾	🥥	🌿	30 MINS
Easy Chicken Bone Broth	72	✓	✓	✓	✓		
Sun-Flour (Sunflower Seed Flour)	74	✓	✓	✓	✓	✓	✓
Coconut Butter	76		✓	✓	✓	✓	✓
Roasted Sunflower Seed Butter	78		✓	✓	✓	✓	✓
Everything Bagel Seasoning	80	✓	✓	✓	✓	✓	✓
Pumpkin Seed Pesto	82	✓	✓	✓		✓	
No-Cook Marinara Sauce	84	✓	✓	✓		✓	✓
Easy Balsamic Glaze	86	✓	✓	✓	✓	✓	✓
Charmoula Sauce	87	✓	✓	✓		✓	✓
Easy Salsa Verde	88	✓	✓	✓		✓	✓
Dairy-Free Caesar Dressing	89	✓	✓		✓		✓
Sesame Ginger Dressing	90	✓	✓		✓		✓
Garlicky Lemon & Tarragon Dressing	91	✓	✓	✓	✓	✓	✓
Tahini Dressing	92	✓	✓	✓	✓	✓	✓
Creamy Sriracha Dipping Sauce	93		✓			✓	✓
Roasted Red Pepper Sauce	94	✓	✓			✓	✓
Dairy-Free Tzatziki	96		✓		✓	✓	✓
All-Purpose Green Sauce	98	✓	✓			✓	✓
Chili-Lime Mayo	100		✓			✓	✓
Sun-Dried Tomato Sauce	102	✓	✓	✓		✓	✓
Dill Caper Tartar Sauce	104		✓		✓	✓	✓
Creamy Garlic Sauce	106	✓	✓	✓	✓	✓	✓
Quick-Pickled Red Onions	108	✓	✓	✓		✓	✓
Olive Salad	110	✓	✓	✓		✓	
Spinach Wraps	112		✓		✓	✓	✓
Fiesta Egg Cups	116	✓	✓				✓
Blueberry Bliss Smoothie Bowl	118		✓	✓	✓		✓
Chorizo & Turnip Hash	120	✓	✓				
Bacon & Caramelized Onion Breakfast Bake	122	✓	✓		✓		
Cinnamon Maple Granola	124		✓		✓	✓	
Crispy Radish Corned Beef Hash	126	✓	✓	✓	✓		✓
Prosciutto & Tomato Omelette	128	✓					✓
Baked Scotch Eggs	130	✓	✓				

RECIPE	PAGE	🚫🥚	🚫🥜	🚫🥛	🚫🍅	🌿	30 min
Breakfast Burrito	132		✓				✓
Eggs in Purgatory	134	✓	✓				
Spicy Sausage & Kale Soup	138	✓	✓	✓			
Roasted Cauliflower & Leek Soup	140	✓		✓	✓		
Curried Turnip & Cauliflower Soup	142		✓	✓		✓	
Chicken & Vegetable Soup	144	✓	✓	✓			
Curried Chicken Salad	146	✓	✓				✓
Easy Tuna Salad	148	✓	✓		✓		✓
Cobb Salad with Warm Bacon Vinaigrette	150	✓	✓				
Simple Egg Salad	152	✓	✓		✓	✓	✓
Spicy Shrimp Salad Sushi Bowl	154		✓				✓
Buffalo Chicken Salad	156	✓	✓				✓
Chef's Salad	158	✓	✓				✓
Hearts of Palm Salad	160	✓	✓	✓		✓	✓
Muffuletta Wrap	162		✓				✓
Chicken Club Wrap	164	✓	✓				✓
Pastrami Roll-Ups	166	✓	✓		✓		✓
Tuscan Chicken with Zoodles	170	✓	✓	✓			✓
Prosciutto-Wrapped Chicken Tenders	172	✓	✓	✓			
Chicken Chop Suey	174		✓	✓			✓
Chicken Korma	176		✓				
Everything Chicken Wings	178	✓		✓	✓		
Sesame Chicken Fingers	180	✓	✓				✓
Simply Roasted Chicken Breasts	182	✓	✓	✓			
Arroz con Pollo	184	✓	✓	✓			
Butter Chicken	186		✓				
Peruvian Chicken	188	✓	✓	✓			
Chicken Jalfrezi	190	✓		✓			✓
Crispy Lemon Chicken	192				✓		✓
Instant Pot Beef Curry	196		✓	✓			
Spanish Rice Hamburger Skillet	198	✓	✓	✓			
Beef Picadillo	200	✓	✓	✓			
Chili Dog Skillet	202		✓				

RECIPE	PAGE	🚫	🚫	🚫	🚫	🌱	30
Sheet Pan Steak Fajitas	204	✓	✓	✓			
Beef Kofta Meatballs	206	✓	✓				✓
Sheet Pan Meatballs with Zoodles	208	✓	✓				✓
Meatloaf Cupcakes	210	✓	✓		✓		✓
Italian-Style Stuffed Peppers	212	✓	✓				
Ginger Beef Stir-Fry	214		✓	✓			✓
Sheet Pan Bacon Burgers	216		✓				
Pork & Pine Nut Eggplant Rollatini	220	✓	✓	✓			
Ham Steaks with Redeye Gravy	222	✓		✓	✓		✓
Bangers & Mash	224	✓					✓
Inside-Out Egg Rolls	226		✓	✓			✓
Slow-Roasted Pork Shoulder	228	✓	✓	✓			
Five-Spice Pork Chops	230	✓	✓	✓			✓
Vindaloo	232		✓	✓			✓
Cajun Pork Tenderloin	234	✓	✓	✓			✓
Sausage-Stuffed Onions with Balsamic Glaze	236	✓	✓	✓	✓		
Shrimp Piccata with Zoodles	240	✓		✓	✓		✓
Oven-Roasted Cajun Shrimp	242	✓	✓	✓			✓
Chilled Seafood Salad	244	✓	✓	✓	✓		
Salmon Burgers	246		✓		✓		✓
Coriander & Wasabi–Crusted Tuna	248		✓	✓	✓		✓
Easy Baked Salmon	250	✓	✓	✓	✓		✓
Fish Curry	252		✓				✓
Fried Calamari	254		✓				✓
Brazilian Shrimp Stew (Moqueca de Camarones)	256		✓	✓			✓
Molcajete Mixto	258	✓	✓	✓			
Mussels in Thai Coconut Broth	260		✓	✓			✓
Crab Cakes	262		✓				✓
Sheet Pan Paella	264	✓	✓	✓			
Spinach-Stuffed Portobello Mushrooms	268	✓			✓	✓	✓
Greek Zucchini Fritters	270	✓	✓		✓	✓	✓
Eggplant & Cauliflower Fritters	272		✓			✓	✓
Roman Fried Artichokes	274	✓	✓	✓	✓	✓	✓

RECIPE	PAGE	⊘	⊘	⊘	⊘	✿	30 MINS
Herbed Mushroom Ragout	276			✓	✓	✓	✓
Easy Vegetable Curry	278		✓	✓		✓	✓
Baked Zucchini Fries	280		✓			✓	
Balsamic Roasted Veggies	282	✓	✓	✓		✓	
Cauliflower & Kale Pilaf	284	✓	✓	✓	✓	✓	✓
Coconut Creamed Spinach	286		✓	✓		✓	✓
Bagna Cauda	288	✓		✓	✓		
Garlic & Chive Cauliflower Mash	290	✓	✓		✓	✓	✓
Oven-Roasted Mushrooms	292	✓		✓	✓	✓	✓
Easy Sesame Broccoli	294	✓		✓	✓	✓	✓
Creamy Coconut Cauliflower Rice	296		✓	✓	✓	✓	
Sautéed Shredded Brussels Sprouts	298	✓	✓	✓	✓	✓	✓
Roasted Bacon-Wrapped Cabbage Wedges	300	✓	✓	✓	✓		
Duchess Cauliflower	302				✓	✓	
Everything Roasted Cauliflower Steaks	304	✓	✓	✓	✓	✓	
Sheet Pan Veggie Burgers	306		✓			✓	
Korean Scallion Pancakes (Pajeon)	308		✓		✓		
Spaghetti Squash Puttanesca	310	✓	✓	✓			✓
Hibiscus Elderberry Tea	314	✓	✓	✓	✓	✓	
Cucumber Mint Cooler	316	✓	✓	✓	✓	✓	✓
Strawberry Lime Refresher	318	✓	✓	✓	✓	✓	✓
Raspberry Green Tea	320	✓	✓	✓	✓	✓	✓
Vanilla Mocha Coconut Creamer	322		✓	✓	✓		✓
Basic Bulletproof Coffee	324			✓	✓		✓
Bulletproof Chai Latte	326			✓	✓		✓
Vanilla Hemp Milk	328	✓	✓	✓	✓	✓	✓
Hemp Milk Cappuccino	330	✓	✓	✓	✓	✓	✓
Green Lemonade	332	✓	✓	✓	✓		✓
Ginger Lemon Detox Drink	334	✓	✓	✓	✓	✓	
Sweet Sesame Coconut Chips	336		✓	✓	✓	✓	
Salty Wasabi Coconut Chips	338		✓	✓	✓		
Baba Ghanoush	340	✓	✓	✓		✓	
Everything Hemp Crackers	342				✓	✓	✓

RECORDS INDEX

Basics

Easy Chicken Bone Broth 72

Sun-Flour (Sunflower Seed Flour) 74

Coconut Butter 76

Roasted Sunflower Seed Butter 78

Everything Bagel Seasoning 80

Pumpkin Seed Pesto 82

No-Cook Marinara Sauce 84

Easy Balsamic Glaze 86

Charmoula Sauce 87

Easy Salsa Verde 88

Dairy-Free Caesar Dressing 89

Sesame Ginger Dressing 90

Garlicky Lemon & Tarragon Dressing 91

Tahini Dressing 92

Creamy Sriracha Dipping Sauce 93

Roasted Red Pepper Sauce 94

Dairy-Free Tzatziki 96

All-Purpose Green Sauce 98

Chili-Lime Mayo 100

Sun-Dried Tomato Sauce 102

Dill Caper Tartar Sauce 104

Creamy Garlic Sauce 106

Quick-Pickled Red Onions 108

Olive Salad 110

Spinach Wraps 112

Breakfast

Fiesta Egg Cups 116

Blueberry Bliss Smoothie Bowl 118

Chorizo & Turnip Hash 120

Bacon & Caramelized Onion Breakfast Bake 122

Cinnamon Maple Granola 124

Crispy Radish Corned Beef Hash 126

Prosciutto & Tomato Omelette 128

Baked Scotch Eggs 130

Breakfast Burrito 132

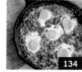
Eggs in Purgatory 134

Soups, Salads & Wraps

Spicy Sausage & Kale Soup — 138

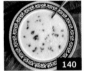
Roasted Cauliflower & Leek Soup — 140

Curried Turnip & Cauliflower Soup — 142

Chicken & Vegetable Soup — 144

Curried Chicken Salad — 146

Easy Tuna Salad — 148

Cobb Salad with Warm Bacon Vinaigrette — 150

Simple Egg Salad — 152

Spicy Shrimp Salad Sushi Bowl — 154

Buffalo Chicken Salad — 156

Chef's Salad — 158

Hearts of Palm Salad — 160

Muffuletta Wrap — 162

Chicken Club Wrap — 164

Pastrami Roll-Ups — 166

Chicken

Tuscan Chicken with Zoodles — 170

Prosciutto-Wrapped Chicken Tenders — 172

Chicken Chop Suey — 174

Chicken Korma — 176

Everything Chicken Wings — 178

Sesame Chicken Fingers — 180

Simply Roasted Chicken Breasts — 182

Arroz con Pollo — 184

Butter Chicken — 186

Peruvian Chicken — 188

Chicken Jalfrezi — 190

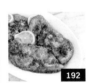
Crispy Lemon Chicken — 192

Beef

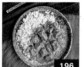
Instant Pot Beef Curry
196

Spanish Rice Hamburger Skillet
198

Beef Picadillo
200

Chili Dog Skillet
202

Sheet Pan Steak Fajitas
204

Beef Kofta Meatballs
206

Sheet Pan Meatballs with Zoodles
208

Meatloaf Cupcakes
210

Italian-Style Stuffed Peppers
212

Ginger Beef Stir-Fry
214

Sheet Pan Bacon Burgers
216

Pork

Pork & Pine Nut Eggplant Rollatini
220

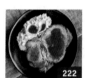
Ham Steaks with Redeye Gravy
222

Bangers & Mash
224

Inside-Out Egg Rolls
226

Slow-Roasted Pork Shoulder
228

Five-Spice Pork Chops
230

Vindaloo
232

Cajun Pork Tenderloin
234

Sausage-Stuffed Onions with Balsamic Glaze
236

Seafood

Shrimp Piccata with Zoodles — 240

Oven-Roasted Cajun Shrimp — 242

Chilled Seafood Salad — 244

Salmon Burgers — 246

Coriander & Wasabi-Crusted Tuna — 248

Easy Baked Salmon — 250

Fish Curry — 252

Fried Calamari — 254

Brazilian Shrimp Stew (Moqueca de Camarones) — 256

Molcajete Mixto — 258

Mussels in Thai Coconut Broth — 260

Crab Cakes — 262

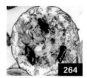
Sheet Pan Paella — 264

Veggie Mains & Sides

Spinach-Stuffed Portobello Mushrooms — 268

Greek Zucchini Fritters — 270

Eggplant & Cauliflower Fritters — 272

Roman Fried Artichokes — 274

Herbed Mushroom Ragout — 276

Easy Vegetable Curry — 278

Baked Zucchini Fries — 280

Balsamic Roasted Veggies — 282

Cauliflower & Kale Pilaf — 284

Coconut Creamed Spinach — 286

Bagna Cauda — 288

Garlic & Chive Cauliflower Mash — 290

Oven-Roasted Mushrooms — 292

Easy Sesame Broccoli — 294

Creamy Coconut Cauliflower Rice — 296

Sautéed Shredded Brussels Sprouts — 298

Roasted Bacon-Wrapped Cabbage Wedges — 300

Duchess Cauliflower — 302

Everything Roasted Cauliflower Steaks — 304

Sheet Pan Veggie Burgers — 306

Korean Scallion Pancakes (Pajeon) — 308

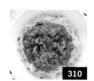
Spaghetti Squash Puttanesca — 310

Drinks & Snacks

Hibiscus Elderberry Tea
314

Cucumber Mint Cooler
316

Strawberry Lime Refresher
318

Raspberry Green Tea
320

Vanilla Mocha Coconut Creamer
322

Basic Bulletproof Coffee
324

Bulletproof Chai Latte
326

Vanilla Hemp Milk
328

Hemp Milk Cappuccino
330

Green Lemonade
332

Ginger Lemon Detox Drink
334

Sweet Sesame Coconut Chips
336

Salty Wasabi Coconut Chips
338

Baba Ghanoush
340

Everything Hemp Crackers
342

DOWNLOADABLE
Charts

On my website, you'll find some handy tools to use during your Squeaky Clean Keto Challenge. Use this QR code to download and print the charts pictured below.

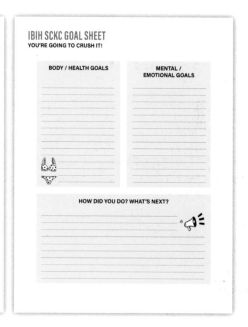

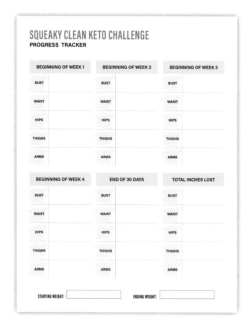

GENERAL INDEX

A

acceptance, as a stage of Squeaky Clean Keto, 20

ahi tuna
Coriander & Wasabi–Crusted Tuna, 248–249

alcohol, 17

All-Purpose Green Sauce recipe, 98–99

anchovies
Bagna Cauda, 288–289
Dairy-Free Caesar Dressing, 89
Spaghetti Squash Puttanesca, 310–311

andouille sausage
Sheet Pan Paella, 264–265

anger, as a stage of Squeaky Clean Keto, 19

apples
Curried Chicken Salad, 146–147
Green Lemonade, 332–333

arm measurement, 23

Arroz con Pollo recipe, 184–185

artichokes
Roman Fried Artichokes, 274–275

asparagus, 31

avocado oil, 46

avocados
Breakfast Burrito, 132–133
Chicken Club Wrap, 164–165
Cobb Salad with Warm Bacon Vinaigrette, 150–151
Hearts of Palm Salad, 160–161
Sheet Pan Bacon Burgers, 216–217
Spicy Shrimp Salad Sushi Bowl, 154–155

B

Baba Ghanoush recipe, 340–341

bacon
about, 39
Bacon & Caramelized Onion Breakfast Bake, 122–123
Chicken Club Wrap, 164–165
Chicken & Vegetable Soup, 144–145
Cobb Salad with Warm Bacon Vinaigrette, 150–151
Roasted Bacon-Wrapped Cabbage Wedges, 300–301
Roasted Cauliflower & Leek Soup, 140–141
Sheet Pan Bacon Burgers, 216–217

Bacon & Caramelized Onion Breakfast Bake recipe, 122–123

Bagna Cauda recipe, 288–289

Baked Scotch Eggs recipe, 130–131

Baked Zucchini Fries recipe, 280–281

bakeware, 52

Balsamic Roasted Veggies recipe, 282–283

Bangers & Mash recipe, 224–225

Basic Bulletproof Coffee recipe, 324–325

basil
Chicken Club Wrap, 164–165
Chicken & Vegetable Soup, 144–145
Eggplant & Cauliflower Fritters, 272–273
Prosciutto & Tomato Omelette, 128–129
Sheet Pan Meatballs with Zoodles, 208–209
Tuscan Chicken with Zoodles, 170–171

bean sprouts
Chicken Chop Suey, 174–175

beef
Beef Kofta Meatballs, 206–207
Beef Picadillo, 200–201
Chili Dog Skillet, 202–203
Easy Beef Bone Broth, 72–73
Ginger Beef Stir-Fry, 214–215
Instant Pot Beef Curry, 196–197
Italian-Style Stuffed Peppers, 212–213
meal prep and, 38–39
Meatloaf Cupcakes, 210–211
Molcajete Mixto, 258–259
Sheet Pan Bacon Burgers, 216–217
Sheet Pan Meatballs with Zoodles, 208–209
Sheet Pan Steak Fajitas, 204–205
Spanish Rice Hamburger Skillet, 198–199
Vindaloo, 232–233

Beef Kofta Meatballs recipe, 206–207

Beef Picadillo recipe, 200–201

bell peppers
Arroz con Pollo, 184–185
Balsamic Roasted Veggies, 282–283
Chicken Chop Suey, 174–175
Chorizo & Turnip Hash, 120–121
Eggplant & Cauliflower Fritters, 272–273
Ginger Beef Stir-Fry, 214–215
Italian-Style Stuffed Peppers, 212–213
Sheet Pan Paella, 264–265
Sheet Pan Steak Fajitas, 204–205
Vindaloo, 232–233

blackberries, 31

blender, 49

Blendtec, 49

blue cheese
	Buffalo Chicken Salad, 156–157

blueberries
	Blueberry Bliss Smoothie Bowl, 118–119
	carbs in, 31

Blueberry Bliss Smoothie Bowl recipe, 118–119

bok choy
	Chicken Chop Suey, 174–175

bologna
	Muffuletta Wrap, 162–163

bone broth, resources for, 344.
	See also Easy Beef Bone Broth recipe; Easy Chicken Bone Broth recipe

Brazilian Shrimp Stew (Moqueca de Camarones) recipe, 256–257

Breakfast Burrito recipe, 132–133

breakfast sausage
	Baked Scotch Eggs, 130–131
	Breakfast Burrito, 132–133
	Sausage-Stuffed Onions with Balsamic Glaze, 236–237

broccoli
	carbs in, 31
	Easy Sesame Broccoli, 294–295
	Ginger Beef Stir-Fry, 214–215
	Sheet Pan Veggie Burgers, 306–307

brown mustard
	Pastrami Roll-Ups, 166–167

brushing teeth, 33

Brussels sprouts
	carbs in, 31
	Sautéed Shredded Brussels Sprouts, 298–299

Buffalo Chicken Salad recipe, 156–157

Bulletproof Chai Latte recipe, 326–327

butter, 32, 36, 48

Butter Chicken recipe, 186–187

buttermilk, 32

C

cabbage
	carbs in, 31
	Inside-Out Egg Rolls, 226–227
	Roasted Bacon-Wrapped Cabbage Wedges, 300–301

cacao butter, resources for, 344

Cajun Pork Tenderloin recipe, 234–235

calamari
	Fried Calamari, 254–255

calcium, 30

capers
	Arroz con Pollo, 184–185
	Beef Picadillo, 200–201
	Dill Caper Tartar Sauce, 104–105
	Olive Salad, 110–111
	Shrimp Piccata with Zoodles, 240–241
	Spaghetti Squash Puttanesca, 310–311

caraway seeds
	Pastrami Roll-Ups, 166–167

Carb Manager, 29

carbs, net, 17

cardamom pods, 33

cauliflower
	Arroz con Pollo, 184–185
	carbs in, 31
	Cauliflower & Kale Pilaf, 284–285
	Chili Dog Skillet, 202–203
	Creamy Coconut Cauliflower Rice, 296–297
	Curried Turnip & Cauliflower Soup, 142–143
	Duchess Cauliflower, 302–303
	Eggplant & Cauliflower Fritters, 272–273
	Everything Roasted Cauliflower Steaks, 304–305
	Fish Curry, 252–253

Garlic & Chive Cauliflower Mash, 290–291
	Italian-Style Stuffed Peppers, 212–213
	microwaving, 302
	riced, 40
	Roasted Cauliflower & Leek Soup, 140–141
	Sheet Pan Paella, 264–265
	Sheet Pan Veggie Burgers, 306–307
	Spanish Rice Hamburger Skillet, 198–199
	Spicy Shrimp Salad Sushi Bowl, 154–155

Cauliflower & Kale Pilaf recipe, 284–285

celery
	Buffalo Chicken Salad, 156–157
	carbs in, 31
	Chicken Chop Suey, 174–175
	Chicken & Vegetable Soup, 144–145
	Easy Beef Bone Broth, 72–73
	Easy Chicken Bone Broth, 72–73
	Green Lemonade, 332–333

chai tea
	Bulletproof Chai Latte, 326–327

Charmoula Sauce recipe, 87

cheddar cheese
	Chili Dog Skillet, 202–203

cheese. See also specific types
	Breakfast Burrito, 132–133
	Fiesta Egg Cups, 116–117

Chef's Salad recipe, 158–159

chest measurement, 23

chicken
	Arroz con Pollo, 184–185
	Buffalo Chicken Salad, 156–157
	Butter Chicken, 186–187
	Chicken Chop Suey, 174–175
	Chicken Club Wrap, 164–165
	Chicken Jalfrezi, 190–191
	Chicken Korma, 176–177

chicken (continued)

Chicken & Vegetable Soup, 144–145

Crispy Lemon Chicken, 192–193

Curried Chicken Salad, 146–147

Easy Chicken Bone Broth, 72–73

Everything Chicken Wings, 178–179

kitchen safety and, 41

meal prep and, 37–38

Peruvian Chicken, 188–189

Prosciutto-Wrapped Chicken Tenders, 172–173

Sesame Chicken Fingers, 180–181

Sheet Pan Paella, 264–265

Sheet Pan Steak Fajitas, 204–205

Simply Roasted Chicken Breasts, 182–183

Tuscan Chicken with Zoodles, 170–171

Vindaloo, 232–233

Chicken Chop Suey recipe, 174–175

Chicken Club Wrap recipe, 164–165

Chicken Jalfrezi recipe, 190–191

Chicken Korma recipe, 176–177

Chicken & Vegetable Soup recipe, 144–145

Chili Dog Skillet recipe, 202–203

Chili-Lime Mayo recipe, 100–101

Chilled Seafood Salad recipe, 244–245

chives

Garlic & Chive Cauliflower Mash, 290–291

Chocolate Hemp Milk recipe, 328–329

chops, 39

chorizo

Chorizo & Turnip Hash, 120–121

Eggs in Purgatory, 134–135

Molcajete Mixto, 258–259

Sheet Pan Paella, 264–265

Chorizo & Turnip Hash recipe, 120–121

chuck roast, 38

cilantro

All-Purpose Green Sauce, 98–99

Arroz con Pollo, 184–185

Beef Kofta Meatballs, 206–207

Beef Picadillo, 200–201

Brazilian Shrimp Stew (Moqueca de Camarones), 256–257

Breakfast Burrito, 132–133

Butter Chicken, 186–187

Charmoula Sauce, 87

Chicken Jalfrezi, 190–191

Chicken Korma, 176–177

Chorizo & Turnip Hash, 120–121

Curried Chicken Salad, 146–147

Easy Salsa Verde, 88

Eggs in Purgatory, 134–135

Fish Curry, 252–253

Inside-Out Egg Rolls, 226–227

Molcajete Mixto, 258–259

Mussels in Thai Coconut Broth, 260–261

Pumpkin Seed Pesto, 82–83

Quick-Pickled Red Onions, 108–109

Spicy Shrimp Salad Sushi Bowl, 154–155

Cinnamon Maple Granola recipe, 124–125

clams

Chilled Seafood Salad, 244–245

clean keto, 12, 14

cleaning

leeks, 140

mussels, 260

club soda

Strawberry Lime Refresher, 318–319

Cobb Salad with Warm Bacon Vinaigrette recipe, 150–151

cocoa butter, 35, 47, 344

cocoa powder

Chocolate Hemp Milk, 328–329

Hemp Milk Cappuccino, 330–331

Vanilla Mocha Coconut Creamer, 322–323

coconut

about, 46

Blueberry Bliss Smoothie Bowl, 118–119

Cinnamon Maple Granola, 124–125

Coconut Butter, 76–77

Salty Wasabi Coconut Chips, 338–339

Sheet Pan Veggie Burgers, 306–307

Sweet Sesame Coconut Chips, 336–337

coconut aminos

about, 47

Butter Chicken, 186–187

Chicken Chop Suey, 174–175

Chili Dog Skillet, 202–203

Chili-Lime Mayo, 100–101

Coriander & Wasabi–Crusted Tuna, 248–249

Crab Cakes, 262–263

Creamy Coconut Cauliflower Rice, 296–297

Creamy Sriracha Dipping Sauce, 93

Easy Vegetable Curry, 278–279

Eggplant & Cauliflower Fritters, 272–273

Ginger Beef Stir-Fry, 214–215

Herbed Mushroom Ragout, 276–277

Inside-Out Egg Rolls, 226–227

Korean Scallion Pancakes (Pajeon), 308–309

Mussels in Thai Coconut Broth, 260–261

resources for, 345

Salty Wasabi Coconut Chips, 338–339

Sheet Pan Veggie Burgers, 306–307

Spicy Shrimp Salad Sushi Bowl, 154–155

Sweet Sesame Coconut Chips, 336–337

Vindaloo, 232–233

Coconut Butter recipe, 76–77

coconut cream, 45

Coconut Creamed Spinach recipe, 286–287

coconut flour

about, 45

Baked Zucchini Fries, 280–281

Crab Cakes, 262–263

Crispy Lemon Chicken, 192–193

Duchess Cauliflower, 302–303

Eggplant & Cauliflower Fritters, 272–273

Everything Hemp Crackers, 342–343

Fried Calamari, 254–255

Korean Scallion Pancakes (Pajeon), 308–309

Salmon Burgers, 246–247

Spinach Wraps, 112–113

coconut milk

about, 35, 45

Blueberry Bliss Smoothie Bowl, 118–119

Brazilian Shrimp Stew (Moqueca de Camarones), 256–257

Butter Chicken, 186–187

Chicken Korma, 176–177

Coconut Creamed Spinach, 286–287

Creamy Coconut Cauliflower Rice, 296–297

Curried Turnip & Cauliflower Soup, 142–143

Dairy-Free Tzatziki, 96–97

Dill Caper Tartar Sauce, 104–105

Easy Vegetable Curry, 278–279

Fish Curry, 252–253

Herbed Mushroom Ragout, 276–277

Instant Pot Beef Curry, 196–197

Mussels in Thai Coconut Broth, 260–261

resources for, 345

Vanilla Mocha Coconut Creamer, 322–323

coconut oil, 46

cod

Fish Curry, 252–253

coffee

about, 34–36

Basic Bulletproof Coffee, 324–325

Ham Steaks with Redeye Gravy, 222–223

Hemp Milk Cappuccino, 330–331

collagen peptides

about, 47

Basic Bulletproof Coffee, 324–325

Blueberry Bliss Smoothie Bowl, 118–119

Bulletproof Chai Latte, 326–327

Vanilla Mocha Coconut Creamer, 322–323

cookware, 52

Coriander & Wasabi-Crusted Tuna recipe, 248–249

corned beef

Crispy Radish Corned Beef Hash, 126–127

cost, 28–29

crab

Chilled Seafood Salad, 244–245

Crab Cakes, 262–263

Crab Cakes recipe, 262–263

cravings, coping with, 18–21

Creamy Coconut Cauliflower Rice recipe, 296–297

Creamy Garlic Sauce recipe, 106–107

Creamy Sriracha Dipping Sauce recipe, 93

Sheet Pan Bacon Burgers, 216–217

Crispy Lemon Chicken recipe, 192–193

Crispy Radish Corned Beef Hash recipe, 126–127

Cronometer, 29

Cucumber Mint Cooler recipe, 316–317

cucumbers

carbs in, 31

Chef's Salad, 158–159

Cucumber Mint Cooler, 316–317

Dairy-Free Tzatziki, 96–97

Green Lemonade, 332–333

Spicy Shrimp Salad Sushi Bowl, 154–155

Curried Chicken Salad recipe, 146–147

Curried Turnip & Cauliflower Soup recipe, 142–143

cutting boards, 51

D

dairy products, 17

Dairy-Free Caesar Dressing recipe, 89

Dairy-Free Tzatziki recipe, 96–97

determination, as a stage of Squeaky Clean Keto, 20

detox, 18

Dijon mustard

Chicken Club Wrap, 164–165

Chili Dog Skillet, 202–203

Cobb Salad with Warm Bacon Vinaigrette, 150–151

Crab Cakes, 262–263

Dairy-Free Caesar Dressing, 89

Simple Egg Salad, 152–153

dill

Chicken Club Wrap, 164–165

Dairy-Free Tzatziki, 96–97

Dill Caper Tartar Sauce, 104–105

dill (continued)
    Greek Zucchini Fritters,
        270–271
Dill Caper Tartar Sauce recipe,
    104–105
dill pickles/dill pickle relish
    Chicken Club Wrap, 164–165
    Pastrami Roll-Ups, 166–167
dirty keto, 12, 13
dressings
    Dairy-Free Caesar Dressing, 89
    Garlicky Lemon & Tarragon
        Dressing, 91
    Sesame Ginger Dressing, 90
    Tahini Dressing, 92
drinks
    Basic Bulletproof Coffee,
        324–325
    Bulletproof Chai Latte,
        326–327
    Cucumber Mint Cooler,
        316–317
    Ginger Lemon Detox Drink,
        334–335
    Green Lemonade, 332–333
    Hemp Milk Cappuccino,
        330–331
    Hibiscus Elderberry Tea,
        314–315
    Raspberry Green Tea, 320–321
    Strawberry Lime Refresher,
        318–319
    Vanilla Mocha Coconut
        Creamer, 322–323
    water, 33
Duchess Cauliflower recipe,
    302–303
    Meatloaf Cupcakes, 210–211

E
Easy Baked Salmon recipe,
    250–251
Easy Balsamic Glaze recipe, 86
    Meatloaf Cupcakes, 210–211
    Sausage-Stuffed Onions with
        Balsamic Glaze, 236–237

Easy Beef Bone Broth recipe, 72–73
    Instant Pot Beef Curry, 196–197
    Roasted Cauliflower & Leek
        Soup, 140–141
Easy Chicken Bone Broth recipe,
    72–73
    Bangers & Mash, 224–225
    Beef Picadillo, 200–201
    Chicken Korma, 176–177
    Chicken & Vegetable Soup,
        144–145
    Curried Turnip & Cauliflower
        Soup, 142–143
    Molcajete Mixto, 258–259
    Sheet Pan Paella, 264–265
    Spanish Rice Hamburger
        Skillet, 198–199
    Spicy Sausage & Kale Soup,
        138–139
Easy Salsa Verde recipe, 88
    Molcajete Mixto, 258–259
Easy Sesame Broccoli recipe,
    294–295
Easy Tuna Salad recipe, 148–149
Easy Vegetable Curry recipe,
    278–279
eggplant
    Baba Ghanoush, 340–341
    Balsamic Roasted Veggies,
        282–283
    Easy Vegetable Curry, 278–279
    Eggplant & Cauliflower
        Fritters, 272–273
    Pork & Pine Nut Eggplant
        Rollatini, 220–221
Eggplant & Cauliflower Fritters
    recipe, 272–273
eggs
    Bacon & Caramelized Onion
        Breakfast Bake, 122–123
    Baked Scotch Eggs, 130–131
    Breakfast Burrito, 132–133
    Chef's Salad, 158–159
    Chorizo & Turnip Hash, 120–121
    Cinnamon Maple Granola,
        124–125

    Cobb Salad with Warm Bacon
        Vinaigrette, 150–151
    Eggs in Purgatory, 134–135
    Everything Hemp Crackers,
        342–343
    Fiesta Egg Cups, 116–117
    Fish Curry, 252–253
    Greek Zucchini Fritters,
        270–271
    kitchen safety and, 42
    Korean Scallion Pancakes
        (Pajeon), 308–309
    Prosciutto & Tomato Omelette,
        128–129
    Sesame Chicken Fingers,
        180–181
    Simple Egg Salad, 152–153
    Spinach Wraps, 112–113
    Spinach-Stuffed Portobello
        Mushrooms, 268–269
Eggs in Purgatory recipe, 134–135
elderberries
    Hibiscus Elderberry Tea,
        314–315
emotional triggers, coping with,
    18–21
emulsifying, 36
equipment, kitchen, 49–53
erythritol
    Cinnamon Maple Granola,
        124–125
espresso
    Hemp Milk Cappuccino,
        330–331
Everything Bagel Seasoning recipe,
    80–81
    Everything Chicken Wings,
        178–179
    Everything Hemp Crackers,
        342–343
    Everything Roasted
        Cauliflower Steaks, 304–305
Everything Chicken Wings recipe,
    178–179
Everything Hemp Crackers recipe,
    342–343

Everything Roasted Cauliflower Steaks recipe, 304–305

exercise, 27

F

FAQ, 26–33

fasting, intermittent, 27

feta cheese
  Greek Zucchini Fritters, 270–271

Fiesta Egg Cups recipe, 116–117

fish and seafood
  Brazilian Shrimp Stew (Moqueca de Camarones), 256–257
  Chilled Seafood Salad, 244–245
  Coriander & Wasabi–Crusted Tuna, 248–249
  Crab Cakes, 262–263
  Easy Baked Salmon, 250–251
  Fish Curry, 252–253
  Fried Calamari, 254–255
  Molcajete Mixto, 258–259
  Mussels in Thai Coconut Broth, 260–261
  Oven-Roasted Cajun Shrimp, 242–243
  Salmon Burgers, 246–247
  Sheet Pan Paella, 264–265
  Shrimp Piccata with Zoodles, 240–241
  Spicy Shrimp Salad Sushi Bowl, 154–155

Fish Curry recipe, 252–253

fish sauce
  Butter Chicken, 186–187
  Chicken Chop Suey, 174–175
  Fish Curry, 252–253
  Ginger Beef Stir-Fry, 214–215
  Inside-Out Egg Rolls, 226–227
  Korean Scallion Pancakes (Pajeon), 308–309
  Salty Wasabi Coconut Chips, 338–339
  Sesame Chicken Fingers, 180–181
  Sesame Ginger Dressing, 90

5-Day Keto Soup Diet Plan, 64–67

Five-Spice Pork Chops recipe, 230–231

food processor, 50

Fried Calamari recipe, 254–255

frother, 50

fruits, 31. *See also specific fruits*

G

garam masala
  Butter Chicken, 186–187

garlic
  All-Purpose Green Sauce, 98–99
  Arroz con Pollo, 184–185
  Baba Ghanoush, 340–341
  Bagna Cauda, 288–289
  Beef Picadillo, 200–201
  Brazilian Shrimp Stew (Moqueca de Camarones), 256–257
  Butter Chicken, 186–187
  Cauliflower & Kale Pilaf, 284–285
  Chicken Chop Suey, 174–175
  Chicken Jalfrezi, 190–191
  Chicken Korma, 176–177
  Chicken & Vegetable Soup, 144–145
  Chilled Seafood Salad, 244–245
  Chorizo & Turnip Hash, 120–121
  Creamy Garlic Sauce, 106–107
  Curried Turnip & Cauliflower Soup, 142–143
  Dairy-Free Caesar Dressing, 89
  Easy Beef Bone Broth, 72–73
  Easy Chicken Bone Broth, 72–73
  Easy Salsa Verde, 88
  Easy Vegetable Curry, 278–279
  Eggs in Purgatory, 134–135
  Garlic & Chive Cauliflower Mash, 290–291
  Garlicky Lemon & Tarragon Dressing, 91

Ginger Beef Stir-Fry, 214–215

Herbed Mushroom Ragout, 276–277

Inside-Out Egg Rolls, 226–227

Instant Pot Beef Curry, 196–197

Molcajete Mixto, 258–259

Mussels in Thai Coconut Broth, 260–261

Olive Salad, 110–111

Peruvian Chicken, 188–189

Pumpkin Seed Pesto, 82–83

Roasted Cauliflower & Leek Soup, 140–141

Roasted Red Pepper Sauce, 94–95

Sautéed Shredded Brussels Sprouts, 298–299

Sheet Pan Paella, 264–265

Sheet Pan Steak Fajitas, 204–205

Sheet Pan Veggie Burgers, 306–307

Spaghetti Squash Puttanesca, 310–311

Spanish Rice Hamburger Skillet, 198–199

Spicy Sausage & Kale Soup, 138–139

Spinach-Stuffed Portobello Mushrooms, 268–269

Sun-Dried Tomato Sauce, 102–103

Tahini Dressing, 92

Tuscan Chicken with Zoodles, 170–171

Vindaloo, 232–233

Garlic & Chive Cauliflower Mash recipe, 290–291
  Bangers & Mash, 224–225

Garlicky Lemon & Tarragon Dressing recipe, 91
  Chef's Salad, 158–159

getting started, 17

ginger
  Butter Chicken, 186–187
  Chicken Jalfrezi, 190–191

ginger *(continued)*

    Chicken Korma, 176–177

    Easy Beef Bone Broth, 72–73

    Easy Chicken Bone Broth, 72–73

    Ginger Beef Stir-Fry, 214–215

    Ginger Lemon Detox Drink, 334–335

    Green Lemonade, 332–333

    Inside-Out Egg Rolls, 226–227

    Instant Pot Beef Curry, 196–197

    Mussels in Thai Coconut Broth, 260–261

    Sesame Ginger Dressing, 90

Ginger Beef Stir-Fry recipe, 214–215

Ginger Lemon Detox Drink recipe, 334–335

grains, 17

grater, 53

Greek Zucchini Fritters recipe, 270–271

green beans

    carbs in, 31

    Chicken & Vegetable Soup, 144–145

    Easy Vegetable Curry, 278–279

green chilis

    Beef Picadillo, 200–201

    Mussels in Thai Coconut Broth, 260–261

    Spanish Rice Hamburger Skillet, 198–199

Green Lemonade recipe, 332–333

grief, as a stage of Squeaky Clean Keto, 19

gum, 32–33

H

habanero peppers

    Instant Pot Beef Curry, 196–197

    Quick-Pickled Red Onions, 108–109

haddock

    Fish Curry, 252–253

ham

    Chef's Salad, 158–159

    Fiesta Egg Cups, 116–117

    Ham Steaks with Redeye Gravy, 222–223

Ham Steaks with Redeye Gravy recipe, 222–223

handheld frother, 50

Hearts of Palm Salad recipe, 160–161

heavy whipping cream, 32

hemp hearts, 44

hemp milk, 36, 345

Hemp Milk Cappuccino recipe, 330–331

hemp seeds

    about, 44

    Beef Kofta Meatballs, 206–207

    Blueberry Bliss Smoothie Bowl, 118–119

    Chocolate Hemp Milk, 328–329

    Cinnamon Maple Granola, 124–125

    Everything Hemp Crackers, 342–343

    Meatloaf Cupcakes, 210–211

    resources for, 345

    Sheet Pan Meatballs with Zoodles, 208–209

    Sheet Pan Veggie Burgers, 306–307

    Strawberry Hemp Milk, 328–329

    Vanilla Hemp Milk, 328–329

Herbed Mushroom Ragout recipe, 276–277

Hibiscus Elderberry Tea recipe, 314–315

high-powered blender, 49

Himalayan pink salt, 80

hips measurement, 23

hot dogs

    Chili Dog Skillet, 202–203

hot sauce

    Buffalo Chicken Salad, 156–157

I

iceberg lettuce

    Chicken Club Wrap, 164–165

if it fits your macros (IIFYM), 13

immersion blender, 49

Inside-Out Egg Rolls recipe, 226–227

Instant Pot Beef Curry recipe, 196–197

intermittent fasting, 27

Italian sausage

    Spicy Sausage & Kale Soup, 138–139

Italian-Style Stuffed Peppers recipe, 212–213

J

jalapeño peppers

    All-Purpose Green Sauce, 98–99

    Easy Salsa Verde, 88

    Easy Vegetable Curry, 278–279

    Molcajete Mixto, 258–259

    Pumpkin Seed Pesto, 82–83

    Sheet Pan Bacon Burgers, 216–217

journaling, 24

K

Kalamata olives

    Greek Zucchini Fritters, 270–271

kale

    Cauliflower & Kale Pilaf, 284–285

    Spicy Sausage & Kale Soup, 138–139

keto breath, 32–33

Keto for Life (Sevigny), 6

kitchen equipment, 49–53

kitchen safety, 41–43

knives, 51

Korean Scallion Pancakes (Pajeon) recipe, 308–309

L

lazy keto, 12, 13
leeks
    cleaning, 140
    Roasted Cauliflower & Leek
      Soup, 140–141
legumes, 17
lemons
    Baba Ghanoush, 340–341
    Beef Kofta Meatballs, 206–207
    Charmoula Sauce, 87
    Chilled Seafood Salad,
      244–245
    Crab Cakes, 262–263
    Creamy Garlic Sauce, 106–107
    Crispy Lemon Chicken,
      192–193
    Cucumber Mint Cooler, 316–317
    Dairy-Free Caesar Dressing, 89
    Dairy-Free Tzatziki, 96–97
    Eggplant & Cauliflower
      Fritters, 272–273
    Fried Calamari, 254–255
    Garlic & Chive Cauliflower
      Mash, 290–291
    Garlicky Lemon & Tarragon
      Dressing, 91
    Ginger Lemon Detox Drink,
      334–335
    Greek Zucchini Fritters,
      270–271
    Green Lemonade, 332–333
    Hearts of Palm Salad, 160–161
    Hibiscus Elderberry Tea,
      314–315
    Oven-Roasted Cajun Shrimp,
      242–243
    Roasted Red Pepper Sauce,
      94–95
    Sautéed Shredded Brussels
      Sprouts, 298–299
    Sheet Pan Paella, 264–265
    Shrimp Piccata with Zoodles,
      240–241
    Simple Egg Salad, 152–153
    Tahini Dressing, 92

lettuce
    Chicken Club Wrap, 164–165
    Pastrami Roll-Ups, 166–167
    Salmon Burgers, 246–247
limes
    All-Purpose Green Sauce,
      98–99
    Arroz con Pollo, 184–185
    Brazilian Shrimp Stew
      (Moqueca de Camarones),
      256–257
    Butter Chicken, 186–187
    Chicken Jalfrezi, 190–191
    Chili-Lime Mayo, 100–101
    Creamy Sriracha Dipping
      Sauce, 93
    Easy Baked Salmon, 250–251
    Easy Salsa Verde, 88
    Instant Pot Beef Curry,
      196–197
    Peruvian Chicken, 188–189
    Pumpkin Seed Pesto, 82–83
    Quick-Pickled Red Onions,
      108–109
    Salmon Burgers, 246–247
    Sesame Ginger Dressing, 90
    Spicy Shrimp Salad Sushi
      Bowl, 154–155
    Strawberry Lime Refresher,
      318–319

M

macros, tracking, 29
Magic Bullet blender, 49
magnesium citrate, 30
marinara sauce, 345
mayonnaise
    All-Purpose Green Sauce,
      98–99
    Baked Zucchini Fries, 280–281
    Beef Kofta Meatballs, 206–207
    Buffalo Chicken Salad, 156–157
    Chicken Club Wrap, 164–165
    Chili Dog Skillet, 202–203
    Chili-Lime Mayo, 100–101
    Crab Cakes, 262–263

    Creamy Sriracha Dipping
      Sauce, 93
    Crispy Lemon Chicken,
      192–193
    Curried Chicken Salad, 146–147
    Dairy-Free Caesar Dressing, 89
    Dairy-Free Tzatziki, 96–97
    Dill Caper Tartar Sauce,
      104–105
    Duchess Cauliflower, 302–303
    Easy Tuna Salad, 148–149
    Eggplant & Cauliflower
      Fritters, 272–273
    Fried Calamari, 254–255
    Garlic & Chive Cauliflower
      Mash, 290–291
    Italian-Style Stuffed Peppers,
      212–213
    Meatloaf Cupcakes, 210–211
    Muffuletta Wrap, 162–163
    Pastrami Roll-Ups, 166–167
    resources for, 345
    Roasted Red Pepper Sauce,
      94–95
    Salmon Burgers, 246–247
    Sesame Ginger Dressing, 90
    Sheet Pan Meatballs with
      Zoodles, 208–209
    Sheet Pan Veggie Burgers,
      306–307
    Simple Egg Salad, 152–153
    Spicy Shrimp Salad Sushi
      Bowl, 154–155
MCT oil, 35
meal plans
    5-Day Keto Soup Diet, 64–67
    Week 1, 56–57
    Week 2, 58–59
    Week 3, 60–61
    Week 4, 62–63
meal prep, tips for, 37–40
measuring, weighing versus, 22
meat, kitchen safety and, 41. *See
    also specific types*
Meatloaf Cupcakes recipe, 210–211
microplane grater, 53

microwaving cauliflower, 302

mint

    chewing, 33

    Cucumber Mint Cooler, 316–317

    Curried Chicken Salad, 146–147

    Inside-Out Egg Rolls, 226–227

    Pork & Pine Nut Eggplant Rollatini, 220–221

    Pumpkin Seed Pesto, 82–83

    Raspberry Green Tea, 320–321

mints, 32–33

Molcajete Mixto recipe, 258–259

moringa, 30

mortadella

    Muffuletta Wrap, 162–163

Muffuletta Wrap recipe, 162–163

multicooker, 53

multivitamin, 30

mushrooms

    about, 40

    Chicken & Vegetable Soup, 144–145

    Herbed Mushroom Ragout, 276–277

    Oven-Roasted Mushrooms, 292–293

    Sheet Pan Veggie Burgers, 306–307

    Spinach-Stuffed Portobello Mushrooms, 268–269

mussels

    cleaning, 260

    Mussels in Thai Coconut Broth, 260–261

    Sheet Pan Paella, 264–265

Mussels in Thai Coconut Broth recipe, 260–261

MyFitnessPal, 29

N

net carbs, 17

No-Cook Marinara Sauce recipe, 84–85

    Sheet Pan Meatballs with Zoodles, 208–209

nori

    Spicy Shrimp Salad Sushi Bowl, 154–155

NutriBullet blender, 49

nuts, 17, 32

O

Olive Salad recipe, 110–111

    Muffuletta Wrap, 162–163

olives

    Arroz con Pollo, 184–185

    Beef Picadillo, 200–201

    Greek Zucchini Fritters, 270–271

    Olive Salad, 110–111

    Spaghetti Squash Puttanesca, 310–311

onions

    Arroz con Pollo, 184–185

    Bacon & Caramelized Onion Breakfast Bake, 122–123

    Balsamic Roasted Veggies, 282–283

    Bangers & Mash, 224–225

    Beef Picadillo, 200–201

    Brazilian Shrimp Stew (Moqueca de Camarones), 256–257

    Butter Chicken, 186–187

    Chicken Jalfrezi, 190–191

    Chicken Korma, 176–177

    Chicken & Vegetable Soup, 144–145

    Chorizo & Turnip Hash, 120–121

    Crispy Radish Corned Beef Hash, 126–127

    Easy Beef Bone Broth, 72–73

    Easy Chicken Bone Broth, 72–73

    Eggs in Purgatory, 134–135

    Herbed Mushroom Ragout, 276–277

    Molcajete Mixto, 258–259

    Olive Salad, 110–111

    Quick-Pickled Red Onions, 108–109

    Sausage-Stuffed Onions with Balsamic Glaze, 236–237

Sheet Pan Bacon Burgers, 216–217

Sheet Pan Paella, 264–265

Sheet Pan Steak Fajitas, 204–205

Spicy Sausage & Kale Soup, 138–139

Vindaloo, 232–233

optimism, as a stage of Squeaky Clean Keto, 19

Oven-Roasted Cajun Shrimp recipe, 242–243

Oven-Roasted Mushrooms recipe, 292–293

P

pantries, essential items for, 44–48

parchment paper, 53

parsley

    Baba Ghanoush, 340–341

    Bacon & Caramelized Onion Breakfast Bake, 122–123

    Bangers & Mash, 224–225

    Beef Kofta Meatballs, 206–207

    Charmoula Sauce, 87

    Chilled Seafood Salad, 244–245

    Crab Cakes, 262–263

    Crispy Lemon Chicken, 192–193

    Eggplant & Cauliflower Fritters, 272–273

    Herbed Mushroom Ragout, 276–277

    Italian-Style Stuffed Peppers, 212–213

    Olive Salad, 110–111

    Salmon Burgers, 246–247

    Sheet Pan Meatballs with Zoodles, 208–209

    Sheet Pan Paella, 264–265

    Shrimp Piccata with Zoodles, 240–241

    Spaghetti Squash Puttanesca, 310–311

Pastrami Roll-Ups recipe, 166–167

peas
Sheet Pan Paella, 264–265
peppermint oil, 33
pepperoncini
Olive Salad, 110–111
personal-sized blender, 49
Peruvian Chicken recipe, 188–189
photos, 25
pine nuts
Pork & Pine Nut Eggplant
Rollatini, 220–221
Spinach-Stuffed Portobello
Mushrooms, 268–269
plateaus, breaking through, 26
poblano peppers
Eggs in Purgatory, 134–135
Sheet Pan Steak Fajitas,
204–205
poppy seeds
Everything Bagel Seasoning,
80–81
porcini mushrooms
Herbed Mushroom Ragout,
276–277
pork
Cajun Pork Tenderloin, 234–235
Five-Spice Pork Chops,
230–231
Inside-Out Egg Rolls, 226–227
meal prep and, 39
Pork & Pine Nut Eggplant
Rollatini, 220–221
Sheet Pan Steak Fajitas,
204–205
Slow-Roasted Pork Shoulder,
228–229
Vindaloo, 232–233
Pork & Pine Nut Eggplant Rollatini
recipe, 220–221
pork sausages
Bangers & Mash, 224–225
portobello mushrooms
Spinach-Stuffed Portobello
Mushrooms, 268–269
potassium, 30
progress, tracking, 22–23

prosciutto
Muffuletta Wrap, 162–163
Prosciutto & Tomato Omelette,
128–129
Prosciutto-Wrapped Chicken
Tenders, 172–173
Prosciutto & Tomato Omelette
recipe, 128–129
Prosciutto-Wrapped Chicken
Tenders recipe, 172–173
prunes
Beef Picadillo, 200–201
psyllium husk powder
about, 46
Cinnamon Maple Granola,
124–125
Eggplant & Cauliflower
Fritters, 272–273
Fried Calamari, 254–255
Korean Scallion Pancakes
(Pajeon), 308–309
resources for, 345
Sheet Pan Veggie Burgers,
306–307
Spinach Wraps, 112–113
Pumpkin Seed Pesto recipe, 82–83
pumpkin seeds
about, 44
Chicken Korma, 176–177
Cinnamon Maple Granola,
124–125
Curried Chicken Salad,
146–147
Pumpkin Seed Pesto, 82–83
resources for, 345

Q
Quick-Pickled Red Onions recipe,
108–109
Chicken Club Wrap, 164–165
Cobb Salad with Warm Bacon
Vinaigrette, 150–151

R
radishes
Beef Picadillo, 200–201

carbs in, 31
Crispy Radish Corned Beef
Hash, 126–127
raspberries
Blueberry Bliss Smoothie Bowl,
118–119
carbs in, 31
Raspberry Green Tea, 320–321
Raspberry Green Tea recipe,
320–321
red chilis
Fish Curry, 252–253
Mussels in Thai Coconut Broth,
260–261
red curry paste
Fish Curry, 252–253
Mussels in Thai Coconut Broth,
260–261
resources, 344–345
rib-eye, 39
Roasted Bacon-Wrapped Cabbage
Wedges recipe, 300–301
Roasted Cauliflower & Leek Soup
recipe, 140–141
Roasted Red Pepper Sauce recipe,
94–95
roasted red peppers
Brazilian Shrimp Stew
(Moqueca de Camarones),
256–257
Roasted Red Pepper Sauce,
94–95
Roasted Sunflower Seed Butter
recipe, 78–79
Cinnamon Maple Granola,
124–125
romaine lettuce
carbs in, 31
Chef's Salad, 158–159
Green Lemonade, 332–333
Roman Fried Artichokes recipe,
274–275

S
SAD (standard American diet),
28–29

safety, kitchen, 41–43

salads
Buffalo Chicken Salad, 156–157
Chef's Salad, 158–159
Cobb Salad with Warm Bacon Vinaigrette, 150–151
Curried Chicken Salad, 146–147
Easy Tuna Salad, 148–149
Hearts of Palm Salad, 160–161
Olive Salad, 110–111
Simple Egg Salad, 152–153
Spicy Shrimp Salad Sushi Bowl, 154–155

salami
Muffuletta Wrap, 162–163

salmon
Easy Baked Salmon, 250–251
Salmon Burgers, 246–247

Salmon Burgers recipe, 246–247

salsa
Breakfast Burrito, 132–133
Chili Dog Skillet, 202–203
Fiesta Egg Cups, 116–117
resources for, 345

salt, 48

Salty Wasabi Coconut Chips recipe, 338–339

sauces
All-Purpose Green Sauce, 98–99
Charmoula Sauce, 87
Creamy Garlic Sauce, 106–107
Creamy Sriracha Dipping Sauce, 93
Dairy-Free Tzatziki, 96–97
Dill Caper Tartar Sauce, 104–105
Easy Salsa Verde, 88
Roasted Red Pepper Sauce, 94–95

sauerkraut, 30

sausage
Baked Scotch Eggs, 130–131
Breakfast Burrito, 132–133
Sausage-Stuffed Onions with Balsamic Glaze, 236–237

Sausage-Stuffed Onions with Balsamic Glaze recipe, 236–237

Sautéed Shredded Brussels Sprouts recipe, 298–299

scallions
Chicken Chop Suey, 174–175
Ginger Beef Stir-Fry, 214–215
Inside-Out Egg Rolls, 226–227
Korean Scallion Pancakes (Pajeon), 308–309
Mussels in Thai Coconut Broth, 260–261
Sesame Ginger Dressing, 90

seafood. See fish and seafood

seltzer
Strawberry Lime Refresher, 318–319

Sesame Chicken Fingers recipe, 180–181

Sesame Ginger Dressing recipe, 90

sesame seeds
Baba Ghanoush, 340–341
Cinnamon Maple Granola, 124–125
Easy Sesame Broccoli, 294–295
Everything Bagel Seasoning, 80–81
Korean Scallion Pancakes (Pajeon), 308–309
Sesame Chicken Fingers, 180–181
Spicy Shrimp Salad Sushi Bowl, 154–155

Sevigny, Mellissa
Keto for Life, 6
personal story of, 5–6

Sheet Pan Bacon Burgers recipe, 216–217

Sheet Pan Meatballs with Zoodles recipe, 208–209

Sheet Pan Paella recipe, 264–265

Sheet Pan Steak Fajitas recipe, 204–205

Sheet Pan Veggie Burgers recipe, 306–307

shopping lists, for meal plans, 57, 59, 61, 63, 67

shrimp
Brazilian Shrimp Stew (Moqueca de Camarones), 256–257
Chilled Seafood Salad, 244–245
cooking, 154
Molcajete Mixto, 258–259
Oven-Roasted Cajun Shrimp, 242–243
Sheet Pan Paella, 264–265
Sheet Pan Steak Fajitas, 204–205
Shrimp Piccata with Zoodles, 240–241
Spicy Shrimp Salad Sushi Bowl, 154–155
Vindaloo, 232–233

Shrimp Piccata with Zoodles recipe, 240–241

silicone kitchen utensils, 51

Simple Egg Salad recipe, 152–153

Simply Roasted Chicken Breasts recipe, 182–183

Slow-Roasted Pork Shoulder recipe, 228–229

snacking, 21

snapper
Fish Curry, 252–253

social life, 28

soups and stews
Chicken & Vegetable Soup, 144–145
Curried Turnip & Cauliflower Soup, 142–143
Easy Beef Bone Broth, 72–73
Easy Chicken Bone Broth, 72–73
Roasted Cauliflower & Leek Soup, 140–141
Spicy Sausage & Kale Soup, 138–139

sour cream
Breakfast Burrito, 132–133